WORKBOOK TO ACCOMPANY

ADMINISTRATIVE MEDICAL ASSISTING

Sixth Edition

Marilyn T. Fordney, CMA-AC

Formerly, Instructor of Medical Insurance, Medical Terminology, Medical Machine Transcription, and Medical Office Procedures

Ventura College, Ventura, California

Linda L. French, CMA-C, NCICS, CPC

Formerly, Instructor and Business Consultant, Administrative Medical Assisting, Medical Terminology, and Medical Insurance Billing and Coding

Simi Valley Adult School and Career Institute, Simi Valley, California
Ventura College, Ventura, California
Oxnard College, Oxnard, California
Santa Barbara Business College, Ventura, California

Joan J. Follis, BS

Formerly, Instructor of Business Education and Medical Office Procedures

Ventura College, Ventura, California

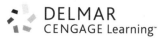

DELMAR
CENGAGE Learning

Australia • Brazil • Japan • Korea • Mexico • Singapore • Spain • United Kingdom • United States

DELMAR
CENGAGE Learning

Workbook to Accompany Administrative Medical Assisting, Sixth Edition
Marilyn T. Fordney, Linda L. French, Joan J. Follis

Vice President, Health Care Business Unit:
  William Brottmiller

Director of Learning Solutions:
  Matthew Kane

Senior Acquisitions Editor: Rhonda Dearborn

Product Manager: Sarah Prime

Marketing Director: Jennifer McAvey

Marketing Coordinator: Andrea Eobstel

Technology Product Manager: Ben Knapp

Technology Project Manager: Erin Pollay

Production Director: Carolyn Miller

Content Project Manager: Brooke Greenhouse

Senior Art Director: Jack Pendleton

For product information and technology assistance, contact us at
Cengage Learning Customer & Sales Support, 1-800-354-9706
For permission to use material from this text or product,
submit all requests online at **www.cengage.com/permissions**
Further permissions questions can be emailed to
permissionrequest@cengage.com

ISBN-13: 978-1-4180-6412-9

ISBN-10: 1-4180-6412-2

Delmar
Executive Woods
5 Maxwell Drive
Clifton Park, NY 12065
USA

Cengage Learning is a leading provider of customized learning solutions with office locations around the globe, including Singapore, the United Kingdom, Australia, Mexico, Brazil, and Japan. Locate your local office at **international.cengage.com/region**

Cengage Learning products are represented in Canada by Nelson Education, Ltd.

For your lifelong learning solutions, visit **delmar.cengage.com**

Visit our corporate website at **www.cengage.com**

Notice to the Reader

Printed in the United States of America
4 5 6 7 8 9 10 12 11 10 09

C O N T E N T S

ACKNOWLEDGMENTS

This *Workbook* has grown to include hundreds of chapter review questions, expanded critical thinking exercises, and more than 100 Job Skills. With this edition, computerized exercises have been developed to incorporate the use of Medical Office Simulated Software (MOSS) so students can be trained in both hands-on and computerized skills. I gratefully acknowledge the work of Cindy Correa, who shared her expertise of MOSS and diligently developed exercises to incorporate the computerized medical office as part of this edition's learning package. These practice exercises will increase students' knowledge of how the computer is used in a medical office, familiarize them with common tasks in commercial medical software, and train them in various job skills—thank you, Cindy, for your invaluable contribution.

I wish to express my gratitude for the help and encouragement provided by friends, colleagues, and family, and the staff of Delmar Learning. And to the people and organizations who so willingly and enthusiastically contributed to the contents of this book, I am ever grateful. Without their expertise, comments, and suggestions, the work would not be as complete as it is.

I extend my sincere thanks to the following people who acted as consultants and assisted in reviewing parts of the manuscript and to the companies who granted permission to use the various forms that are an integral part of this *Workbook*. The realistic forms allow students to complete and master Job Skills so they are ready to enter the workforce. This is our ultimate goal!

Hal Buntley, LVN, CMA, EMT
Administrative Medical Assisting Instructor
San Antonio College
San Antonio, Texas

George S. Conomikes and Staff
President
Conomikes Association, Inc.
Los Angeles, California

Deluxe Corporation
500 Main Street
Groton, Massachusetts

Cynthia L. Hotta
Executive Senior Managed Care Representative
GalaxoSmithKline
Pittsburgh, Pennsylvania

Medical Arts Press
100 Schelten Road
Lincolnshire, Illinois

Carolyn Talesfore
Advertising and Promotion Manager
Bibbero Systems, Inc.
Petaluma, California

Barbara Warfield
Ted Hernandez
Rhino Graphics
Port Hueneme, California

INTRODUCTION TO THE *WORKBOOK*

PERFORMANCE OBJECTIVES

1. Use medical terminology, decode abbreviations, and spell terms accurately.
2. Define job duties and name the interpersonal skills required of an administrative medical assistant.
3. Understand human behavior and work as a team member.
4. Name types of health care settings and handle patient referrals to hospitals and physician specialists.
5. Maintain confidentiality, ensure patient integrity, and follow medicolegal rules.
6. Communicate using various styles and body language, noting unique qualities of other cultures.
7. Perform duties as a receptionist exhibiting a professional demeanor.
8. Use correct telephone etiquette and triage patient medical complaints.
9. Schedule surgery and office appointments efficiently and complete outpatient requisition forms.
10. File Medical records using standardized alphabetic rules.
11. Create charts; prepare and maintain patient medical records.
12. Use a Physician's Desk Reference, translate prescriptions, and record prescription information.
13. Compose and key letters; abstract information from written communication; edit, annotate, and proofread.
14. Process incoming mail; prepare and classify outgoing mail.
15. Prepare and send statements and utilize effective collection techniques.
16. Code diagnoses and procedures and complete health insurance claim forms.
17. Write checks, make deposits, and perform banking procedures.
18. Post figures accurately and compute totals while performing bookkeeping procedures.
19. Conduct an office meeting, replenish office supplies, and manage inventory.
20. Perform payroll procedures; generate and analyze accounting reports.
21. Compose a resumé and perform functions to seek a job as a medical assistant.

INSTRUCTIONS TO THE STUDENT

This *Workbook* has been prepared for those who use *Administrative Medical Assisting* as a text. The *Workbook* Job Skills combined with the theory learned in the textbook meet the educational entry-level competencies outlined by the Commission on Accreditation of Allied Health Education Programs (CAAHEP) and the Accrediting Bureau of Health Education Schools (ABHES) as well as the educational components of the American Association of Medical Assistants Role Delineation Study of 2003.

The following components have been developed to make the *Workbook* a complete learning tool, which allows practical application of job skills that will be performed in a physician's office. An asterisk (*) indicates features new to or enhanced for this edition.

Part I: Chapter Exercises*

- **Objectives** are clearly stated for all Job Skills.
- **Focus on Certification*** summarizes content listed by the (1) American Association of Medical Assistants for the Certified Medical Assistant Certification/Recertification Examination, (2) Registered Medical Assistant Certification Examination Competencies and Construction Parameters, and (3) Certified Medical Administrative Specialist Competencies and Examination Specifications listed by the American Medical Technologists.

- **Abbreviation and Spelling Review** incorporates medical terminology into a short chart note for each chapter, giving students an opportunity to write definitions for abbreviations and spell medical terms.

- **Review Questions** cover key points in chapters and address areas not covered by the exam-style review questions in the textbook. Review questions help students prepare for a multiple-choice theory test on each chapter studied. Answers are found in the Instructor's Manual.

- **Critical Thinking Exercises*** have been expanded and enhanced to offer students an opportunity to address situations and solve problems realistic to an office setting.

- **Job Skills*** have been enhanced to include up-to-date forms and technical information and have been expanded to cover all competencies listed by CAAHEP and ABHES. They have been redesigned to include a Performance Evaluation Checklist with the directions, thus eliminating the need for a separate form to grade each Job Skill.

Read through each Job Skill entirely before attempting to begin the assignment. Follow the directions in the *Workbook* where noted and refer to the Procedure in the textbook for step-by-step directions. These directions are comprehensive and written to assist students with the office task, not just the Job Skill in the *Workbook*. Where noted, refer to the textbook figures for visual examples.

Performance objectives are stated for each exercise. Your instructor will indicate which standards are expected, the time frame for the completion of each exercise, and the accuracy required for individual exercises. Points are assigned for each Job Skill for the first, second, and third attempt according to the steps required and difficulty of the task. These may be adjusted by your instructor.

Part II: Forms*

Blank forms are realistic and similar to those found in medical offices. They are easily removed and require completion for a variety of Job Skills. With this edition, the Form File is also found online at www.delmarlearning.com/companions. Click "Allied Health" from the left menu, and then click on this book's title, *Administrative Medical Assisting, Sixth Edition*. The *Workbook* forms may be used to complete many of the Job Skills on a computer.

Part III: Competency Grids*

Competency grids are included in this edition with reference numbers that correlate text and assignments by chapters to:

- CAAHEP Competency Standards for Medical Assisting Educational Programs

- ABHES Competencies for Medical Assisting Programs

- AAMA Certification Examination Content Outline for the CMA

- AMT Competencies and Construction Parameters for the RMA

- AMT Competencies and Examination Specifications for the CMAs

- AAMA Role Delineation Study for the CMA

These are included to assist students in studying for certification examinations and to assist instructors in complying with educational standards set by regulatory bodies.

Part IV: Appendix for Practon Medical Group, Inc.

Important information is listed in the Practon Medical Group, Inc., reference file, which has been expanded to include detailed office protocols. Before beginning the Job Skills, tear out the appendix, place it in a three-ring binder, and add section indexes so you can access information quickly to help you complete the *Workbook* Job Skills. The appendix includes (1) medical practice reference material; (2) office policies, including information about the daily routine in the office, office hours, appointment protocols, information regarding telephone calls, and filing routines; (3) payment policies and health insurance guidelines; and (4) directions for using the office fee schedule. A mock fee schedule is provided, which lists procedure codes, descriptions of services, and fees you will need when answering questions that patients might ask and for posting to ledgers and completing insurance forms. Also included are (5) a listing of *CPT* code modifiers with brief descriptions and (6) a sample listing of Medicare *Level II HCPCS* codes with fees.

Part V: Abbreviation Tables*

Abbreviation tables that appear in the textbook are listed to help decode abbreviations and locate medical definitions when completing Abbreviation and Spelling Review, answering questions, and performing Job Skills.

Additional Items Needed

If you do not have a background in medical terminology, you need to obtain and use a good medical dictionary. In addition to the blank forms included in this *Workbook*, you will need the following items. Check them off as you obtain them for your course work.

_____   1 three-ring binder with index tabs

_____   1 folder with pockets to hand in assignments

_____   3 manila file folders

_____   3 name labels for manila folders

_____   50 sheets of 8½″ by 11″ white typing or computer paper

_____   60 3″ by 5″ white file cards

_____   2 white number 10 envelopes (9½″ by 4″)

_____   rubber bands, paper clips, pens, highlighter pen set (5 colors), pencils, transparent tape

Optional items:

_____   7 white number 10 envelopes (large)

_____   7 white number 6 envelopes (small)

Notebook Content Suggestions

It is a good idea to remove the reference appendix (Part IV) and the Abbreviation Tables (Part V) from the *Workbook* and place them in a notebook. You may want to remove the blank forms (Part II), which may be photocopied prior to use. The forms may also be printed from the online companion that accompanies this book. To access it, go to www.delmarlearning.com/companions. Click on "Allied Health" from the left menu, and then click on this book's title. Following are several items from the textbook that you may want to also include.

List of Evaluation and Management *CPT* Codes	Tables 16-5 and 16-6
Comprehensive List of *CPT* Modifiers	Table 16-7
Insurance Form Template for Medicare	Figure 16-3
Insurance Form Template for Medicare/Medigap	Figure 16-6
Insurance Form Template for TRICARE	Figure 16-9
CMS-1500 Claim Form Field-by-Field Instructions	Appendix A
Commercial Insurance Template	Figure A-1
Glossary	Pages G1–G14

Portfolio

Saving your completed work in a portfolio is strongly suggested. You may wish to bring it to a job interview in order to present the type of job skills you have acquired and the level of work you have performed during your course of study. You will need a three-ring binder with indexes, and you should add items to this folder as you progress through the course. You should organize the material and develop a table of contents. There are several ways to accomplish this, but a simple way would be according to job duties (e.g., appointment scheduling, telephone techniques, insurance coding and claim forms, letter composition, bookkeeping, payroll, and so forth). Your instructor may suggest additional items to include or a specific arrangement of all items.

The content of this portfolio is evidence of your administrative skills and is a good indication of your organizational abilities as well as the neatness and completeness of your work.

WORKBOOK JOB SKILL EXERCISES

Chapter Exercises

- Objectives
- Focus on Certification
- Abbreviation and Spelling Review
- Review Questions
- Critical Thinking Exercises
- Job Skills with Performance Evaluation Checklists

C H A P T E R **1**

A Career As an Administrative Medical Assistant

OBJECTIVES

After completing the exercises, the student will be able to:

1. Enhance knowledge of medical terminology, interpret abbreviations, and accurately spell medical words.

2. List the duties of an administrative medical assistant.

3. Name specialty areas that utilize administrative skills.

4. State important interpersonal skills for medical assistants.

5. List attributes for good team interaction.

6. Name the stages of dying.

7. Complete a self-assessment of present job skills and personal and professional attributes to identify strengths and weaknesses.

8. Use the Internet to obtain information about certification and/or registration.

9. Use the Internet to perform a self-test of anatomy and physiology or medical terminology.

10. Develop a medical practice survey.

FOCUS ON CERTIFICATION*

CMA Content Summary
- Medical terminology
- Understanding emotional behavior
- Professionalism
- Empathy

RMA Content Summary
- Medical terminology
- Scope of practice
- Credentialing requirements
- Ethics
- Professional development and conduct
- Interpersonal skills
- Instructing patients

CMAS Content Summary
- Medical terminology
- Professionalism
- Community referral resources

Review Questions

Review the objectives, glossary, and chapter information before completing the following review questions.

1. In a customer service–oriented practice, the elements of customer service are demonstrated by the <u>physician</u>, <u>management team</u>, and <u>all employees</u>.

2. True or False: Each employee and patient has the same idea about what "good" service means. <u>False</u>

3. Define "flextime." <u>scheduling so the office has complete coverage.</u>

4. Name some specialty areas in which administrative skills may be used in a health care career.
   a. <u>anesthesiologist assistant</u>
   b. <u>dental assistant</u>
   c. <u>cardiovascular technologist</u>
   d. <u>cytotechnologist</u>
   e. <u>opthalmalic technician</u>

5. A medical transcriptionist is now also known as a <u>medical language specialist</u> or <u>speech recognition technician</u>

6. Of the duties an administrative medical assistant might perform,
   a. List two that require interpersonal skills.
      <u>Collecting fees</u>
      <u>greeting patients</u>

   b. List five that require keyboard input skills (assume you work in a computerized office).
      <u>Scheduling appointments.</u>
      <u>Making contact notes.</u>
      <u>submitting insurance claims.</u>
      <u>Researching referral info.</u>
      <u>Faxing information to patients.</u>

*This *Workbook* and accompanying textbook meet the entry-level administrative and general competencies for the CMA outlined by the AAMA Examination Content Outline and Role Delineation Study and for the RMA and CMAS outlined by the AMT Competencies and Examination Specifications (see Competency Grid in textbook Appendix B).

c. List five that require basic math skills.

collecting fees

billing patients

submitting pre-auths

scheduling appointments

writing checks

d. List five that require other clerical skills.

maintaining records

correspondence

taking notes/messages

writing memos

transcribing letters

7. In addition to the many duties that an administrative medical assistant performs, there are various interpersonal skills required. Name four that you would like to be known for.

a. greeting patients

b. showing interest + concern

c. having a positive attitude

d. taking initiative

8. When trying to understand a viewpoint or evaluating a patient's behavior, it is important to **listen** show empathy and **be professional**.

9. An emergency has occurred in Dr. Practon's office. Name the behavior the medical assistant must exhibit to patients.

a. professionalism

b. respect

c. courtesy

d. empathy

e. concern

10. List some attributes an employee needs for good team interaction.

a. integrity

b. openness

c. respect for others

d. dedication

e. warmth + sensitivity

f. a positive attitude

11. What must a health care worker be aware of and understand in order to avoid work-related emotional and psychological problems? that stress needs to be taken care of before it leads to burnout

12. When patients receive unfortunate news about themselves or loved ones, how should medical assistants act, and what are some things that can be done to help? show empathy, check for understanding + give patients proper info about resources

13. List the stages of dying.

    a. _denial_

    b. _anger_

    c. _bargaining_

    d. _depression_

    e. _acceptance_

14. What is the name of the national foundation that offers medical care and support to patients and family members dealing with a terminal illness or the loss of a loved one? _Hospice foundation of America_

15. Define "stress", and name one thing that has caused stress in your life. _Stress is a condition comprising physical, psychological, + emotional reactions to time constraints, irritating circumstances_

16. How does a medical assistant's excellent grooming reflect the image and management of the medical office? _Shows a professional image and sets the standard for professionalism_

17. Give the names of two national organizations that certify or register medical assistants trained in both clinical and administrative areas.

    a. _American Association of Medical Assistants_   AAMA

    b. _Commission of Accreditation of Allied Health Programs_

18. Name five ways a medical assistant can keep knowledge of research and new techniques current.

    a. _read professional publications_

    b. _attend seminars_

    c. _research information on internet_

    d. _join a local chapter of certified worker_

    e. _network with peers at workshops_

✗ Critical Thinking Exercises

1. Another medical assistant in the office criticizes a patient behind his or her back for wearing bizarre clothes. What would your response be? _That it is not professional to criticize fashion choices of patients_

2. Following are some questions that will help you do a self-assessment. Read each of them carefully and try to answer them honestly. After you have completed them, identify and mark your strengths with an *S* and your weaknesses with a *W*. This will not only help you to know what areas you need to work on but will help you determine which type of job you may be best suited.

    _S_ a. Are you considerate of others?

    _S_ b. Do you treat people with respect?

    _S_ c. Do you have a kind, friendly, and good-natured manner?

    _S_ d. Do you have the ability to be discreet and keep information confidential?

    _S_ e. Do you have a positive attitude?

_____ S   f. Can you smile easily?

_____ S   g. Can you listen instead of talking all the time?

_____ S   h. Are you polite?

_____ S   i. Can you be sympathetic and empathetic and discern the difference?

_____ S   j. Are you reliable and dependable?

_____ S   k. Are you honest and trustworthy?

_____ S   l. Can you accept responsibility?

_____ S   m. Can you remain calm during an emergency?

_____ S   n. Are you well groomed, with a neat appearance?

_____ S   o. Are you a team player?

_____ S   p. Are you patient?

_____ S   q. Do you reserve judgment of others?

_____ S   r. Do you have good judgment?

_____ S   s. Are you willing to learn?

_____ S   t. Do you accept criticism?

_____ S   u. Are you sensitive to the feelings of others?

_____ S   v. Can you remain free from bias?

JOB SKILL 1–1
Interpret and Accurately Spell Medical Terms and Abbreviations

Name _____ Date _____ Score _____

Performance Objective

Task: Decode abbreviations.

Conditions: Use pen or pencil. Refer to Procedure 1-1 in the textbook for step-by-step directions.

Standards: Complete all steps listed in this skill in _____ minutes with a minimum score of _____.
                (Time element and accuracy criteria may be given by instructor.)

Time: **Start:** _____ **Completed:** _____ **Total:** _____ minutes

Scoring: One point for each step performed satisfactorily unless otherwise listed or weighted by instructor.

Directions with Performance Evaluation Checklist

Read the following patient's chart note and write the meanings for the abbreviations listed below the note. To decode any abbreviations you do not understand or that appear unfamiliar to you, refer to the list of abbreviations in Part V of this *Workbook*. Medical terms in the chart note are *italicized;* study them for spelling. Use your medical dictionary to look up their definitions. Your instructor may give a test for the spelling and definition of the words and abbreviations. Note: Although abbreviations are not presented in Chapter 1 of the textbook, they appear throughout the text, and a chart note with medical terms and abbreviations is presented at the beginning of each chapter of the *Workbook* entitled "Abbreviation and Spelling Review" to offer students the opportunity to learn these terms. Refer back to Procedure 1-1 in the textbook while doing these.

Bart J. Stephens

September 15, 20XX Routine PE. Ht 6 ft. Wt 163 lb. P 70. BP 130/70. Pt s̄ complaints. *Systemic* Ex neg. except for Grade I *pulmonic murmur*. EKG, CBC, UA, & chest x-ray films neg. IMP: No disease. Rx: *Tetanus toxoid* booster, 0.5 ml. Ret p.r.n.

Fran Practon, MD
Fran Practon, MD

1st Attempt	2nd Attempt	3rd Attempt	
_____	_____	_____	Gather materials (equipment and supplies) listed under "Conditions."
_____	_____	_____	1. PE *Physical Examination*
✓	_____	_____	2. Ht *height*
✓	_____	_____	3. ft *foot, feet*
✓	_____	_____	4. wt *weight*
✓	_____	_____	5. lb *pound*
_____	_____	_____	6. P *pulse*
✓	_____	_____	7. BP *Blood pressure*
✓	_____	_____	8. pt *patient*
_____	_____	_____	9. s̄ *without*
✓	_____	_____	10. Ex *examination*
✓	_____	_____	11. neg. *negative*
_____	_____	_____	12. EKG *electrocardiogram*
_____	_____	_____	13. CBC *complete blood count*
_____	_____	_____	14. UA *urinalysis*

JOB SKILL 1-1 *(continued)*

_____	_____	_____	15. IMP	*impression*	
_____	_____	_____	16. Rx	*perscription*	
_____	_____	_____	17. ml	*milliliters*	
_____	_____	_____	18. ret	*return*	
_____	_____	_____	19. p.r.n.	*as necessary*	
_____	_____	_____	Complete within specified time.		
___/21	___/21	___/21	**Total points earned** (To obtain a percentage score, divide the total points earned by the number of points possible.)		

Comments:

Evaluator's Signature: _____ **Need to Repeat:** _____

National Curriculum Competency: CAAHEP: III.C.3.c(1)(a)	ABHES: VI.B.1.a.2(g)

JOB SKILL 1–2
Use the Internet to Obtain Information on Certification and/or Registration

Name _____ Date _____ Score _____

Performance Objective

Task: Research certification and/or registration via the Internet.

Conditions: Computer with Internet connection and references from Table 1-1 in the textbook.

Standards: Complete all steps listed in this skill in _____ minutes with a minimum score of _____.
(Time element and accuracy criteria may be given by instructor.)

Time: **Start:** _____ **Completed:** _____ **Total:** _____ minutes

Scoring: One point for each step performed satisfactorily unless otherwise listed or weighted by instructor.

Directions with Performance Evaluation Checklist

1st Attempt	2nd Attempt	3rd Attempt	
_____	_____	_____	Gather materials (equipment and supplies) listed under "Conditions."
_____	_____	_____	1. Study Table 1-1 to determine what areas of certification or registration interest you.
_____	_____	_____	2. Access the Internet via cable or modem.
_____	_____	_____	3. Type in the Web site address from the column on the right side of the table for the organization(s) you have selected (e.g., Certified Bookkeeper = http://www.aipb.org).
_____	_____	_____	4. Select key terms ("certification," "registration," or "about" the program).
____/4	____/4	____/4	5. Print the information to read and share with your class, and label a file folder to keep it for future reference.
_____	_____	_____	Complete within specified time.
____/10	____/10	____/10	**Total points earned** (To obtain a percentage score, divide the total points earned by the number of points possible.)

Comments:

Evaluator's Signature: _____ **Need to Repeat:** _____

National Curriculum Competency: CAAHEP: III.C.3.c(4)(c)   ABHES: VI.B.1.a.2(h), VI.B.1.a.2(n), VI.B.1.a.3(d)

JOB SKILL 1–3
Use the Internet to Test Your Knowledge of Anatomy and Physiology or Medical Terminology

Name _____ Date _____ Score _____

Performance Objective

Task: Test your knowledge of anatomy and physiology or medical terminology via the Internet. If you have not completed your course of study in anatomy and physiology or medical terminology, you may use this job skill to test your knowledge at a later time.

Conditions: Computer with Internet connection.

Standards: Complete all steps listed in this job skill in _____ minutes with a minimum score of _____. (Time element and accuracy criteria may be given by instructor.)

Time: **Start:** _____ **Completed:** _____ **Total:** _____ minutes

Scoring: One point for each step performed satisfactorily unless otherwise listed or weighted by instructor.

Directions with Performance Evaluation Checklist

1st Attempt	2nd Attempt	3rd Attempt	
_____	_____	_____	Gather materials (equipment and supplies) listed under "Conditions."
_____	_____	_____	1. Access the Internet via cable or modem.
_____	_____	_____	2. Type in the Web site address for the American Association of Medical Assistants: http://www.aama-ntl.org
_____	_____	_____	3. Scroll down to "AAMA CMA Practice Exams."
_____	_____	_____	4. Select either "anatomy and physiology" or "medical terminology."
_____	_____	_____	5. Read the instructions and download, open, and print the answer form.
_____	_____	_____	6. Read each question and mark the answer.
___/50	___/50	___/50	7. Compare your answers with the answer key, which is listed directly after the questions.
_____	_____	_____	8. Make note of the questions you need to study.
_____	_____	_____	Complete within specified time.
___/59	___/59	___/59	**Total points earned** (To obtain a percentage score, divide the total points earned by the number of points possible.)

Comments:

Evaluator's Signature: _____ **Need to Repeat:** _____

National Curriculum Competency: CAAHEP: III.C.3.c(1)	ABHES: VI.B.1.a.2(g), VI.B.1.a.2(n), VI.B.1.a.3(d)

JOB SKILL 1–4
Develop a Medical Practice Survey

Name _____ Date _____ Score _____

Performance Objective

Task: Design a patient satisfaction survey form.

Conditions: White 8½ × 11 paper, pen or pencil, and computer if available.

Standards: Complete all steps listed in this skill in _____ minutes with a minimum score of _____.
(Time element and accuracy criteria may be given by instructor.)

Time: **Start:** _____ **Completed:** _____ **Total:** _____ minutes

Scoring: One point for each step performed satisfactorily unless otherwise listed or weighted by instructor.

Directions with Performance Evaluation Checklist

1st Attempt	2nd Attempt	3rd Attempt	
_____	_____	_____	Gather materials (equipment and supplies) listed under "Conditions."
____/5	____/5	____/5	1. Design your own survey form using the reference material on Practon Medical Group, Inc., found in Part IV of this *Workbook*.
____/5	____/5	____/5	2. Formulate at least five questions that address patient satisfaction.
_____	_____	_____	Complete within specified time.
____/12	____/12	____/12	**Total points earned** (To obtain a percentage score, divide the total points earned by the number of points possible.)

Comments:

Evaluator's Signature: _____ **Need to Repeat:** _____

National Curriculum Competency: CAAHEP: III.C.3.c(1)	ABHES: VI.B.1.a.2(j), VI.B.1.a.2(n), VI.B.1.a.2(o)

CHAPTER 2

The Health Care Environment: Past, Present, and Future

OBJECTIVES

After completing the exercises, the student will be able to:

1. Identify contributions of historic medical pioneers.
2. List the benefits of using managed care and a traditional health care system.
3. Differentiate the types of health care settings.
4. Make referral decisions regarding appropriate hospital departments.
5. Refer patients to the correct specialist.
6. Decode abbreviations for physician specialists and medical health care professionals.
7. Catalog skills needed by the administrative medical assistant.

FOCUS ON CERTIFICATION*

CMA Content Summary

- Medical terminology
- Working as a team
- Patient instruction
- Appropriate referrals
- Prepaid HMO, PPO, POS

*This *Workbook* and accompanying textbook meet the entry-level administrative and general competencies for the CMA outlined by the AAMA Examination Content Outline and Role Delineation Study and for the RMA and CMAS outlined by the AMT Competencies and Examination Specifications (see Competency Grid in textbook Appendix B).

RMA Content Summary
- Medical terminology
- Patient instruction

- Insurance terminology (HMO, PPO, EPO)

CMAS Content Summary
- Medical terminology

- Prepare information for referrals

Abbreviation and Spelling Review

Read the following patient's chart note and write the meanings for the abbreviations listed below the note. To decode any abbreviations you do not understand or that appear unfamiliar to you, refer to the list of abbreviations in Part V of this *Workbook*. Step-by-step directions for this exercise are in Procedure 1–1 of Chapter 1 in the textbook. Medical terms in the chart note are italicized; study them for spelling. Use your medical dictionary to look up their definitions. Your instructor may give a spelling and definition test that includes these words and abbreviations.

Troy Wenzlau

36-year-old W male seen as E for Fx L *humerus*. Pt DNS for re-exam last month as scheduled. Pt has been on SD X 3 mo for back pain and was determined P&S from a previous back injury last yr. Given I of *Demerol* 50 mg IM for pain, x-ray L arm ordered. Cast and return to ofc in 2 wks.

Gerald Practon, MD

Gerald Practon, MD

W	*white*	X	
E		mo	
Fx		P&S	
L		yr	
Pt		I	
DNS		mg	
re-exam		IM	
SD		ofc	
		wks	

Review Questions

Review the objectives, glossary, and chapter information before completing the following review questions.

1. Briefly describe the contribution of each of the following:
   a. Imhotep *physician who attended the pharaohs*

   b. Edward Jenner *Englishman who invented the process of vaccination + the smallpox vaccine*

   c. Frederick Banting *Canadian physician who discovered insulin*

   d. Anton van Leeuwenhoek *Dutch lens maker who developed first lens strong enough to see bacteria*

e. Pierre and Marie Curie _French researchers who discovered_
and worked with radium

f. Paul Ehrlich _German physician who developed_
chemotherapy + developed drug to fight syphilis

2. Match the pioneer in medicine in the left column with the appropriate item in the right column by writing the letters in the blanks.

_____ Ignaz Phillip Semmelweis		a. father of modern anatomy
_____ Joseph Lister		b. father of medicine
_____ Louis Pasteur		c. founder of nursing
_____ Jonas Edward Salk		d. discovered the x-ray
_____ Clara Barton		e. developed the first lens strong enough to see bacteria
_____ Aesculapius		f. discovered how yellow fever is transmitted
_____ Ambrose Pare		g. father of bacteriology
_____ Walter Reed		h. discovered the vaccine against polio
_____ William Harvey		i. Greek god of healing
_____ Wilhem C. Roentgen		j. founded the American Red Cross
_____ Hippocrates		k. father of sterile surgery
_____ Andraes Vesalius		l. father of modern surgery
_____ James Marion Sims		m. fought against puerperal fever
_____ Florence Nightingale		n. demonstrated circulation of blood
_____ Alexander Fleming		o. invented the vaginal speculum
		p. discovered insulin
		q. discovered penicillin

3. Name several factors that contributed to the rise of health care costs as medicine advanced. _malpractice_
suits + health insurance rates, high rents
new electronic equipment + medical records

4. List the benefits of using a managed care organization (MCO) and a traditional health care system as you compare and contrast their similarities and differences.

Traditional	**Managed Care**
a. _choose where to get tested_	a. _no deductible_
b. _no pre-auth_	b. _small co-pay_
c. _see whatever specialist_	c. _pre-auth required_
d. _go to whatever hospital_	d. _referral required_
e. _patients choose who they see_	e. _most meds covered_
f. _fee for service_	f. _most tests covered_

5. In a health maintenance organization (HMO), what is a treating physician called? _PCP_
Primary Care Physician 'Gatekeeper'

6. In a preferred provider organization (PPO), what is the health care provider called and what incentive is there for the patient to use this provider?

a. _____

b. _____

7. In an independent practice association (IPA), how is the physician paid? _____

8. Why is an exclusive provider organization (EPO) called *exclusive*? _____

9. What choice of care do patients have when belonging to a point-of-service plan? _____

   _____

10. A variety of specialists practicing medicine together is called: _____

    _____ .

11. List three services urgent care centers provide that most other practices do not offer.

    a. _____

    b. _____

    c. _____

12. Why should the medical assistant meet the hospital personnel where his or her physician is on staff?

    _____

13. Name several types of nonprofit hospitals.

    a. _____   d. _____

    b. _____   e. _____

    c. _____

14. Name three important factors to consider when choosing a reliable laboratory.

    a. _____

    b. _____

    c. _____

Critical Thinking Exercise

1. Choose the type of health care *setting* you would like to work in and list the *reasons* for your choice.

   Setting: _____

   Reasons: _____

   _____

   _____

JOB SKILL 2–1
Direct Patients to Specific Hospital Departments

Name _____ Date _____ Score _____

Performance Objective

Task: Make determinations to direct patients to specific hospital departments.

Conditions: Use pen or pencil. Refer to textbook Figures 2–5A and B (hospital departments) and Procedure 2–1 for step-by-step directions.

Standards: Complete all steps listed in this skill in _____ minutes with a minimum score of _____. (Time element and accuracy criteria may be given by instructor.)

Time: Start: _____ Completed: _____ Total: _____ minutes

Scoring: One point for each step performed satisfactorily unless otherwise listed or weighted by instructor.

Directions with Performance Evaluation Checklist

In many situations, the administrative medical assistant will be interacting with the hospital. A knowledge of various hospital departments and the services they offer is helpful in order to expediently schedule tests, arrange surgery, obtain test results, and refer patients. In the following scenario, you are the administrative assistant in Dr. Gerald Practon's office. A patient, Reiko Kimon, was discharged from the hospital last week and has various questions. List the correct hospital department you would direct the patient to.

1st Attempt	2nd Attempt	3rd Attempt	
_____	_____	_____	Gather materials (equipment and supplies) listed under "Conditions."
_____	_____	_____	1. Where does she go to pick up a copy of her operative report? _____
_____	_____	_____	2. Where can she attend a nutritional education class? _____
_____	_____	_____	3. Where does she go for a urinalysis? _____
_____	_____	_____	4. She has a question about the medication that was given to her when she left the hospital. _____
_____	_____	_____	5. Should she use a bronchodilator before she goes to have a pulmonary function test? _____
_____	_____	_____	6. She would like to personally tell the hospital president how wonderfully she was cared for during her hospital stay. _____
_____	_____	_____	7. She would like to speak to the physician who admitted her when she first arrived by ambulance at the hospital. _____
_____	_____	_____	8. She would like to know whether anyone has found a convalescent hospital for her mother, who is an inpatient and soon to be discharged._____
_____	_____	_____	9. She would like to schedule occupational therapy. _____
_____	_____	_____	10. She does not understand a hospital bill and would like it explained._____
_____	_____	_____	11. She would like the name of the new OB-GYN doctor from San Francisco who is performing deliveries at the hospital. _____
_____	_____	_____	12. She has a question regarding the contrast media that will be given to her before a bone scan. _____
_____	_____	_____	13. She would like to pick up a preparation kit for a barium enema._____
_____	_____	_____	14. She has a question regarding an old refund that should have been sent to her by now. _____
_____	_____	_____	15. She would like to speak to the utilization review nurse who was assigned to her case. _____

JOB SKILL 2–1 *(continued)*

_____ _____ _____ 16. She would like to know if she can wear her wedding ring in the MRI
machine. _____

_____ _____ _____ 17. She would like to know how to dress for the treadmill test._____

_____ _____ _____ 18. She would like to know the preparation for a sigmoidoscopy that is
scheduled._____

_____ _____ _____ 19. She would like to know what time to arrive for a blood transfusion._____

_____ _____ _____ Complete within specified time.

___/21 ___/21 ___/21 **Total points earned** (To obtain a percentage score, divide the total points earned
by the number of points possible.)

Comments:

Evaluator's Signature: _____ **Need to Repeat:** _____

JOB SKILL 2–2
Refer Patients to the Correct Physician Specialist

Name _____ Date _____ Score _____

Performance Objective

Task: Match the correct specialist with the patient's complaint.

Conditions: Use pen or pencil. Refer to textbook Table 2-3 for a list of medical specialties with descriptions and Procedure 2–2 for step-by-step directions.

Standards: Complete all steps listed in this skill in _____ minutes with a minimum score of _____. (Time element and accuracy criteria may be given by instructor.)

Time: Start: _____ Completed: _____ Total: _____ minutes

Scoring: One point for each step performed satisfactorily unless otherwise listed or weighted by instructor.

Directions with Performance Evaluation Checklist

In many situations, administrative medical assistants deal with the authorization referral process. They may also handle patients being referred by primary care physicians to specialists. To enhance understanding of these processes, consider the patients' problems and match their complaints with the correct specialist.

1st Attempt	2nd Attempt	3rd Attempt	Patient Complaint	Specialist
_____	_____	_____	Gather materials (equipment and supplies) listed under "Conditions."	
_____	_____	_____	1. _____ Pregnant	A. Allergist
_____	_____	_____	2. _____ Operation	B. Dermatologist
_____	_____	_____	3. _____ Microbiology report	C. Neonatologist
_____	_____	_____	4. _____ Bladder and kidney problems	D. Neurologist
_____	_____	_____	5. _____ Chronic runny nose from dust	E. Nuclear medicine
_____	_____	_____	6. _____ Severe depression	F. Obstetrician
_____	_____	_____	7. _____ Face lift	G. Ophthalmologist
_____	_____	_____	8. _____ Premature infant	H. Orthopedic surgeon
_____	_____	_____	9. _____ Infant DPT injection	I. Otolaryngologist
_____	_____	_____	10. _____ Ear discharge	J. Pathologist
_____	_____	_____	11. _____ X-rays	K. Pediatrician
_____	_____	_____	12. _____ Fractured bone	L. Physiatrist
_____	_____	_____	13. _____ Rehabilitation for chronic back pain	M. Plastic surgeon
_____	_____	_____	14. _____ Multiple sclerosis (disease of nervous system)	N. Psychiatrist
_____	_____	_____	15. _____ Glaucoma (increased pressure in eye)	O. Radiologist
_____	_____	_____	16. _____ Severe case of skin psoriasis	P. Surgeon
_____	_____	_____	17. _____ Bone scan (radionuclear)	Q. Urologist
_____	_____	_____	Complete within specified time.	
___/19	___/19	___/19	**Total points earned** (To obtain a percentage score, divide the total points earned by the number of points possible.)	

JOB SKILL 2–2 *(continued)*

Comments:

JOB SKILL 2–3
Define Abbreviations for Health Care Professionals

Name _____ Date _____ Score _____

Performance Objective

Task: Match terms for health care professionals with correct abbreviations.

Conditions: Use pen or pencil. Refer to Table 2-4 in the textbook for a list of physician specialists, health care professionals, and abbreviations. See Procedure 1-1 in Chapter 1 of the textbook for step-by-step directions.

Standards: Complete all steps listed in this skill in _____ minutes with a minimum score of _____. (Time element and accuracy criteria may be given by instructor.)

Time: Start: _____ **Completed:** _____ **Total:** _____ minutes

Scoring: One point for each step performed satisfactorily unless otherwise listed or weighted by instructor.

Directions with Performance Evaluation Checklist

Read the following scenario, decode the abbreviations for the appropriate physician specialists and health care professionals, and write the correct term on the line provided.

Laverne M. Stinowski   May 15, 20XX

Mrs. Stinowski was brought by ambulance to the hospital and was cared for by an EMT. In the emergency room she was treated by a DEM. During her hospital stay she was seen daily by the MD, who was also a FACS. After discharge, Mrs. Stinowski visited the physician's private office and was processed in by a CMA. An LVN drew her blood and escorted her to the treatment room. The physician was out of the office, so an RNP saw Mrs. Stinowski. An order was given for her to see an RPT. The blood test was read in the laboratory by an MT(ASCP). The patient's record was typed by a CMT, and her insurance claim was processed by a CPC. The patient went home, and the PA-C was in charge of ordering the patient a VN for the following day.

Gerald M. Practon, MD
_____
Gerald M. Practon, MD

1st Attempt	2nd Attempt	3rd Attempt		
_____	_____	_____	Gather materials (equipment and supplies) listed under "Conditions."	
_____	_____	_____	1. EMT	_____
_____	_____	_____	2. DEM	_____
_____	_____	_____	3. MD	_____
_____	_____	_____	4. FACS	_____
_____	_____	_____	5. CMA	_____
_____	_____	_____	6. LVN	_____
_____	_____	_____	7. RNP	_____
_____	_____	_____	8. RPT	_____
_____	_____	_____	9. MT (ASCP)	_____
_____	_____	_____	10. CMT	_____
_____	_____	_____	11. CPC	_____
_____	_____	_____	12. PA-C	_____
_____	_____	_____	13. VN	_____
_____	_____	_____	Complete within specified time.	
____/15	____/15	____/15	**Total points earned** (To obtain a percentage score, divide the total points earned by the number of points possible.)	

JOB SKILL 2–3 (*continued*)

Comments:

JOB SKILL 2–4
Determine Basic Skills for the Administrative Medical Assistant

Name _____ Date _____ Score _____

Performance Objective

Task: Review job requirements and determine basic skills necessary for the administrative medical assistant.

Conditions: Use pen or pencil. Refer to the list of medical specialties and administrative medical assistant job requirements found in Table 2–3 of the textbook.

Standards: Complete all steps listed in this skill in _____ minutes with a minimum score of _____. (Time element and accuracy criteria may be given by instructor.)

Time: **Start:** _____ **Completed:** _____ **Total:** _____ minutes

Scoring: One point for each step performed satisfactorily unless otherwise listed or weighted by instructor.

Directions with Performance Evaluation Checklist

Record some basic skills the administrative medical assistant needs. You will see these skills occurring repetitiously under the different specialties listed in Table 2–3.

1st Attempt	2nd Attempt	3rd Attempt	
_____	_____	_____	Gather materials (equipment and supplies) listed under "Conditions."
_____	_____	_____	1. _____
_____	_____	_____	2. _____
_____	_____	_____	3. _____
_____	_____	_____	4. _____
_____	_____	_____	5. _____
_____	_____	_____	6. _____
_____	_____	_____	7. _____
_____	_____	_____	8. _____
_____	_____	_____	Complete within specified time.
___/10	___/10	___/10	**Total points earned** (To obtain a percentage score, divide the total points earned by the number of points possible.)

Comments:

Evaluator's Signature: _____ **Need to Repeat:** _____

National Curriculum Competency: Skills listed are part of CAAHEP and ABHES competencies.

CHAPTER 3

Medicolegal and Ethical Responsibilities

OBJECTIVES

After completing the exercises, the student will be able to:

1.   Write meanings for chart note abbreviations.

2.   Enhance spelling skills by learning new medical words.

3.   Use critical thinking skills to answer legal questions.

4.   Compose a letter of withdrawal.

FOCUS ON CERTIFICATION*

CMA Content Summary

- Medical (legal) terminology
- Performing within ethical boundaries
- Maintaining confidentiality
- Medical practice acts
- Federal compliance with right to privacy and HIPAA

- Release medical information
- Physician-patient relationships
- Office policies and procedures compliance plan

RMA Content Summary

- Medical (legal) terminology
- Medical law
- Medical ethics
- Understand and maintain patient confidentiality during check-in procedures

- Employ effective written communication skills adhering to ethics and laws of confidentiality
- Prepare and release private health information as required, adhering to state and federal guidelines

*This *Workbook* and accompanying textbook meet the entry-level administrative and general competencies for the CMA outlined by the AAMA Examination Content Outline and Role Delineation Study and for the RMA and CMAS outlined by the AMT Competencies and Examination Specifications (see Competency Grid in textbook Appendix B).

CMAS Content Summary

- Apply principles of medical law and ethics to the health care setting
- Know basic laws pertaining to medical practice
- Know and observe disclosure laws
- Know the principles of medical ethics established by the AMA

- Recognize unethical practices and identify ethical responses for situations in the medical office
- Understand and employ risk management and quality assurance concepts

Abbreviation and Spelling Review

Read the following patient's chart note and write the meanings for the abbreviations listed below the note. To decode any abbreviations you do not understand or that appear unfamiliar to you, refer to the list of abbreviations in Part V of this *Workbook*. Step-by-step directions for this exercise are in Procedure 1-1 of Chapter 1 in the textbook. Medical terms in the chart note are italicized; study them for spelling. Use your medical dictionary to look up their definitions. Your instructor may give a spelling and definition test that includes these words and abbreviations.

David K. Chung

September 20, 20XX HX: *Diarrhea* 3 days. T 99°F. No A. Cough producing yellow *sputum. Wheezing* in lt base. Moderate PND. Rec *vaporizer* and *amoxicillin* 250 mg p.o. q.8h. Diag URI. Etiol. unknown. Ordered CXR, CBC, & UA. Retn 2 wks.

Gerald Practon, MD
_____
Gerald Practon, MD

HX	_____	h.	_____
T	_____	diag	_____
F	_____	URI	_____
A	_____	etiol.	_____
lt	_____	CXR	_____
PND	_____	CBC	_____
rec	_____	UA	_____
mg	_____	retn	_____
p.o.	_____	wks	_____
q.	_____		

Review Questions

Review the objectives, glossary, and chapter information before completing the following review questions.

1. Match the terms in the left column with the definitions in the right column by writing the letters in the blanks.

_____ Oath of Hippocrates

_____ medical ethics

_____ bioethics

_____ privileged information

_____ medical etiquette

a. information in a medical record

b. code of conduct, courtesy, and manners customary in the medical profession

c. moral principles and standards in the medical profession

d. modern code of ethics

_____ Principles of Medical Ethics

    e. branch of ethics concerning moral issues, questions, and problems that arise in the practice of medicine and in biomedical research

    f. first standards of medical conduct and ethics

2. HIPAA stands for _____ .

3. What are the three items a one-time signed consent form covers?

    a. _____

    b. _____

    c. _____

4. What form must be obtained for use and disclosure of protected health information not included in the consent form? _____

5. Information about a patient's past, present, or future health condition that contains personal identifying data is called _____ .

6. What does the privacy rule provide? _____

_____

_____

7. State the definition of a compliance plan. _____

_____

_____

8. What is the common term for litigation? _____

9. The phrase used today for medical malpractice is _____ .

10. Name two types of medical professional liability insurance.

    a. _____

    b. _____

11. A physician is legally responsible for any act you perform while in his employ. The legal phrase used to describe this responsibility is _____ , and it means _____ .

12. Define *tort*. _____

_____

_____

13. Match the words in the left column with the definitions in the right column by writing the letters in the blanks.

    _____ malfeasance   a. carelessness or negligence by a professional person

    _____ misfeasance   b. lawful treatment done in the wrong way

    _____ nonfeasance   c. failure of the physician to do anything

    _____ malpractice   d. reckless disregard for the safety of another; being indifferent to an injury that could occur

    _____ criminal negligence   e. wrongful treatment of the patient

14. Name the three principal defenses in a malpractice lawsuit.

    a. _____

    b. _____

    c. _____

15. Name three alternatives to the litigation process.

    a. _____

    b. _____

    c. _____

16. Name three types of bonding.

    a. _____

    b. _____

    c. _____

17. Name three circumstances in which a minor may become emancipated.

    a. _____

    b. _____

    c. _____

Critical Thinking Exercises

1. A subpoena is served on Dr. Bradley in regard to patient Teri Sanchez. In this instance, is a patient release-of-information form necessary? _____

2. Mrs. Marinacci states she wishes to donate her kidneys for transplant when she dies. How does she legally record her wishes? _____

   _____

   _____

3. A sales representative from the Hope Surgical Company brings a case of bourbon for your physician. Can your physician ethically accept this gift? Why or why not?

   _____

4. Betty Harper is given a booklet on the office policies that explains charges for missed appointments, telephone calls, and insurance form completion. She brings two insurance forms, and you bill her for this service. Is this ethical?

   _____

   _____

5. You overhear Linda Mason telling another patient in the reception room that another physician is treating her for her stomach ulcer. You know Dr. Practon is also treating her for this same condition in addition to her high blood pressure. What should you do? _____

   _____

   _____

6. Martin P. Finley is examined, and the physician discovers a wart recurring on the patient's thumb. Mr. Finley asks the physician to remove it. In this instance, what kind of contract exists?

   _____

7. A tow truck has a head-on collision on a rural highway 25 miles out of town. Dr. O'Halloran is driving along and notices the accident. He stops, finds a victim of the accident bleeding profusely, and renders first aid. Will he be held liable for any medical complication in aiding this victim? _____

   Name the law that governs this situation. _____

8. Candice Goodson, a 15-year-old, comes into the office and requests an examination for her and her baby. Can the physician care for the infant and Candice without Candice's parents' consent? _____

   Why or why not? _____

9. Gary Ryan has an outstanding bill of $200. You receive a signed authorizaion form for release-of-information from Dr. Homer's office requesting a copy of his progress notes since surgery. Can you ethically withhold this information until Mr. Ryan pays his bill?

_____

10. Dr. Rodriguez examines Mr. Garcia and diagnoses a gallstone. He reports this to the patient and recommends surgery. The patient says he agrees to the surgery. Are all conditions of informed consent present in this case?

_____

    If not, name any that might be missing. _____

_____

11. An insurance company sends Dr. Practon a request for the records of Jerry Osborne. A signed authorization accompanies the request. The medical record indicates that the physician discussed HIV testing, and the patient refused the test. What would you do? _____

_____

_____

12. Dr. Gerald Practon receives a request from a social worker for medical records on a minor who is a ward of the court. The minor has signed a release. What would you do? _____

_____

_____

JOB SKILL 3-1
Compose a Letter of Withdrawal

Name _____ Date _____ Score _____

Performance Objective

Task: Compose a letter of withdrawal from Dr. Gerald Practon to a patient who has failed to pay his medical bill.

Conditions: White paper (8½″ × 11″), computer or typewriter. Refer to Part IV of the *Workbook* for letterhead reference information. Refer to Figure 3-11 in the textbook for an illustration of a letter and sample wording.

Standards: Complete all steps listed in this skill in _____ minutes with a minimum score of _____. (Time element and accuracy criteria may be given by instructor.)

Time: **Start:** _____ **Completed:** _____ **Total:** _____ minutes

Scoring: One point for each step performed satisfactorily unless otherwise listed or weighted by instructor.

Directions with Performance Evaluation Checklist

Patrick C. Pieper of 697 Williams Street, Woodland Hills, XY 12345 has received medical services amounting to $525. He provided insurance information at the time services were rendered but he is not eligible for medical coverage or benefits under the plan. He has received four statements and made over the telephone two promises to pay, which he has not kept. Dr. Gerald Practon would now like to send a letter of withdrawal and is allowing Mr. Pieper 30 days to locate another physician. He will be referred to the Ventura County Medical Society, (555) 676-5544, if he is unable to locate a new physician. Compose a personal letter of withdrawal on Dr. Practon's letterhead stating the above information.

1st Attempt	2nd Attempt	3rd Attempt	
_____	_____	_____	Gather materials (equipment and supplies) listed under "Conditions."
_____/5	_____/5	_____/5	1. Using a computer or typewriter, prepare a letterhead that contains the Practon group name, street address, city, state, zip, and telephone number.
_____	_____	_____	2. Format the letter in block style (everything aligned to the left) or modified block style (as in Figure 3-11).
_____	_____	_____	3. Include current date.
_____	_____	_____	4. Include inside address.
_____	_____	_____	5. Include salutation.
____/20	____/20	____/20	6. Compose letter including reason for withdrawing from patient's care, number of days Dr. Practon will be available to attend to Mr. Pieper, referral source for finding a physician, and release of medical record information.
_____/2	_____/2	_____/2	7. Include closing and Dr. Practon's typed and signed signature.
_____	_____	_____	8. Include initials of letter composer.
_____	_____	_____	9. Include list of items that are enclosed with letter.
_____	_____	_____	Complete within specified time.
____/35	____/35	____/35	**Total points earned** (To obtain a percentage score, divide the total points earned by the number of points possible.)

JOB SKILL 3-1 *(continued)*

Comments:

Evaluator's Signature: _____ **Need to Repeat:** _____

National Curriculum Competency: CAAHEP: III.C.3.c(1)	ABHES: VI.B.1.a2(j), VI.B.1.a2(n), VI.B.1.a3(a), VI.B.1.a3(d), VI.B.1.a5(b), VI.B.1.a5(c), VI.B.1.a5(d)

C H A P T E R **4**

The Art of Communication

OBJECTIVES

After completing the assignments, the student will be able to:

1. Write the meaning for chart note abbreviations.
2. Enhance spelling skills by learning new medical terms.
3. Answer questions relating to all aspects of the communication cycle.
4. Demonstrate body language.
5. Name unique qualities of other cultures.

FOCUS ON CERTIFICATION*

CMA Content Summary
- Medical terminology
- Psychology
- Individual self-worth, social and emotional behavior
- Maslow's hierarchy
- Hereditary, cultural, and environmental influences on behavior

- Defense mechanisms
- Adapting communication
- Verbal and nonverbal communication
- Evaluating understanding of communication

RMA Content Summary
- Medical terminology
- Human/Interpersonal relations
- Age-specific responses/support

- Communication methods
- Active listening

*This *Workbook* and accompanying textbook meet the entry-level administrative and general competencies for the CMA outlined by the AAMA Examination Content Outline and Role Delineation Study and for the RMA and CMAS outlined by the AMT Competencies and Examination Specifications (see Competency Grid in textbook Appendix B).

CMAS Content Summary
- Medical terminology
- Human relations/behaviors
- Oral communication

Abbreviation and Spelling Review

Read the following patient's chart note and write the meanings for the abbreviations listed below the note. To decode any abbreviations you do not understand or that appear unfamiliar to you, refer to the list of abbreviations in Part V of this *Workbook*. Step-by-step directions for this exercise are found in Procedure 1-1 of Chapter 1 in the textbook. Medical terms in the chart note are italicized; study them for spelling. Use your medical dictionary to look up their definitions. Your instructor may give a spelling and definition test that includes these words and abbreviations.

32-year-old Cauc female came in for init visit. CO chr pelvic pain, HA, and slt shortness of breath. No ALL. Performed H & P. PMH revealed FUO, PID and *chronic* UTI. Ordered lab. work and M. Patient NYD. Pt to have re ch in approx 3 days. R/O STD.

Gerald Practon, MD

Gerald Practon, MD

Cauc	_____	PID	_____
init	_____	UTI	_____
CO	_____	lab.	_____
chr	_____	M	_____
HA	_____	NYD	_____
slt	_____	Pt	_____
ALL	_____	re ch	_____
H & P	_____	approx	_____
PMH	_____	R/O	_____
FUO	_____	STD	_____

Review Questions

Review the objectives, glossary, and chapter information before completing the following review questions.

1. Of all the professionals that make up a health care team, who has the most interaction with the patient?

   _____

2. Name the basic elements of the communication cycle.

   a. _____

   b. _____

   c. _____

   d. _____

   e. _____

3. List, in order of importance, the top three ways humans communicate messages.

   a. _____

   b. _____

   c. _____

4. Name four forms of communication, including the most productive.

   a. _____

   b. _____

   c. _____

   d. _____

5. When interviewing a patient, what is the key to obtaining accurate information and what should you avoid?

   a. key: _____

   b. avoid: _____

6. What is the number one reason for failure of relationships? _____

7. When does trust begin to develop between the physician and the patient? _____

   _____

   _____

8. What is the term used when a patient refuses to follow the doctor's treatment plan? _____

9. Describe defensive behavior. _____

   _____

   _____

10. Briefly name and describe the five levels of needs according to Maslow's hierarchy theory.

    a. _____

       _____

    b. _____

       _____

    c. _____

       _____

    d. _____

       _____

    e. _____

       _____

11. How can the meaning of spoken words change? _____

    _____

12. What is a "double message"? _____

    _____

13. What is a "comfort zone" and why does it vary? _____

    _____

14. Why do we all need to feel as if we are being listened to? _____

    _____

15. What is the difference between active listening and reflective listening? _____

    _____

16. When trying to encourage a patient to open up and talk, what type of feedback is recommended and why?

    _____

    _____

17. A silent pause may be used to:

    a. _____

    b. _____

    c. _____

    d. _____

    e. _____

    f. _____

    g. _____

18. Why is a professional health care interpreter preferred over a family member when translation is needed?

    _____

    _____

    _____

    _____

19. Why is it important to keep an open mind when dealing with patients of varied ethnic backgrounds?

    _____

    _____

20. The following suggestions are made for special needs patients. State the type of impairment that would match the recommendation listed.

    a. use verbal descriptions _____

    b. use simple words and short phrases, allowing plenty of time for the patient to digest what you have said

    _____

    c. eliminate background noises _____

    d. look directly at the patient when you are speaking _____

21. Name three of the "outward" signs of anxiety.

    a. _____

    b. _____

    c. _____

Critical Thinking Exercises

1. Name one or more common colloquialisms that may confuse a message. _____

    _____

    _____

2. Think about and describe one circumstance in which a person's body language did not match what he or she was saying. _____

    _____

    _____

3. The physician has asked you to convey the following message to a patient. Translate the message into layman's terms so it can be understood. Note: You may need to look up some terms in a medical dictionary. "The patient's chronic diverticulosis has caused acute gastritis, which is resolving. The patient's cystitis and urethritis are unrelated and the Ciprofloxacin will help clear that up."

_____

_____

_____

_____

4. What are some environmental elements in your classroom that may interfere with active listening and

communication? _____

_____

5. Suggestions are listed in the textbook for how to deal with an angry patient. Can you think of a time when you were really angry and the person dealing with you:

a. made the matter worse? Describe how. _____

_____

b. was able to help you dissipate your anger? Describe how. _____

_____

6. In this chapter you have read this powerful statement:

> *In their research, psychologists have learned that the manner in which the medical staff interacts with a sick person can foster wellness or it can unintentionally aggravate a physical condition . . . that the patient's mental state is often more important than performing expert medical skills.*

What do you feel your responsibility is as a member of a health care team, and how does communication play a role in this?

_____

_____

_____

_____

_____

7. Respond to the following situations:

a. A patient, Mrs. Takuchi, stops at your desk on the way out, complaining that the physician wanted to give her an injection but she will not let anybody jab a needle into her and put something into her body. What would you say?

_____

_____

_____

b. The clinical medical assistant, Susan Owens, complains that you did not order the supplies she had requested in time. What would your response be?

_____

_____

_____

JOB SKILL 4-1
Demonstrate Body Language

Name _____ Date _____ Score _____

Performance Objective

Task: Demonstrate positive and negative body language.

Conditions: Two or more persons; props may be used. Note: This exercise may be performed as a "role playing" exercise by dividing the class into teams of two or more. One person or team demonstrates the body language, and the other person or team guesses what feelings the first is trying to display.

Standards: Complete all steps listed in this skill in _____ minutes with a minimum score of _____. (Time element and accuracy criteria may be given by instructor.)

Time: **Start:** _____ **Completed:** _____ **Total:** _____ minutes

Scoring: One point for each step performed satisfactorily unless otherwise listed or weighted by instructor.

Directions with Performance Evaluation Checklist

1st Attempt	2nd Attempt	3rd Attempt	
_____	_____	_____	Gather materials (equipment and supplies) listed under "Conditions."
_____	_____	_____	1. Study the various types of body language described in the textbook under "Nonverbal Communication."
____/10	____/10	____/10	2. Without speaking, use body language to convey the way you are feeling or may feel at times.
____/12	____/12	____/12	**Total points earned** (To obtain a percentage score, divide the total points earned by the number of points possible.)

Comments:

Evaluator's Signature: _____ **Need to Repeat:** _____

National Curriculum Competency: CAAHEP: III.C.3.c(1)(c)   ABHES: VI.B.1.a.2(i), VI.B.1.a.2(k), VI.B.1.a.2(l)

JOB SKILL 4-2
Name Unique Qualities of Other Cultures

Name _____ Date _____ Score _____

Performance Objective

Task: Research and discover unique qualities of other cultures in order to help you understand and serve patients in your geographical area.

Conditions: This will vary according to region but could include library and Internet research, personal interviews, or personal reports (see Resources at the end of Chapter 4).

Standards: Complete all steps listed in this skill in _____ minutes with a minimum score of _____. (Time element and accuracy criteria may be given by instructor.)

Time: **Start:** _____ **Completed:** _____ **Total:** _____ minutes

Scoring: One point for each step performed satisfactorily unless otherwise listed or weighted by instructor.

Directions with Performance Evaluation Checklist

1st Attempt	2nd Attempt	3rd Attempt	
_____	_____	_____	Gather materials (equipment and supplies) listed under "Conditions."
_____	_____	_____	1. Determine which culture you will be researching and what method you will use to discover unique qualities. If you live in an area where there is little ethnic diversity, you may want to look at the migration statistics for your state.
_____	_____	_____	2. Determine which unique features would have an impact on communication.
_____	_____	_____	3. Determine which unique features would have an impact on the delivery of health care.
_____	_____	_____	4. Select one quality that you admire from a culture that is different from yours.
____/5	____/5	____/5	5. Write a one-page summary of unique qualities and be prepared to present it orally to your class.
____/10	____/10	____/10	**Total points earned** (To obtain a percentage score, divide the total points earned by the number of points possible.)

Comments:

Evaluator's Signature: _____ **Need to Repeat:** _____

National Curriculum Competency: CAAHEP: III.C.3.c(3)(b)	ABHES: VI.B.1.a.2(b), VI.B.1.a.2(m)

CHAPTER 5

The Receptionist

OBJECTIVES

After completing the exercises, the student will be able to:

1. Write meanings for chart note abbreviations.
2. Enhance spelling skills by learning new medical words.
3. Respond to situations in a medical office.
4. Supervise filling in a patient information form.
5. Prepare an application form for a disabled person placard.
6. Research materials for in-office resources and patient education.

FOCUS ON CERTIFICATION*

CMA Content Summary

- Medical terminology
- Social and environmental influences on behavior
- Professional attitude
- Confidentiality
- Promoting competent patient care
- General office policies

- Health maintenance and disease prevention instruction
- Community resources
- Professional communication/behavior
- Interviews (registration)
- Office emergencies
- Physician delays

RMA Content Summary

- Medical terminology
- Professional conduct
- Communication methods
- Patient brochures/informational materials
- Patient instruction

- Receiving and greeting patients
- Basic emergency triage
- Patient demographics
- Confidentiality
- Assisting patients

*This *Workbook* and accompanying textbook meet the entry-level administrative and general competencies for the CMA outlined by the AAMA Examination Content Outline and Role Delineation Study and for the RMA and CMAS outlined by the AMT Competencies and Examination Specifications (see Competency Grid in textbook Appendix B).

CMAS Content Summary

- Medical terminology
- Human relations
- Health histories
- Medical emergencies
- Screening visitors/vendors
- Examination room flow

- Patient information and community resources
- Confidentiality
- Biohazardous waste, hazardous chemicals, office safety
- Maintaining facility and environment

Abbreviation and Spelling Review

Read the following patients' chart notes and write the meanings for the abbreviations listed below the note. To decode any abbreviations you do not understand or that appear unfamiliar to you, refer to the list of abbreviations in Part V of this *Workbook*. Step-by-step directions for this exercise are found in Procedure 1-1 of Chapter 1 in the textbook. Medical terms in the chart note are italicized; study them for spelling. Use your medical dictionary to look up their definitions. Your instructor may give a spelling and definition test that includes these words and abbreviations.

DATE	PROGRESS
10/1/20XX	Maria D. Gomez, well-developed Hispanic ♀ fell on sharp object at 9 a.m. *Laceration* of L lower lip 0.5 cm. Tr.: cleaned, *sutured*, & drained. DTaP inj. Retn in 5 days. Fran Practon, MD

♀ _____   Tr. _____

a.m. _____   DTaP _____

L _____   inj. _____

cm _____   retn _____

DATE	PROGRESS
10/1/20XX	Barry K. Wesson This white ♂ had severe pain Ⓛ *sternoclavicular* area. Chest clear to P&A, EKG, ō. AP&L chest XR–N. Demerol 75mg for pain Dx *neuralgia*. Fran Practon, MD

♂ _____   AP&L _____

Ⓛ _____   XR _____

P&A _____   N _____

EKG _____   mg _____

ō _____   Dx _____

Review Questions

Review the objectives, glossary, and chapter information before completing the following review questions.

1. Why are first impressions so important in a medical setting? _____

_____

2. What benefits are attained by patients and the physician when the receptionist is attentive to patients' needs?

   _____

   _____

3. Name several things that are necessary for a person to be successful when multitasking.

   a. _____

   b. _____

   c. _____

   d. _____

4. If you are asked in the evening to pull the records of all patients who will be seen the following day, in what order should they be organized? _____

   _____

   _____

5. What should you check for in each chart after pulling it to be sure the chart is complete and ready for the physician prior to the patient's arrival? _____

   _____

   _____

6. What safeguard can be taken against the mispronunciation of a patient's name? _____

   _____

   _____

7. When greeting patients, what is the easiest way to customize requests and comments to prevent sounding like a broken record? _____

   _____

8. Is calling out a patient's name who is seated in the reception area a violation of HIPAA? Why or why not?

   _____

   _____

9. When addressing patients, when should surnames be used? _____

   _____

10. List alternatives to using a standard patient sign-in log so patient names and "reason for visit" are not viewed by others.

    a. _____

    b. _____

    c. _____

    d. _____

    e. _____

11. List typical ways patients can be registered or preregistered in a medical office.

    a. _____

    b. _____

    c. _____

12. Does a primary care physician with a managed care plan need an authorization prior to seeing a new patient?

    _____

13. What steps need to be taken before releasing PHI to a patient's family member? _____
_____
_____

14. You are the receptionist and have just found out the doctor will be an hour late. Name three options that can be given to waiting patients.

    a. _____

    b. _____

    c. _____

15. List six special considerations that the office staff can provide a disabled or geriatric patient.

    a. _____

    b. _____

    c. _____

    d. _____

    e. _____

    f. _____

16. If your office has an open reception area, what are three things you need to take into consideration on a daily basis?

    a. _____

    b. _____

    c. _____

17. When you visit a physician's office, what are some things that have favorably impressed you in the reception area? _____
_____
_____
_____

18. The medical receptionist needs to maintain a _____ attitude, react _____, and follow _____ _____ in a situation that demands immediate attention, such as an office emergency.

Critical Thinking Exercises

Study the office situations. Use critical thinking skills, tact, and consideration to determine and record your responses. Indicate the situations you have difficulty handling by circling the corresponding numbers in red and bringing them to class for discussion.

1. An impatient Mr. Griffin complains about being kept waiting. How would you respond? _____
_____
_____
_____
_____
_____

2. A patient, Mr. Avery, invites you to have lunch with him. What would you do? _____

_____

_____

_____

_____

_____

_____

3. Despite a "No Smoking" sign, a patient in the waiting room, Mrs. Wilson, lights a cigarette. What would you do or say? _____

_____

_____

_____

_____

_____

_____

_____

4. An overtalkative patient, Mrs. Crowe, is bothering you while you are trying to complete a number of tasks before the next patient arrives. What would you do? _____

_____

_____

_____

_____

_____

_____

5. A patient, Mr. Mendez, comes into the reception room, arrives at your desk or window, and asks your advice about some medication he has seen advertised. What would be your response? _____

_____

_____

_____

_____

_____

6. A patient, Mrs. Jeffers, asks you when she will be through with her treatment. She has just finished seeing the physician and comes to your desk to make her return appointment. What would be your response? _____

_____

_____

_____

_____

7. Mrs. Jones comes up to your desk and asks you if you think cigarette smoking is harmful. What would you say?

_____

_____

_____

_____

8. A friend of yours stops in to see you at the office and wants to "visit." She remains at your desk for 15 minutes talking. The reception room is full of patients. What would you say? _____

_____

_____

_____

_____

_____

9. Mr. Carson, a blind patient, comes to your office for medical care. How would you handle this patient during his visit? _____

_____

_____

_____

_____

_____

10. A patient, Mrs. Jesse Bacon, has just had an appointment and thinks that the physician is withholding information from her. She stops by your desk and inquires, "What do you think the chances are of my returning to work on Monday?" How would you respond? _____

_____

_____

_____

_____

11. An eldery female patient, accompanied by her husband, has arrived for an emergency appointment. She seems to be in pain and is barely able to walk. What should be your immediate response? _____

_____

_____

_____

_____

_____

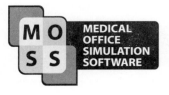

Computer Competency

Go to the Online Companion for this book at www.delmarlearning.com/companions to complete Medical Office Simulation Software activities for this chapter.

JOB SKILL 5-1
Prepare a Patient Registration Form

Name _____ Date _____ Score _____

Performance Objective

Task: Become familiar with questions on a patient registration form. Interview a classmate, friend, or family member and ask him or her to write the information requested on the form as one would when visiting a medical office for the first time. Ask for an insurance card and photocopy it if possible. Proofread the form after completion and make corrections or additions to verify that all information is complete.

Conditions: Use Form 1 found in *Workbook* Part II and a pen. Refer to Figure 5-5 and Procedure 5-2 in the textbook for an illustration and step-by-step directions.

Standards: Complete all steps listed in this skill in _____ minutes with a minimum score of _____. (Time element and accuracy criteria may be given by instructor.)

Time: Start: _____ Completed: _____ Total: _____ minutes

Scoring: One point for each step performed satisfactorily unless otherwise listed or weighted by instructor.

Directions with Performance Evaluation Checklist

1st Attempt	2nd Attempt	3rd Attempt	
_____	_____	_____	Gather materials (equipment and supplies) listed under "Conditions."
_____	_____	_____	1. Select a classmate, friend, or family member to interview.
_____	_____	_____	2. Direct the person to fill out all areas on the Patient Resgistration form and put N/A in areas that do not apply.
_____	_____	_____	3. Obtain an photocopy insurance card(s) for the file (if possible).
_____	_____	_____	4. Proofread form for legibility.
____/7	____/7	____/7	5. Verify that the header information (date, account number, isurance number co-payment, work injury, auto accident, date of injury) at the top of the form was completed.
____/20	____/20	____/20	6. Verify patient's personal information section is completed and all nonapplicable blanks are marked N/A.
____/20	____/20	____/20	7. Verify patient's responsible party information section is completed and all nonapplicable blanks are marked N/A.
____/20	____/20	____/20	8. Verify patient's insurance information section is completed and all nonapplicable blanks are marked N/A.
____/3	____/3	____/3	9. Verify patient's referral information section is completed and all nonapplicable blanks are marked N/A.
____/5	____/5	____/5	10. Verify emergency contact section is completed and all nonapplicable blanks are marked N/A.
____/4	____/4	____/4	11. Verify the assignment of benefits name is filled in, the financial agreement is dated and signed, and method of payment indicated.
_____	_____	_____	Complete within specified time.
____/85	____/85	____/85	**Total points earned** (To obtain a percentage score, divide the total points earned by the number of points possible.)

JOB SKILL 5-1 (continued)

Comments:

Evaluator's Signature: _____ **Need to Repeat:** _____

National Curriculum Competency: CAAHEP: III.C.3.a(1)(a), III.C.3.c(3)(a)   ABHES: VI.B.1.a(3)(a), VI.B.1.a(7)(a)

JOB SKILL 5-2
Prepare an Application Form for a Disabled Person Placard

Name _____ Date _____ Score _____

Performance Objective

Task: 1. Ask a student, family member, or friend to complete an application form for a disabled person placard, making up a medical condition that is either permanent or temporary; review and verify its completion.
2. Complete physician portion for physician review and signature.

Conditions: Use Form 2 found in *Workbook* Part II, pen, and the Medical Practice Reference Material found in Part IV for physician information. Refer to Figure 5-8 and Procedure 5-3 in the textbook for an illustration and step-by-step directions.

Standards: Complete all steps listed in this skill in _____ minutes with a minimum score of _____.
(Time element and accuracy criteria may be given by instructor.)

Time: Start: _____ **Completed:** _____ **Total:** _____ minutes

Scoring: One point for each step performed satisfactorily unless otherwise listed or weighted by instructor.

Directions with Performance Evaluation Checklist

1st Attempt	2nd Attempt	3rd Attempt	
_____	_____	_____	Gather materials (equipment and supplies) listed under "Conditions."
_____	_____	_____	1. Check to see that correct box was marked at top of form.
____/10	____/10	____/10	2. Complete the applicant's information.
____/2	____/2	____/2	3. Verify that the applicant signed and dated the form.
_____	_____	_____	4. Indicate the reason the patient is applying (1 through 7).
_____	_____	_____	5. Complete the type of disability (temporary, moderate, permanent).
____/7	____/7	____/7	6. Complete the physician's information.
_____	_____	_____	7. Proofread document before physician review and signature.
_____	_____	_____	Complete within specified time.
____/26	____/26	____/26	**Total points earned** (To obtain a percentage score, divide the total points earned by the number of points possible.)

Comments:

Evaluator's Signature: _____ **Need to Repeat:** _____

National Curriculum Competency: CAAHEP: III.C.3.a(1), III.C.3.c(2)(e), III.C.3.c(3)(b)	ABHES: VI.B.1.a.2(f), VI.B.1.a.2(m), VI.B.1.a.3(a), VI.B.1.a.7(b)

JOB SKILL 5-3
Research Materials for In-Office Resources and/or Patient Education

Name _____ Date _____ Score _____

Performance Objective

Task: Research to determine what materials are available for in-office resources or patient education using the Internet, telephone, or U.S. mail, and order sample items to share with the class.

Conditions: Computer with Internet connection, telephone, or your own stationery and envelope prepared with Practon Medical Group letterhead (Medical Practice Reference Material found in Part IV of the *Workbook*); resources listed at end of textbook chapter.

Standards: Complete all steps listed in this skill in _____ minutes with a minimum score of _____. (Time element and accuracy criteria may be given by instructor.)

Time: **Start:** _____ **Completed:** _____ **Total:** _____ minutes

Scoring: One point for each step performed satisfactorily unless otherwise listed or weighted by instructor.

Directions with Performance Evaluation Checklist

1st Attempt	2nd Attempt	3rd Attempt	
_____	_____	_____	Gather materials (equipment and supplies) listed under "Conditions."
_____	_____	_____	1. Read resource list at end of chapter in the textbook.
_____	_____	_____	2. Determine if you would like to research materials for office resources or patient education and select a specific topic.
_____	_____	_____	3. Decide whether you will use the Internet, telephone, or a letter to make a request for resource or patient education material.
____/4	____/4	____/4	4. Contact the appropriate source and determine what resources are available.
_____	_____	_____	5. Request a sample of the item(s) selected.
_____	_____	_____	Complete within specified time.
____/10	____/10	____/10	**Total points earned** (To obtain a percentage score, divide the total points earned by the number of points possible.)

Comments:

Evaluator's Signature: _____ **Need to Repeat:** _____

National Curriculum Competency: CAAHEP: III.C.3.c(1)(a), III.C.3.c(1)(d), III.C.3.c(3)(c), III.C.3.c(3)(d)	ABHES: VI.B.1.a.2(e), VI.B.1.a.3(f), VI.B.1.a.7(c)

CHAPTER 6

Telephone Procedures

OBJECTIVES

After completing the exercises, the student will be able to:

1. Write meanings for chart note abbreviations.

2. Enhance spelling skills by learning new medical words.

3. Screen telephone calls and determine the person(s) the calls should be transferred to.

4. Triage patient medical complaints.

5. Prepare telephone message forms.

FOCUS ON CERTIFICATION*

CMA Content Summary

- Medical terminology
- Professional attitude
- Confidentiality
- Verbal communication
- Patient instruction
- Professional tact, diplomacy, courtesy
- Interview techniques
- Receive, organize, prioritize, and transmit information

- Telephone techniques
- Medical records
- Release medical information
- Telephone services and use
- Patient information booklet
- Patient education
- Personnel manual

*This *Workbook* and accompanying textbook meet the entry-level administrative and general competencies for the CMA outlined by the AAMA Examination Content Outline and Role Delineation Study and for the RMA and CMAS outlined by the AMT Competencies and Examination Specifications (see Competency Grid in textbook Appendix B).

RMA Content Summary

- Medical terminology
- Disclosure laws
- Communication methods
- Patient instruction

- Document patient encounters
- Telephone communication
- Chart information

CMAS Content Summary

- Medical terminology
- Human relation skills
- Basic charting
- Medical emergencies
- Effective oral communication

- Incoming telephone calls
- Telephone technique
- Telephone emergency protocols
- Paper charting methods
- Confidentiality

Abbreviation and Spelling Review

Read the following patient's chart note and write the meanings for the abbreviations listed below the note. To decode any abbreviations you do not understand or that appear unfamiliar to you, refer to the list of abbreviations in Part V of this *Workbook*. Step-by-step directions for this exercise are in Procedure 1-1 of Chapter 1 in the textbook. Medical terms in the chart note are italicized; study them for spelling. Use your medical dictionary to look up their definitions. Your instructor may give a spelling and definition test that includes these words and abbreviations.

John F. Mason

October 15, 20XX Pt comes in PO complaining of *anorexia, nausea, & stomatitis.* CBC reveals RBC 80–90, WBC 60–80, Hgb 17 g/100ml. Applied $AgNO_3$. Wound healing well. Cont. med. Ordered BUN. Retn 3 days. RO *uremia.*

Gerald Practon, MD

Gerald Practon, MD

Pt	_____	ml	_____
PO	_____	$AgNO_3$	_____
CBC	_____	Cont.	_____
RBC	_____	med.	_____
WBC	_____	BUN	_____
Hgb	_____	retn	_____
g	_____	RO	_____

Review Questions

Review the objectives, glossary, and chapter information before completing the following review questions.

1. What are three voice components to consider when practicing telephone technique and cultivating a cheerful and calm voice?

   a. _____ b. _____ c. _____

2. What are the two basic things to consider when choosing a telephone system?

   a. _____

   b. _____

3. All incoming calls should be answered before the _____ ring.

4. When speaking to an elderly caller, you should be prepared to_____

_____ .

5. When placing outgoing calls, you should always plan your conversation and _____

_____ .

6. Give four reasons the physician might choose to use a cellular telephone.

   a. _____

   b. _____

   c. _____

   d. _____

7. Name five ways to assure confidentiality when leaving a message in a voice mail system.

   a. _____

   b. _____

   c. _____

   d. _____

   e. _____

8. How does an answering service assist the medical office? _____

_____

9. List five telephone procedures that might be discussed in an information booklet presented to a patient on his or her first visit to the office.

   a. _____

   b. _____

   c. _____

   d. _____

   e. _____

10. Name and define two types of critical situations requiring medical care.

   a. _____

   _____

   b. _____

   _____

11. When telephone lines are busy and calls have to be placed on hold, list several things to consider and actions to take.

   a. _____

   b. _____

   c. _____

   d. _____

   e. _____

   f. _____

   g. _____

12. Name five things that should be included when recording information on a telephone message slip.

    a. _____

    b. _____

    c. _____

    d. _____

    e. _____

13. If no action has been taken on a patient call during the day, what should you do so that the call will not be overlooked in a telephone log? _____

    _____

    _____

14. Define "conference call" and discuss the procedures for setting up this type of call. _____

    _____

    _____

Critical Thinking Exercises

1. Dr. Practon reproaches you for having forgotten to make a telephone call he asked you to make. What would you say? _____

   _____

   _____

   _____

   _____

   _____

2. A patient, Mrs. Braun, wishes to use the physician's telephone. You know she is a talkative person. How would you handle this situation? _____

   _____

   _____

   _____

   _____

   _____

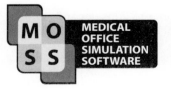

Computer Competency

Go to the Online Companion for this book at www.delmarlearning.com/companions to complete Medical Office Simulation Software activities for this chapter.

JOB SKILL 6-1
Screen Incoming Telephone Calls

Name _____ Date _____ Score _____

Performance Objective

Task: To screen incoming telephone calls and determine the person or persons the calls should be transferred to.

Conditions: Pen or pencil.

Standards: Complete all steps listed in this skill in _____ minutes with a minimum score of _____. (Time element and accuracy criteria may be given by instructor.)

Time: Start: _____ Completed: _____ Total: _____ minutes

Scoring: One point for each step performed satisfactorily unless otherwise listed or weighted by instructor.

Directions with Performance Evaluation Checklist

Refer to the Telephone Decision Grid (Table 6-1) in the textbook to aid in determining how the receptionist would screen and transfer incoming telephone calls. Members of the staff are doctor (MD), office manager (OM), certified medical assistant (CMA), insurance supervisor (INS), and bookkeeper (BK). Write the abbreviations of all those who would be appropriate to receive each telephone call in the space provided. If a message slip would be appropriate, place a check mark on the line (✓).

1st Attempt	2nd Attempt	3rd Attempt	Transfer Call to	Telephone Call Description
			MD OM CMA INS BK	
_____	_____	_____		Gather materials (equipment and supplies) listed under "Conditions."
_____	_____	_____	1. _____	Daughter wants to talk to her father, the physician, and he is with a patient.
_____	_____	_____	2. _____	Doctor is on another telephone and a nurse is at the hospital telephones regarding a patient. After determining urgency, call should be directed to whom?
_____	_____	_____	3. _____	New patient, ill, wants to speak to physician about recently prescribed medication.
_____	_____	_____	4. _____	Patient requests laboratory test results.
_____	_____	_____	5. _____	Insurance carrier requests patient information.
_____	_____	_____	6. _____	Doctor's wife calls to inquire about time of medical association dinner, and doctor is involved with an emergency situation.
_____	_____	_____	7. _____	Patient telephones about a recent bill.
_____	_____	_____	8. _____	Pharmacy telephones regarding a new prescription.
_____	_____	_____	9. _____	Attorney telephones doctor regarding malpractice matter.
_____	_____	_____	10. _____	Professional society member calls for physician.
_____	_____	_____	11. _____	A mother calls about a child who has sunburn.
_____	_____	_____	12. _____	Pharmacy requests Rx refill for patient.
_____	_____	_____	13. _____	Family member asks for information about a child who is under the doctor's care.
_____	_____	_____	14. _____	Patient requests telephone consultation with physician, who is out of the office.
_____	_____	_____	15. _____	Pharmaceutical representative asks to make an appointment with physician for sales presentation.

JOB SKILL 6-1 *(continued)*

_____	_____	_____	16.	_____	Another doctor desires to talk to physician, who is available.
_____	_____	_____	17.	_____	OSHA representative calls about making visit to do inspection.
_____	_____	_____	18.	_____	Established patient asks to talk to physician, who is unable to take the call.
_____	_____	_____	19.	_____	Accountant telephones regarding tax records.
_____	_____	_____	20.	_____	Established patient requests Rx refill.
_____	_____	_____	21.	_____	Established patient calls to report chest pain.
_____	_____	_____	22.	_____	Nurse at convalescent home calls regarding a patient refusing all medication.
_____	_____	_____	23.	_____	Telephone referral request is received from another physician, and doctor is with a patient.
_____	_____	_____	24.	_____	Dentist calls to ask if doctor's patient is taking a new drug.
_____	_____	_____	25.	_____	Former office employee telephones to request a recommendation for a job.
____/5	____/5	____/5	26.	_____	Put check mark by those needing message slips.
_____	_____	_____			Complete within specified time.
____/32	____/32	____/32			**Total points earned** (To obtain a percentage score, divide the total points earned by the number of points possible.)

Comments:

Evaluator's Signature: _____ **Need to Repeat:** _____

National Curriculum Competency: CAAHEP: III.C.3.c(1)(d)	ABHES: VI.B.1.a.2(e), VI.B.1.a.2(h), VI.B.1.a.4(e)

JOB SKILL 6-2
Prepare Telephone Message Forms

Name _____ Date _____ Score _____

Performance Objective

Task: Evaluate the following incoming telephone calls and determine action to be taken on each call. Complete message forms for all calls that require the transfer of information to message slips.

Conditions: Message slips (Forms 3 through 6 in Part II of the *Workbook*), and pen or pencil.

Standards: Complete all steps listed in this skill in _____ minutes with a minimum score of _____. (Time element and accuracy criteria may be given by instructor.)

Time: Start: _____ Completed: _____ Total: _____ minutes

Scoring: One point for each step performed satisfactorily unless otherwise listed or weighted by instructor.

Directions with Performance Evaluation Checklist

It is the morning of Tuesday, November 6, (current year) and both physicians (Fran Practon, MD, and Gerald Practon, MD) are at the hospital and will not be in the office until 1 p.m. Determine which calls may be taken care of immediately (e.g., by making an appointment) and which calls need information transferred to a message slip. Then, indicate what action has been taken on each telephone call and write it on the line following the call (message FP, made appt., or other action). If a message should be taken, record the necessary information (name of patient and caller, telephone number, if chart is attached, and so forth) on the left portion of the form. Be sure to indicate the date and time of the call and your initials.

On the right portion of the form, record who the message is for (i.e., G.P. or F.P.) and compose the message in a complete but brief statement or question. Refer to call No. 1 for an example:

EXAMPLE

1. (9:15) Marguerite Houston (Mrs. C. F.) calls and sounds upset. She wants to ask Dr. Gerald Practon if she can discontinue the medication he prescribed Friday because she thinks she is allergic to it; she now has a rash on her face. You have told her that the doctor is not in the office and that you will ask him to call her (678-7892) as soon as he comes in.

EXAMPLE

	Name of Caller	**Tel. #**	**Reason for Call**	**Action Taken**
Call No. 1	*Marguerite Houston*	*678-7892*	*Can she discontinue medication? Rash on face.*	*Message GP*

PRIORITY ☐		TELEPHONE RECORD 📞
PATIENT Marguerite Houston AGE	MESSAGE G.P.	
CALLER " "	Rash on face - possibly allergic to newly prescribed medication - call asap.	
TELEPHONE 678-7892		
REFERRED TO		TEMP ALLERGIES
CHART #	RESPONSE	
CHART ATTACHED ☒ YES ☐ NO		
DATE Nov. 6, 20XX TIME 9:15 REC'D BY B.C.		
Copyright © 1978 Bibbero Systems, Inc. Printed in the U.S.A.	PHY/RN INITIALS DATE / / TIME HANDLED BY	

Figure 6-1

JOB SKILL 6-2 (*continued*)

1st Attempt	2nd Attempt	3rd Attempt	
_____	_____	_____	Gather materials (equipment and supplies) listed under "Conditions."
____/10	____/10	____/10	1. (9:35) Donald Eggert (765-3145) asks to speak to Dr. Fran Practon. He wants to make an appointment for an injection next week.
____/10	____/10	____/10	2. (9:40) A person calls and refuses to identify himself. He requests information on a patient, Marilyn Turner.
____/10	____/10	____/10	3. (9:55) A patient, Bruce Jeffers (486-2468), calls to cancel his appointment with Dr. Gerald Practon that is scheduled for this afternoon because he has to leave on a flight to New York tomorrow (N.Y. phone 542-671-0121). He will make another appointment upon his return late next week. He would like to know what to do about the series of daily injections he has been receiving from Dr. Practon.
____/10	____/10	____/10	4. (9:58) Phyllis Sperry (678-1162) wants to know the results of the Pap test taken last week by Dr. Fran Practon. (You can find these results in the file and they are normal.)
____/10	____/10	____/10	5. (10:15) Mr. G. W. Witte (678-5478) represents the General Surgical Supply Company and wants to show the doctors a new instrument. You have suggested he call the next day when you will let him know whether either of the physicians will be able to talk to him or schedule an appointment.
____/10	____/10	____/10	6. (10:20) Midway Pharmacy (649-3762) calls Dr. Fran Practon and wants to know if there can be a refill on Philip Stevenson Jr.'s prescription for sleeping pills, No. 8711342.
____/10	____/10	____/10	7. (10:25) Sylvia Cone (411-8215) calls and asks to speak to Dr. Gerald Practon. She refuses to leave a message and says that it is urgent.
____/10	____/10	____/10	8. (10:55) Charles Jones (487-6650) calls to ask if the Practons can recommend an eye, ear, and nose specialist. (There is a reference sheet near the telephone.)
____/10	____/10	____/10	9. (11:00) Mary Lu Practon, the Practons' 14-year-old daughter, calls to report that she is going to Disneyland with the Cone family for the day. She will return home about 9:00 p.m. (Cone's cell phone is 555-678-9000).
____/10	____/10	____/10	10. (11:05) Betty Knott (678-0076) calls to ask if Dr. Gerald Practon will donate time to give flu injections next Sunday from either 9 to 12 or 1 to 3. She needs to know as soon as possible. She is calling from the Reseda Red Cross office on Sepulveda Boulevard, where the injections are to be given.

JOB SKILL 6-2 *(continued)*

_____/10 _____/10 _____/10 11. (11:18) Alan Becker (486-9993) calls and is upset about the bill he received today from Dr. Fran Practon. He thinks the amount is exorbitant, and he asks to speak to Dr. Practon or someone in authority.

_____

_____/10 _____/10 _____/10 12. (11:20) Patricia Papakostikus (687-4512) telephones the office to make an appointment. She is having daily headaches.

_____

_____/10 _____/10 _____/10 13. (11:30) Dr. Martin Laird (643-1108) calls to ask if Dr. Gerald Practon would like a ride to the AMA meeting tonight. Dr. Practon should let Dr. Laird know before 4:00 p.m.

_____

_____/10 _____/10 _____/10 14. (11:45) Elizabeth Montague (411-0068) calls to ask if she should continue her medication. She feels fine now. Dr. Gerald Practon is her physician.

_____

_____/10 _____/10 _____/10 15. (11:50) Alyson Pierce (Mrs. D. M.) (765-9077) calls to ask if Dr. Fran Practon can stop by on her way home tonight at 562 Lynnbrook Avenue, Agoura, to look at her little girl, Courtney, aged 3, who has a high fever (103° F). Alyson has no means of transportation. You tell her you will check with the doctor as soon as possible and will let her know if this home visit can be worked out.

_____

_____/10 _____/10 _____/10 Wrote message forms legibly.

_____ _____ _____ Complete within specified time.

____/162 ____/162 ____/162 **Total points earned** (To obtain a percentage score, divide the total points earned by the number of points possible.)

Comments:

Evaluator's Signature: _____ **Need to Repeat:** _____

National Curriculum Competency: CAAHEP: III.C.3.c(1)(d), III.C.3.c(1)(e)	ABHES: VI.B.1.a.2(e), VI.B.1.a.2(h), VI.B.1.a.2(j), VI.B.1.a.3(a), VI.B.1.a.5(b)

JOB SKILL 6-3
Document Telephone Messages and Physician Responses

Name _____ Date _____ Score _____

Performance Objective

Task: Document telephone messages and physician responses on telephone message slips. Separate slips and attach to file page for insertion in medical record.

Conditions: One sheet of colored paper, two sheets of telephone message forms (Forms 7 and 8), scissors, cellophane adhesive tape or glue, and pen or pencil. Refer to Figures 6-5 and 6-7 in the textbook for visual illustrations.

Standards: Complete all steps listed in this skill in _____ minutes with a minimum score of _____. (Time element and accuracy criteria may be given by instructor.)

Time: **Start:** _____ **Completed:** _____ **Total:** _____ minutes

Scoring: One point for each step performed satisfactorily unless otherwise listed or weighted by instructor.

Directions with Performance Evaluation Checklist

This exercise is for patient Krista Lee Carlisle, Record Number 1181. You will be preparing her chart in Chapter 9 (Patients' Medical Records). On a sheet of colored paper, type the patient's name and record number in the upper right corner. In the upper left corner, type "Telephone Messages." Insert the following data on the telephone message slips. When completed, cut apart the message forms and tape or glue them to the sheet of colored paper; retain it for future use.

1st Attempt	2nd Attempt	3rd Attempt	
_____	_____	_____	Gather materials (equipment and supplies) listed under "Conditions."
____/15	____/15	____/15	1. On February 28, 20XX, at 3:00 p.m., Mrs. Robyn Carlisle called Dr. Gerald Practon stating Krista Lee, age 17, is in bed with flu symptoms. She cancelled her appointment for 3/1/XX. Patient's telephone number is 849-7730. Dr. Practon telephoned Mrs. Carlisle at 4:40 p.m. to recommend that Krista Lee drink plenty of fluids; he will prescribe medication if flu symptoms worsen.
____/15	____/15	____/15	2. On March 2, 20XX, at 3:10 p.m., Robyn Carlisle called Dr. Gerald Practon about her daughter, Krista Lee, who has a temperature of 100.2 degrees F. She said Krista is having chest congestion and a persistent dry cough. She asked for a prescription of cough syrup. The family pharmacy is Long's Drug Store (telephone 849-2221). Dr. Practon asks you to fax an order to the pharmacy for Robitussin-PE, 2 teaspoons, every 4 hours. You ordered the medication from the pharmacy and called Mrs. Carlisle at 4:05 p.m. to give her the information.
____/15	____/15	____/15	3. On March 3, 20XX, at 9 a.m., you receive another call from Robyn Carlisle about Krista Lee. She says she thinks Krista has a possible allergy to the medication because she has a rash on her chest; she is continuing to cough and her temperature is 100 degrees F. Dr. Practon returns call at 11:15 a.m. He tells Robyn to discontinue the Robitussin and suggests an appointment be made for the next day, March 4.
____/15	____/15	____/15	4. Krista Lee sees Dr. Practon on March 4, 20XX, and he prescribes a different cough medication. Dr. Practon asks Mrs. Carlisle to report back in a day or two regarding the rash and cough. Robyn Carlisle calls on March 6, 20XX, at 3:30 p.m., saying Krista's rash has disappeared but she still has a cough, which is now producing discolored phlegm; temperature of 100.3 degrees F. Dr. Practon returns her call at 4:15 p.m. and orders a chest x-ray at College Hospital the following morning and a return appointment the afternoon of March 7. Krista Lee's chart is updated to indicate that she is allergic to codeine.

JOB SKILL 6-3 *(continued)*

____/4   ____/4   ____/4   Wrote message forms legibly.

_____   _____   _____   Complete within specified time.

___/66   ___/66   ___/66   **Total points earned** (To obtain a percentage score, divide the total points earned by the number of points possible.)

Comments:

Evaluator's Signature: _____ **Need to Repeat:** _____

National Curriculum Competency: CAAHEP: III.C.3.a(1)(c), III.C.3.c(1)(e)   ABHES: VI.B.1.a.2(e), VI.B.1.a.2(h), VI.B.1.a.2(j), VI.B.1.a.3(a), VI.B.1.a.5(b)

CHAPTER 7

Appointments

OBJECTIVES

After completing the exercises, the student will be able to:

1. Write meanings for chart note abbreviations.

2. Enhance spelling skills by learning new medical words.

3. Set up three appointment sheets, block the schedule, and record the physician's personal appointments, meetings, and hospital visits.

4. Schedule and record patient appointments using proper abbreviations and coordinating physician and patient availability.

5. Prepare a daily appointment reference for the physician and photocopy the daily appointment schedule.

6. Complete appointment cards.

7. Abstract information and complete a hospital/surgery scheduling form.

8. Transfer surgery scheduling information into a form letter.

9. Complete requisition forms for outpatient diagnostic tests.

FOCUS ON CERTIFICATION*

CMA Content Summary

- Medical abbreviations and symbols
- Disease abbreviations
- Appointment abbreviations
- Appointment office policies
- Telephone technique
- Computerized appointments
- Scheduling and monitoring appointments

*This *Workbook* and accompanying textbook meet the entry-level administrative and general competencies for the CMA outlined by the AAMA Examination Content Outline and Role Delineation Study and for the RMA and CMAS outlined by the AMT Competencies and Examination Specifications (see Competency Grid in textbook Appendix B).

RMA Content Summary

- Abbreviations and symbols
- Interpersonal skills with vendors and business associates
- Patient education
- Appointment documentation

- Medical terminology applications
- Scheduling systems
- Managing various appointments
- Telephone etiquette

CMAS Content Summary

- Medical terminology and abbreviations
- Human relation skills and professionalism
- Charting
- Appointment scheduling and monitoring
- Appointment cancellations, no-shows, referrals, recalls

- Hospital admissions and outside appointments
- Appointment flow
- Telephone technique
- Patient chart documentation
- Computerized appointments

Abbreviation and Spelling Review

Read the following patient's chart note and write the meanings for the abbreviations listed below the note. To decode any abbreviations you do not understand or that appear unfamiliar to you, refer to the list of abbreviations in Part V of this *Workbook*. Step-by-step directions for this exercise are in Procedure 1-1 of Chapter 1 in the textbook. Medical terms in the chart note are italicized; study them for spelling. Use your medical dictionary to look up their definitions. Your instructor may give a spelling and definition test that includes these words and abbreviations.

Dan F. Goodson

September 3, 20XX IV *chemotherapy* started in hospital. Daily hosp PO exams. See op. report giving dx: *superficially infiltrating transitional* cell Ca Class III. Pt DC from hosp 11-1-20XX. Retn for OV 3 p.m. Friday. PT to be started in 1 mo.

Gerald Practon, MD
Gerald Practon, MD

IV _____	DC _____
hosp _____	retn _____
PO _____	OV _____
op. _____	p.m. _____
dx _____	PT _____
Ca _____	mo _____
Pt _____	

Review Questions

Review the objectives, glossary, and chapter information before completing the following review questions.

1. Describe an appointment template. _____

_____

2. In a typical office, what time intervals are usually assigned for the following types of patients?

   Initial visits: _____ Follow-up examinations: _____

3. What is the name of the sheet used to track the number of patients seen daily for various types of appointments in order to determine a scheduling system? _____

   _____

4. What five factors should be taken into consideration when an appointment book is being selected?

   a. _____ d. _____

   b. _____ e. _____

   c. _____

5. Why is it advantageous to schedule patient appointments one right after the other? _____

   _____

6. What is the benefit of having a medical assistant make confirmation telephone calls to patients scheduled to be seen within one or two days? _____

   _____

7. Which patient flow technique do most physician offices use? _____

8. Describe true wave scheduling. _____

   _____

   _____

9. What are long wait times equated with? _____

10. List four actions the medical assistant might take when an emergency telephone call indicates an immediate response.

    a. _____

    b. _____

    c. _____

    d. _____

11. When might an appointment be scheduled for a patient who is habitually late? _____

    _____

12. Besides having a written record of all appointments, why is it important to keep accurate and permanent information? _____

    _____

    _____

13. What systems or devices might a physician use to keep track of out-of-office appointments?

    a. _____

    b. _____

    c. _____

    d. _____

    e. _____

14. Why should postcards not be sent to remind patients of upcoming appointments? _____

    _____

15. Explain what an appointment reference sheet is and what purpose it serves. _____
_____
_____

Critical Thinking Exercises

1. Mrs. Bettle, who has arrived for her appointment an hour early, is sure that she has come at the right time. What would you say to her? _____
_____
_____
_____
_____

2. After seeing the physician, Mrs. Hall stops at your desk for a new appointment. What do you say to her?
_____
_____
_____
_____
_____

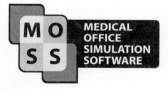

Computer Competency

Go to the Online Companion for this book at www.delmarlearning.com/companions to complete Medical Office Simulation Software activities for this chapter.

JOB SKILL 7-1
Prepare Appointment Sheets

Name _____ Date _____ Score _____

Performance Objective

Task: Set up three appointment pages, labeling each and blocking segments of time.

Conditions: Three appointment records, Forms 9, 10, and 11; pen or pencil. Refer to Procedure 7-1 in the textbook for step-by-step directions.

Standards: Complete all steps listed in this skill in _____ minutes with a minimum score of _____.
                (Time element and accuracy criteria may be given by instructor.)

Time: **Start:** _____ **Completed:** _____ **Total:** _____ minutes

Scoring: One point for each step performed satisfactorily unless otherwise listed or weighted by instructor.

Directions with Performance Evaluation Checklist

1st Attempt	2nd Attempt	3rd Attempt	
_____	_____	_____	Gather materials (equipment and supplies) listed under "Conditions."
____/6	____/6	____/6	1. Set up three appointment sheets for Dr. Gerald Practon (left column) and Dr. Fran Practon (right column).
____/2	____/2	____/2	2. Label the first sheet Monday, October 27, 20XX.
____/2	____/2	____/2	3. Label the second sheet Tuesday, October 28, 20XX.
____/2	____/2	____/2	4. Label the third sheet Wednesday, October 29, 20XX.
____/6	____/6	____/6	5. Refer to the Office Hours section of Office Policies in Part IV of this *Workbook* to determine when the physicians are in the office. Circle the opening and closing hours of the office for each day.
____/9	____/9	____/9	6. Block off all periods when the physicians are not in the office, i.e., lunch hours, afternoons off, and surgery/hospital responsibility time.
____/2	____/2	____/2	7. Record Dr. G. Practon's plans to visit Donald Pierce at the hospital at 9:00 a.m. on Tuesday morning and at noon on Wednesday.
____/2	____/2	____/2	8. Record Dr. F. Practon's one-hour dental appointment with Dr. Bryce Crowe at 2:30 p.m. on Wednesday. She will need to leave the office at 2:15 p.m.
____/9	____/9	____/9	9. Indicate which appointment times are reserved for unscheduled patients (work-ins, emergences, and so forth).
_____	_____	_____	Complete within specified time.
____/42	____/42	____/42	**Total points earned** (To obtain a percentage score, divide the total points earned by the number of points possible.)

Comments:

Evaluator's Signature: _____ **Need to Repeat:** _____

National Curriculum Competency: CAAHEP: III.C.3.a(1)(a)	ABHES: VI.B.1.a.3(c)

JOB SKILL 7-2
Schedule Appointments

Name _____ Date _____ Score _____

Performance Objective

Task: Record patient appointments accurately using acceptable abbreviations on appointment sheets. Adjust to individual patient preferences, medical needs, and unexpected changes.

Conditions: Use the three appointment records from Job Skill 7-1 (Forms 9, 10, and 11), *Workbook* Table 7-1 for appointment reference information, and textbook Table 7-1 (also found in Part V of this *Workbook* (Abbreviation Tables), if you need help decoding appointment and patient care abbreviations. Step-by-step directions are in textbook Procedure 7-2. Use pen or pencil.

Standards: Complete all steps listed in this skill in _____ minutes with a minimum score of _____. (Time element and accuracy criteria may be given by instructor.)

Time: **Start:** _____ **Completed:** _____ **Total:** _____ minutes

Scoring: One point for each step performed satisfactorily unless otherwise listed or weighted by instructor.

Directions with Performance Evaluation Checklist

All patients are established unless otherwise indicated. An asterisk (*) by a patient's name indicates a patient of Dr. Fran Practon; all others are patients of Dr. Gerald Practon. Refer to the Appointment section of Office Policies in Part IV of this *Workbook* to determine the amount of time for each appointment. Schedule an appointment for each patient appearing in this exercise. It may help to use a ruler as you go down the list of names in *Workbook* Table 7-1 and check them off as you schedule.

1st Attempt	2nd Attempt	3rd Attempt	
_____	_____	_____	Gather materials (equipment and supplies) listed under "Conditions."
_____/5	_____/5	_____/5	1. Schedule an appointment for: *Melissa Jones.
_____/5	_____/5	_____/5	2. Schedule an appointment for: *Marsha MacFadden.
_____/5	_____/5	_____/5	3. Schedule an appointment for: Wendy Snow.
_____/5	_____/5	_____/5	4. Schedule an appointment for: Phyllis Dayton.
_____/5	_____/5	_____/5	5. Schedule an appointment for: *Rebecca Martinez.
_____/5	_____/5	_____/5	6. Schedule an appointment for: *Jane Call.
_____/5	_____/5	_____/5	7. Schedule an appointment for: *Mary Fay Jeffers.
_____/5	_____/5	_____/5	8. Schedule an appointment for: *Philip Stevenson Jr.
_____/5	_____/5	_____/5	9. Schedule an appointment for: *Shirley Van Alystine.
_____/5	_____/5	_____/5	10. Schedule an appointment for: Courtney Pierce.
_____/5	_____/5	_____/5	11. Schedule an appointment for: Paul Stone.
_____/5	_____/5	_____/5	12. Schedule an appointment for: *Alan Becker.
_____/5	_____/5	_____/5	13. Schedule an appointment for: *Marguerite Houston.
_____/5	_____/5	_____/5	14. Schedule an appointment for: *Paul Frenzel.
_____/5	_____/5	_____/5	15. Schedule an appointment for: Elizabeth Montgomery, RN.
_____/5	_____/5	_____/5	16. Schedule an appointment for: Lu Chung.
_____/5	_____/5	_____/5	17. Schedule an appointment for: Jerry Calhoun.
_____/5	_____/5	_____/5	18. Schedule an appointment for: Cathy Martinez.
_____/5	_____/5	_____/5	19. Schedule an appointment for: Lloyd Wix.
_____/5	_____/5	_____/5	20. Schedule an appointment for: Bruce Jeffers.
_____/5	_____/5	_____/5	21. Schedule an appointment for: *Ashley Jones.
_____/5	_____/5	_____/5	22. Schedule an appointment for: *David Martinez.
_____/5	_____/5	_____/5	23. Schedule an appointment for: Carl Freeburg.
_____/5	_____/5	_____/5	24. Schedule an appointment for: *Anne Rule.
_____/5	_____/5	_____/5	25. Schedule an appointment for: Charles Jones.

JOB SKILL 7-2 (*continued*)

_____/5	_____/5	_____/5	26. Schedule an appointment for: Robert LaRue.
_____/5	_____/5	_____/5	27. Schedule an appointment for: *Phyllis Sperry.
_____/5	_____/5	_____/5	28. Schedule an appointment for: Sylvia Cone.
_____/5	_____/5	_____/5	29. Schedule an appointment for: *Pat Wochesky.
_____/5	_____/5	_____/5	30. Schedule an appointment for: Sheila Haley.
_____/5	_____/5	_____/5	31. Schedule an appointment for: Frank Elder.
_____/5	_____/5	_____/5	32. Schedule an appointment for: *Donald Eggert.
_____	_____	_____	Complete within specified time.
___/162	___/162	___/162	**Total points earned** (To obtain a percentage score, divide the total points earned by the number of points possible.)

TABLE 7-1. Information Necessary for the Student to Prepare Appointment Schedules for Drs. Fran T. Practon and Gerald M. Practon

Name	Phone Number	Complaint or Procedure	Appointment Preference
*Melissa Jones	487-6650	Pap, estrogen inj.	Tues., p.m.
*Marsha MacFadden	487-0027	ECG, brief OV	Tues., a.m.
Wendy Snow	765-6626	Cast ck, leg	Mon.
Phyllis Dayton	411-2244	Pap, limited exam	Mon.
*Rebecca Martinez	765-0008	Measles inj.	Wed.
*Jane Call	678-0134	Smallpox vac.	Wed.
*Mary Fay Jeffers	486-2468	MMR	Mon. after school
*Philip Stevenson Jr.	457-1133	BP, UA	Mon.
*Shirley Van Alystine	678-4421	IUD, BP	Tues.
Courtney Pierce	765-9077	Fever, cough	Tues. p.m.
Paul Stone	411-7206	F/U	Late Tues.
*Alan Becker	486-9993	Face infection, ltd. exam	Mon.
*Marguerite Houston	678-7892	Inj. for allergy	Tues. around 3:00 p.m.
*Paul Frenzel	765-8897	Dressing change	Early Wed., a.m.
Elizabeth Montgomery, RN	411-0068	BP	Tues. a.m. (see F. P.?)
Lu Chung	678-4455	Allergy complaint	Mon.
Jerry Calhoun	678-8771	N/P, CPX, CBC	Late as possible Tues.
Cathy Martinez	765-0008	Excise lesion on back	Wed.
Lloyd Wix	678-5529	Consult	Tues. 10:30 a.m.—must see G. P. (Wed.?)
Bruce Jeffers	486-2468	Remove glass from eye	Early Wed.
*Ashley Jones	487-6650	Suture removal	Mon. after 2:30 p.m.
*David Martinez	765-0008	Remove splinter from leg	Wed. a.m.
Carl Freeburg	486-0011	Aspirate left elbow	Late Wed.
*Anne Rule	457-9001	N/P, CPX	Mon. a.m.
Charles Jones	487-6650	Audiogram, ear lavage	Mon. p.m.
Robert LaRue	487-3355	Brief OV, VDRL	Must have Tues. a.m. (see F. P.?)
*Phyllis Sperry	678-1162	N/P, CPX	Tues. p.m.
Sylvia Cone	411-8215	HA, N/P	Wed. after lunch
*Pat Wochesky	765-3446	New OB	Wed. a.m.
Sheila Haley	678-6669	Tetanus	Wed. a.m.
Frank Elder	486-0918	N/P, pain in side, BUN, CBC	Mon.
*Donald Eggert	765-3145	Sore elbow, ltd. exam	Early Mon. p.m.

*Asterisks indicate Dr. Fran T. Practon's patients.

Comments:

Evaluator's Signature: _____ **Need to Repeat:** _____

National Curriculum Competency: CAAHEP: III.C.3.a(1)(a)   ABHES: VI.B.1.a.3(c)

JOB SKILL 7-3
Prepare an Appointment Reference Sheet

Name _____ Date _____ Score _____

Performance Objective

Task: Key or type the names of patients who are to be seen by the physician on a given day for a reference sheet. Make a photocopy of the appointment sheet for comparison or to use as an alternative reference.

Conditions: One sheet of white paper, computer (word processor) or typewriter, and photocopy machine.

Standards: Complete all steps listed in this skill in _____ minutes with a minimum score of _____. (Time element and accuracy criteria may be given by instructor.)

Time: **Start:** _____ **Completed:** _____ **Total:** _____ minutes

Scoring: One point for each step performed satisfactorily unless otherwise listed or weighted by instructor.

Directions with Performance Evaluation Checklist

1st Attempt	2nd Attempt	3rd Attempt	
_____	_____	_____	Gather materials (equipment and supplies) listed under "Conditions."
_____	_____	_____	1. Abstract information from Dr. Gerald Practon's schedule for Day 3 listed in Job Skill 7-1 and 7-2.
____/3	____/3	____/3	2. Center and bold-face the following information as the title for the appointment reference sheet: Wednesday, October 29, 20XX, Dr. Gerald Practon.
____/3	____/3	____/3	3. Make three columns and title them in capital letters: TIME, NAME, REASON FOR VISIT.
____/15	____/15	____/15	4. Key a single-spaced list of appointment times, patient names (last name first), and reason for visit to let Dr. G. Practon know who is expected the morning of Wednesday, October 29, 20XX.
_____	_____	_____	5. Photocopy the appointment page for Wednesday, October 29, 20XX, and compare it with the typed list. Additional copies would generally be made for office staff.
_____	_____	_____	Complete within specified time.
____/25	____/25	____/25	**Total points earned** (To obtain a percentage score, divide the total points earned by the number of points possible.)

Comments:

Evaluator's Signature: _____ **Need to Repeat:** _____

National Curriculum Competency: CAAHEP: III.C.3.a(1)(a)   ABHES: VI.B.1.a.3(c)

JOB SKILL 7-4
Complete Appointment Cards

Name _____ Date _____ Score _____

Performance Objective

Task: Write accurate and legible appointment cards.

Conditions: Use appointment cards (Form 12) and pen or pencil.

Standards: Complete all steps listed in this skill in _____ minutes with a minimum score of _____.
                 (Time element and accuracy criteria may be given by instructor.)

Time: Start: _____ **Completed:** _____ **Total:** _____ minutes

Scoring: One point for each step performed satisfactorily unless otherwise listed or weighted by instructor.

Directions with Performance Evaluation Checklist

Write the patient's name at the top of the card, check the correct physician, circle the day of the week, and write the appointment date and time for the following patients.

1st Attempt	2nd Attempt	3rd Attempt	
_____	_____	_____	Gather materials (equipment and supplies) listed under "Conditions."
____/5	____/5	____/5	1. Charles Jones, Wednesday, October 29, at 2:00 p.m.
____/5	____/5	____/5	2. *Marguerite Houston, Tuesday, November 12, at 3:00 p.m.
____/5	____/5	____/5	3. Carl Freeburg, Wednesday, November 6, at 2:45 p.m.
____/5	____/5	____/5	4. *Pat Wochesky, Monday, December 2, at 9:00 a.m.
_____	_____	_____	Complete within specified time.
____/22	____/22	____/22	**Total points earned** (To obtain a percentage score, divide the total points earned by the number of points possible.)

Comments:

Evaluator's Signature: _____ **Need to Repeat:** _____

JOB SKILL 7-5
Abstract Information and Complete a Hospital/Surgery Scheduling Form

Name _____ Date _____ Score _____

Performance Objective

Task: Review a patient's medical record and then abstract and key or type the required information on the hospital/surgery scheduling form.

Conditions: Wayne G. Weather's patient information (*Workbook* Figure 7-1), one hospital/surgery scheduling form (Form 13), pen or pencil, and correction fluid. Refer to Procedure 7-4 in the textbook for step-by-step directions.

Standards: Complete all steps listed in this skill in _____ minutes with a minimum score of _____. (Time element and accuracy criteria may be given by instructor.)

Time: **Start:** _____ **Completed:** _____ **Total:** _____ minutes

Scoring: One point for each step performed satisfactorily unless otherwise listed or weighted by instructor.

Directions with Performance Evaluation Checklist

Using Mr. Wayne Weather's "Patient Information for Medical Records" found in *Workbook* Figure 7-1, abstract data to complete the hospital/surgical scheduling form. Use the following additional information: Mr. Weather was referred to Dr. Gerald Practon by Dr. Mary Hill (597 Moran Road, Woodland Hills, XY 12345) and is to be admitted to College Hospital for a three-day stay on Tuesday, October 28, 20XX, at 5:30 a.m. His diagnosis is lumbar herniated nucleus pulposus, and a second opinion is not required. His preadmission testing of CBC, EKG, and chest x-ray was performed on October 27, 20XX. He has not been previously hospitalized. Mr. Weather is a smoker and prefers a ward room. The elective lumbar (L4-L5) laminectomy is scheduled for Tuesday, October 28, 20XX, at 7:30 a.m. Preadmission operation instructions as well as insurance and financial arrangements have been discussed.

Dr. Clarence Cutler (55011 Paxton Blvd., Woodland Hills, XY 12345) will be the assistant surgeon and Dr. Harold Barker (621 W. Elm Street, Woodland Hills, XY 12345) will give general anesthesia. The surgery, scheduled by hospital employee Robert Slye, should take approximately one hour to complete. Kevin Raye of Aetna Casualty & Security Company provided the authorization number, 8036981, and the scheduling was completed and reported to the patient on October 24. Susan Smith at the referring physician's office has been notified and all arrangements have been posted in the appointment book.

1st Attempt	2nd Attempt	3rd Attempt	
_____	_____	_____	Gather materials (equipment and supplies) listed under "Conditions."
_____	_____	_____	1. Section 1: Indicate patient name.
_____	_____	_____	2. Section 1: Indicate procedure.
_____	_____	_____	3. Section 1: Indicate status of surgery.
_____	_____	_____	4. Section 1: Indicate diagnosis.
_____	_____	_____	5. Section 1: Indicate facility.
_____	_____	_____	6. Section 1: Indicate admitting status.
_____	_____	_____	7. Section 1: Indicate assistant surgeon.
_____	_____	_____	8. Section 1: Indicate anesthesiologist.
_____	_____	_____	9. Section 1: Indicate referring physician.
_____/3	_____/3	_____/3	10. Section 2: Indicate patient's age, date of birth, smoking status.
_____	_____	_____	11. Section 2: Indicate type of room preferred.
_____/2	_____/2	_____/2	12. Section 2: Indicate telephone numbers.
_____/2	_____/2	_____/2	13. Section 2: Indicate insurance information.
_____	_____	_____	14. Section 2: Indicate second opinion requirements.
_____/3	_____/3	_____/3	15. Section 2: Indicate emergency contact.

JOB SKILL 7-5 *(continued)*

_____	_____	_____	16.	Section 2: Indicate previous admitting information.
_____/3	_____/3	_____/3	17.	Section 2: Indicate preadmission testing.
_____	_____	_____	18.	Section 2: Indicate admission procedures reported.
_____	_____	_____	19.	Section 2: Indicate instructions given to patient.
_____	_____	_____	20.	Section 2: Indicate insurance/financial discussion.
_____/2	_____/2	_____/2	21.	Section 3: Indicate operating room reservation.
_____	_____	_____	22.	Section 3: Indicate hospital surgical scheduling person.
_____	_____	_____	23.	Section 3: Indicate assistant surgeon notified.
_____	_____	_____	24.	Section 3: Indicate anesthesiologist notified.
_____	_____	_____	25.	Section 3: Indicate referring physician notified.
_____	_____	_____	26.	Section 3: Indicate admission and preadmission tests confirmed.
_____	_____	_____	27.	Section 3: Indicate prior authorization obtained.
_____	_____	_____	28.	Section 3: Indicate appointment book data posted.
_____	_____	_____	29.	Section 3: Indicate patient advised.
_____	_____	_____	30.	Section 3: Indicate H & P done.
_____/2	_____/2	_____/2	31.	Section 3: Indicate name of office scheduler and date scheduled.
_____	_____	_____		Complete within specified time.
____/43	____/43	____/43		**Total points earned** (To obtain a percentage score, divide the total points earned by the number of points possible.)

Comments:

Evaluator's Signature: _____ **Need to Repeat:** _____

National Curriculum Competency: CAAHEP: III.C.3.a(1)(b)	ABHES: VI.B.1.a.3(h)

JOB SKILL 7-5 *(continued)*

PATIENT INFORMATION FOR MEDICAL RECORDS *(Please Print)*				DATE: 10/24/XX		

PATIENT (MR.) MRS. MISS

LAST NAME	FIRST NAME	MIDDLE
Weather	Wayne	G

PATIENT ADDRESS

STREET	CITY	STATE	ZIP	HOME PHONE
6304 Fracture Road	Woodland Hills, XY 12345		555/965-2110	

SOCIAL SECURITY NUMBER	DATE OF BIRTH	AGE	DRIVER'S LICENSE NO.
072-XX-5334	1-6-43		G-0073-121

PATIENT EMPLOYER	OCCUPATION
Bu T. Floor Coverings	carpet layer

EMPLOYER'S ADDRESS

STREET	CITY	STATE	ZIP	BUS. PHONE
3100 Rug Street,	Woodland Hills,	XY	12345	555/861-0122

SPOUSE'S NAME	MARITAL STATUS	REFERRED BY
Nancy B. Weather (M) S D W SEP.		Employer

SPOUSE'S EMPLOYER

STREET	CITY	STATE	ZIP	BUS. PHONE
Superior Optical Co. 25 E. Main St.,	Woodland Hills, XY		12345-0000	555/761-0811

IN CASE OF EMERGENCY CONTACT:

NAME	ADDRESS	CITY	STATE	ZIP	TELEPHONE
Jolly B. Rosen (stepbrother)	3641 Hope St,	Woodland Hills,	XY	12345	555/876-6025

◄ MEDICAL INSURANCE INFORMATION

COMPANY	POLICY NUMBER
Aetna Casualty and Security Co. 2412 Wilshire Blvd., Woodland Hills, XY 12345-0000	
N/A	3201

◄ IF SOMEONE OTHER THAN PATIENT IS RESPONSIBLE FOR PAYMENT PLEASE COMPLETE THIS SECTION

RESPONSIBLE PARTY MR. MRS. MISS

LAST NAME	FIRST NAME	MIDDLE	RELATION

ADDRESS	STREET	CITY	STATE	ZIP	TELEPHONE

OCCUPATION	EMPLOYED BY

EMPLOYER'S ADDRESS	STREET	CITY	STATE	ZIP	BUS. PHONE

I hereby authorize Dr. *Gerald Praston* to furnish to the above insurance company(s) or to a designated attorney, all information which said insurance company(s) or attorney may request. I hereby assign to Dr. *Gerald Praston* all money to which I am entitled for medical and/or surgical expense relative to the service rendered by him, but not to exceed my indebtedness to said physician and/or surgeon. It is understood that any money received from the above named insurance company, over and above my indebtedness will be refunded to me when my bill is paid in full. I understand I am financially responsible to said doctor(s) for charges not covered by this assignment. I further agree in the event of non-payment, to bear the cost of collection, and/or Court cost and reasonable legal fees should this be required.

_____
INSURED OR GUARDIAN SIGNATURE

Wayne G. Weather
PATIENT'S SIGNATURE

_____

58-8409   © 1976 BIBBERO SYSTEMS, INC., SAN FRANCISCO

Figure 7-1

JOB SKILL 7-6
Transfer Surgery Scheduling Information to a Form Letter

Name _____ Date _____ Score _____

Performance Objective

Task: Use surgical scheduling information and fill in a form letter to be mailed to persons involved in the procedure.

Conditions: Use hospital/surgery scheduling form (Form 13) for reference. Duplicate Form 14 using photocopy machine; one copy will be sent to the patient, and the other will be retained in Dr. Practon's files. Use pen or pencil.

Standards: Complete all steps listed in this skill in _____ minutes with a minimum score of _____. (Time element and accuracy criteria may be given by instructor.)

Time: **Start:** _____ **Completed:** _____ **Total:** _____ minutes

Scoring: One point for each step performed satisfactorily unless otherwise listed or weighted by instructor.

Directions with Performance Evaluation Checklist

1st Attempt	2nd Attempt	3rd Attempt	
_____	_____	_____	Gather materials (equipment and supplies) listed under "Conditions."
_____	_____	_____	1. Read the surgical scheduling form letter to determine what information needs to be abstracted from the hospital/surgery scheduling form (Form 13).
____/3	____/3	____/3	2. Fill in the date and complete the inside address.
____/10	____/10	____/10	3. Fill in the information in the body of the letter.
____/4	____/4	____/4	4. Sign the letter and fill in the information for the physicians involved.
_____	_____	_____	Complete within specified time.
____/20	____/20	____/20	**Total points earned** (To obtain a percentage score, divide the total points earned by the number of points possible.)

Comments:

Evaluator's Signature: _____ **Need to Repeat:** _____

National Curriculum Competency: CAAHEP: III.C.3.a(1)(b)	ABHES: VI.B.1.a.3(h)

JOB SKILL 7-7
Complete Requisition Forms for Outpatient Diagnostic Tests

Name _____ Date _____ Score _____

Performance Objective

Task: Handwrite information on requisition forms to be given to patients to have outpatient diagnostic tests performed.

Conditions: Use Laboratory Requisition (Form 15) and X-Ray Request (Form 16) and pen. Refer to Procedure 7-5 in textbook for step-by-step directions. Refer to Medical Practice Reference Material (Part IV of the *Workbook*) for physician data.

Standards: Complete all steps listed in this skill in _____ minutes with a minimum score of _____. (Time element and accuracy criteria may be given by instructor.)

Time: **Start:** _____ **Completed:** _____ **Total:** _____ minutes

Scoring: One point for each step performed satisfactorily unless otherwise listed or weighted by instructor.

Directions with Performance Evaluation Checklist

Read the following case scenario, abstract information, and complete two requisition forms.

An HMO patient, Ted N. Thatcher, comes to the office complaining of neck and right shoulder pain. After an examination, Dr. Fran Practon orders fasting laboratory tests (arthritis profile, uric acid, and urinalysis). Comprehensive cervical spine x-rays and a complete shoulder series are scheduled for March 4, 20XX, at 11:00 a.m. Diagnosis is acute cervical arthritis (*ICD-9-CM* code 721.0) and shoulder pain (*ICD-9-CM* code 719.41). Patient to return in one week.

Mr. Thatcher's Social Security number is 450-XX-9509; birthdate: 5/8/73; address: 870 N. Seacrest St., Woodland Hills, XY 12345-0846; telephone number: (555) 987-4589; insurance: HMO Net, 4390 Main Street, Woodland Hills, XY 12345-0846, policy no. 459-0987-0. For this particular managed care plan, the outside services that Dr. Practon ordered do not require preauthorization. Today's date: February 28, 20XX.

1st Attempt	2nd Attempt	3rd Attempt	
_____	_____	_____	Gather materials (equipment and supplies) listed under "Conditions."
_____	_____	_____	1. List what type of diagnostic tests are to be performed.
_____	_____	_____	2. List the date the patient has agreed upon.
_____	_____	_____	3. List the name of the insurance carrier.
_____	_____	_____	4. Telephone the diagnostic facility (ABC Radiology) and schedule the tests. List the time the tests are scheduled.
____/20	____/20	____/20	5. Abstract information from the case scenario and fill in the Laboratory Requisition form; hand the form to the patient and record information in chart.
____/15	____/15	____/15	6. Abstract information from the case scenario and fill in the X-Ray Request form; hand to the patient and record information in chart.
_____	_____	_____	Complete within specified time.
____/41	____/41	____/41	**Total points earned** (To obtain a percentage score, divide the total points earned by the number of points possible.)

Comments:

Evaluator's Signature: _____ Need to Repeat: _____

National Curriculum Competency: CAAHEP: III.C.3.a(1)(b)   ABHES: VI.B.1.a.3(h)

CHAPTER **8**

Filing Procedures

OBJECTIVES

After completing the exercises, the student will be able to:

1. Enhance knowledge of medical terminology, interpret abbreviations, and accurately spell medical words.

2. Determine filing units.

3. Index and file names alphabetically.

4. File patient and business names alphabetically.

5. Index names on file folder labels and arrange file cards in alphabetical order.

6. Color code file cards.

FOCUS ON CERTIFICATION*

CMA Content Summary

- Medical terminology and abbreviations
- Release of patient information
- Priority of incoming and outgoing data
- Medical records and personal records
- Release of medical information
- Computerized storage devices
- Computer security and passwords
- File maintenance
- Needs, purposes, and terminology of filing systems
- Process for filing documents
- Patient record organization
- Filing guidelines
- Retaining and purging medical records

*This *Workbook* and accompanying textbook meet the entry-level administrative and general competencies for the CMA outlined by the AAMA Examination Content Outline and Role Delineation Study and for the RMA and CMAS outlined by the AMT Competencies and Examination Specifications (see Competency Grid in textbook Appendix B).

RMA Content Summary

- Filing terminology
- Receive, process, and document results received from outside providers
- Manage patient medical record system
- Record diagnostic test results in patient charts
- File patient and physician communication in charts

- File material according to proper systems
- Protect, store, and retain medical records according to proper conventions and HIPAA privacy regulations
- Prepare and release private health information

CMAS Content Summary

- Manage medical record systems
- Manage and file paper and electronic documents
- File records alphabetically, numerically, by subject, and by color
- Employ indexing rules
- Arrange contents of patients' charts and employ chart management

- Store, protect, retain, and destroy records appropriately
- Observe and maintain confidentiality of records, charts, test results, and protected health information

Abbreviation and Spelling Review

Read the following patient's chart note and write the meanings for the abbreviations listed below the note. To decode any abbreviations you do not understand or that appear unfamiliar to you, refer to the list of abbreviations in Part V of this *Workbook*. Step-by-step directions for this exercise are in Procedure 1-1 of Chapter 1 in the text. Medical terms in the chart note are italicized; study them for spelling. Use your medical dictionary to look up their definitions. Your instructor may give a spelling and definition test that includes these words and abbreviations.

DATE	PROGRESS
12-3-20XX	Doris A Waxman PC: *occipital* headaches PX: HEENT NO *diplopia*, no *tinnitus*. See PI TPR neg., CV: no chest pain, *palpitation*, *orthopnea*, *dyspnea* or *exertion* or *hemoptysis*. GI: one episode of *emesis* last night. Some belching & intolerance to fried foods. RUQ abdom pain; no *hematemesis* or *melena*. GU: no frequency or *dysuria*. GYN: no abnormal bleeding. Ordered oral *cholecystography* Dx: rule out GB disease. Fran Practon, MD

PC _____

PX _____

HEENT _____

PI _____

TPR _____

neg. _____

CV _____

GI _____

RUQ _____

abdom _____

GU _____

GYN _____

Dx _____

GB _____

Review Questions

Review the objectives, glossary, and chapter information before completing the following review questions.

1. Why is it important for all members of the office staff to follow a general office filing system and obey filing rules? _____

    _____

2. When determining the choice of a medical filing system, what must be considered?

    a. _____

    b. _____

    c. _____

    d. _____

    e. _____

    f. _____

3. Name three advantages of using an alphabetic color-coded file system.

    a. _____

    b. _____

    c. _____

4. Name several types of information that may be filed in a subject file.

    a. _____

    b. _____

    c. _____

    d. _____

5. Why is numeric filing considered an indirect method? _____

    _____

    _____

6. Where are numeric filing systems primarily used? _____

    _____

7. In a chronological filing system, numbers are used based on _____ .

8. What type of filing system can organize, retrieve, and store information so that it is readily available?

    _____

9. Guarding files so that information is not lost in a computerized system requires _____ .

10. What is the purpose of a tickler file? _____

11. A person's first name is also called the _____ ,

    and the last name is the _____ .

12. A married woman may legally write her name three different ways. Give three examples of the way a name can be written.

    a. _____

    b. _____

    c. _____

13. What considerations should be made when selecting filing equipment?

    a. _____

    b. _____

    c. _____

    d. _____

    e. _____

14. Name two purposes served by file guides.

    a. _____

    b. _____

15. What steps would you take when a patient's chart cannot be located?

    a. _____

    b. _____

    c. _____

    d. _____

    e. _____

    f. _____

    g. _____

    h. _____

16. To purge files, what two procedures can solve the problem of determining when to transfer patient files from active to inactive status?

    a. _____

    b. _____

17. Name three space-saving, quick, and easy retrieval methods of storing large volumes of medical records.

    a. _____

    b. _____

    c. _____

Critical Thinking Exercise

1. State at least two circumstances that might require cross-referencing of names in alphabetic files.

    a. _____

    b. _____

JOB SKILL 8-1
Determine Filing Units

Name _____ Date _____ Score _____

Performance Objective

Task: Designate filing units so that names can be filed alphabetically in an office file.

Conditions: Assemble 50 names and pen or pencil. Refer in the textbook to alphabetic filing rules (Chapter 8) used for indexing and Procedure 8-5 for step-by-step directions.

Standards: Complete all steps listed in this skill in _____ minutes with a minimum score of _____. (Time element and accuracy criteria may be given by instructor.)

Time: **Start:** _____ **Completed:** _____ **Total:** _____ minutes

Scoring: One point for each step performed satisfactorily unless otherwise listed or weighted by instructor.

Directions with Performance Evaluation Checklist

Study each name and designate units using pen or pencil to underline. Use one line for the first unit, two lines for the second unit, three lines for the third unit, and four lines for the fourth unit. Study the example below before beginning.

EXAMPLE

1st Attempt	2nd Attempt	3rd Attempt	
			Underline each unit of name: <u>A.</u> <u>Marsha</u> <u>Moore</u>
_____	_____	_____	Gather materials (equipment and supplies) listed under "Conditions."
_____	_____	_____	1. Underline each unit of name: Rebecca Rodene Rochester.
_____	_____	_____	2. Underline each unit of name: Wm. John Taylor Kelly.
_____	_____	_____	3. Underline each unit of name: Jamie Trethorn.
_____	_____	_____	4. Underline each unit of name: Dan A. DeLeon.
_____	_____	_____	5. Underline each unit of name: E. Mary LeVan.
_____	_____	_____	6. Underline each unit of name: Amy Kay M'Oeters.
_____	_____	_____	7. Underline each unit of name: Shelby C. St. John.
_____	_____	_____	8. Underline each unit of name: Robert F. MacGregor.
_____	_____	_____	9. Underline each unit of name: S. J. VanderLinder.
_____	_____	_____	10. Underline each unit of name: Kelly Saint Thomas.
_____	_____	_____	11. Underline each unit of name: Priscilla Ruby DuMont.
_____	_____	_____	12. Underline each unit of name: Peter deWinter.
_____	_____	_____	13. Underline each unit of name: Sister Mary Beth.
_____	_____	_____	14. Underline each unit of name: Mayor Bill A. King.
_____	_____	_____	15. Underline each unit of name: Dr. John J. Jackson.
_____	_____	_____	16. Underline each unit of name: Mary-Kay deVille.
_____	_____	_____	17. Underline each unit of name: Sji Mulzono.
_____	_____	_____	18. Underline each unit of name: Mark Philip-DeGeer.
_____	_____	_____	19. Underline each unit of name: Pope John Paul.
_____	_____	_____	20. Underline each unit of name: Maj. Steve Royal Smith.
_____	_____	_____	21. Underline each unit of name: Mrs. Noreen J. Cline.
_____	_____	_____	22. Underline each unit of name: Charles T. Lloyd Jr.
_____	_____	_____	23. Underline each unit of name: Charles T. Lloyd II.
_____	_____	_____	24. Underline each unit of name: Peter L. Morrison, MD.

JOB SKILL 8-1 (*continued*)

_____	_____	_____	25. Underline each unit of name: Sarah May Dennis-Brit.
_____	_____	_____	26. Underline each unit of name: C. Ngyume.
_____	_____	_____	27. Underline each unit of name: Paul Wm. SeValle.
_____	_____	_____	28. Underline each unit of name: Foster Memorial Community Hospital.
_____	_____	_____	29. Underline each unit of name: Ft. Benning Convalescent Home.
_____	_____	_____	30. Underline each unit of name: A-1 Pharmacy.
_____	_____	_____	31. Underline each unit of name: American Medical Corp.
_____	_____	_____	32. Underline each unit of name: Dr. Spock's Clinic.
_____	_____	_____	33. Underline each unit of name: St. Jude's Hospital.
_____	_____	_____	34. Underline each unit of name: Russ Wilder Ambulance Service.
_____	_____	_____	35. Underline each unit of name: Mt. Blanc Druggist.
_____	_____	_____	36. Underline each unit of name: Century 21 Medical Supply.
_____	_____	_____	37. Underline each unit of name: College of St. Catherine.
_____	_____	_____	38. Underline each unit of name: Washington School, St. Paul, MN.
_____	_____	_____	39. Underline each unit of name: Mary Cain Pharmacy, Waco, TX.
_____	_____	_____	40. Underline each unit of name: Mary Cain Pharmacy, Inc.
_____	_____	_____	41. Underline each unit of name: Riverside County Public Library.
_____	_____	_____	42. Underline each unit of name: St. Joseph's Community Hospital, Austin, TX.
_____	_____	_____	43. Underline each unit of name: University of California–Los Angeles.
_____	_____	_____	44. Underline each unit of name: University of California–Davis.
_____	_____	_____	45. Underline each unit of name: St. Louis Publications.
_____	_____	_____	46. Underline each unit of name: Father Buechner.
_____	_____	_____	47. Underline each unit of name: Sister Sue Ellen.
_____	_____	_____	48. Underline each unit of name: C. R. Toll.
_____	_____	_____	49. Underline each unit of name: Rebecca Toll (Mrs. John).
_____	_____	_____	50. Underline each unit of name: Mrs. John A. Peterson.
_____	_____	_____	Complete within specified time.
____/52	____/52	____/52	**Total points earned** (To obtain a percentage score, divide the total points earned by the number of points possible.)

Comments:

Evaluator's Signature: _____   **Need to Repeat:** _____

JOB SKILL 8-2
Index and File Names Alphabetically

Name _____ Date _____ Score _____

Performance Objective

Task: Demonstrate a knowledge of standarized alphabetic rules to competently file and retrieve medical records; apply this knowledge as you alphabetize names for class discussion.

Conditions: Assemble 18 groups of names and pen or pencil. Refer to alphabetic filing rules (textbook Chapter 8) used for indexing and Procedure 8-5 for step-by-step directions.

Standards: Complete all steps listed in this skill in _____ minutes with a minimum score of _____. (Time element and accuracy criteria may be given by instructor.)

Time: **Start:** _____ **Completed:** _____ **Total:** _____ minutes

Scoring: One point for each step performed satisfactorily unless otherwise listed or weighted by instructor.

Directions with Performance Evaluation Checklist

Underline the first, second, and third units of each name to show proper indexing order, placing one line under the surname, two lines under the given name, and three lines under the third name or initial. Alphabetize each group of three names, writing the corresponding letters, in order, in the answer column.

EXAMPLE

Units underlined: (a) J. T. Jefferson (b) John Thompson (c) Mrs. T. J. Brown (Marsha)

Units in correct order: (a) Jefferson, J. T. (b) Thompson, John (c) Brown, Marsha (Mrs. T. J.)

Correct filing order: c a b (c) Brown, Marsha (Mrs. T. J.) (a) Jefferson, J. T. (b) Thompson, John

1st Attempt	2nd Attempt	3rd Attempt		
_____	_____	_____		Gather materials (equipment and supplies) listed under "Conditions."
____/3	____/3	____/3	1. _____	(a) Henrietta S. Lamar (b) Greta Lee Mason (c) Mary Lou LaMotte
____/3	____/3	____/3	2. _____	(a) Raymond Lorenzana (b) R. Lorenzo (c) Tony Lorenzen
____/3	____/3	____/3	3. _____	(a) Roger N. Stephens (b) Garland N. St. John (c) Robert Sprague
____/3	____/3	____/3	4. _____	(a) Walter E. Johnston (b) Willard L. Johnson (c) Geo. W. Johnstone
____/3	____/3	____/3	5. _____	(a) Hugh M. MacAdoo (b) Bruce T. McCall (c) Robert A. Macall
____/3	____/3	____/3	6. _____	(a) Lt. Margaret Kim (b) Margaret LaForgeaus (c) Mrs. M. LeMaster (Loretta)
____/3	____/3	____/3	7. _____	(a) H. King IV (b) H. M. King Jr. (c) Mrs. H. M. King (Alice)
____/3	____/3	____/3	8. _____	(a) Mrs. Tina Simmons (Leonard) (b) Richard K. Simmons (c) R. K. Simons-Steele
____/3	____/3	____/3	9. _____	(a) J. W. Winn, MD, 1404 Rosealea Rd., Cleveland, Ohio (b) James W. Winn, 1203 Venetta Drive, Cleveland, Ohio (c) J. W. Winn, 18 Maple St., Cleveland, Ohio
____/3	____/3	____/3	10. _____	(a) Mary Sue Shelton (b) Martha Lee Shelton-Alston (c) Sheila-Lynn Alston (Mrs. Shelton A.)
____/3	____/3	____/3	11. _____	(a) Willard Champs, 1072 Main St. (b) Willard Champs, 290 Main St. (c) Wilfred Champs, 10234 Main St.
____/3	____/3	____/3	12. _____	(a) Jas. E. McBean (b) J. L. MacBeen (c) Jason McBean
____/3	____/3	____/3	13. _____	(a) W. L. Arthur-Davis (b) Carolyn Archer (Mrs. David) (c) Sister Arletta-Marie

JOB SKILL 8-2 *(continued)*

____/3   ____/3   ____/3   14. _____ (a) Grace Ayers (b) A. Joseph Almonzaz (c) Mrs. Anthony Ayers (Gloria)

____/3   ____/3   ____/3   15. _____ (a) Norman Gilliam (b) N. Gilliam (c) Mrs. N. R. Gilliam (Norma)

____/3   ____/3   ____/3   16. _____ (a) Matthew Kuboushek (b) Toshi Kubota (c) I. M. Kuchenber

____/3   ____/3   ____/3   17. _____ (a) Dr. Vincent DeLucca (b) Victoria Deems (c) Dr. Carl Deams Jr.

____/3   ____/3   ____/3   18. _____ (a) Mrs. Loretta Maggio (b) Bokker T. Magallon Sr. (c) B. L. Magill, Rev.

_____   _____   _____   Complete within specified time.

____/56   ____/56   ____/56   **Total points earned** (To obtain a percentage score, divide the total points earned by the number of points possible.)

Comments:

Evaluator's Signature: _____ **Need to Repeat:** _____

National Curriculum Competency: CAAHEP: III.C.3.a(1)(d)	ABHES: VI.B.1.a.3(i)

JOB SKILL 8-3
File Patient and Business Names Alphabetically

Name _____ Date _____ Score _____

Performance Objective

Task: Sort patient names and business names in alphabetic order according to standardized alphabetic filing rules. Note: This is an advanced exercise.

Conditions: Assemble 10 groups of names and pen or pencil. Refer in the textbook to alphabetic filing rules (Chapter 8) used for indexing and Procedure 8-5 for step-by-step directions.

Standards: Complete all steps listed in this skill in _____ minutes with a minimum score of _____. (Time element and accuracy criteria may be given by instructor.)

Time: Start: _____ Completed: _____ Total: _____ minutes

Scoring: One point for each step performed satisfactorily unless otherwise listed or weighted by instructor.

Directions with Performance Evaluation Checklist

After each group of four names, indicate by letter the order in which the names would be arranged in a file.

1st Attempt	2nd Attempt	3rd Attempt		
_____	_____	_____	Gather materials (equipment and supplies) listed under "Conditions."	
____/4	____/4	____/4	1. _____	a. Mrs. Allene Baker b. A. Baker c. A. Barker, MD d. Dr. Barker
____/4	____/4	____/4	2. _____	a. The Apple Advertising Co. b. Apple-Cornwall, Inc. c. Appling Health Care d. Allan Applesey Corp.
____/4	____/4	____/4	3. _____	a. Brother Brian Advertising b. The Bonita Rehab Facility c. B and B Clinic d. Bonita Rd. Care
____/4	____/4	____/4	4. _____	a. Larue-McGuire Canyon Hospital b. Los Angeles Community Care c. Laruem Medical Clinic d. Las Robles Medical Center
____/4	____/4	____/4	5. _____	a. Fortieth St. Convalescent Center b. The Forrest Hospital c. The Frew-Forrest Medical Group d. Forrest Medical Facility
____/4	____/4	____/4	6. _____	a. Professor Sam A. Zimmer b. Zimmer-Kliev Agency c. Prof. A. Zimmer d. Z and Z Druggists
____/4	____/4	____/4	7. _____	a. Robin Persy-Doerr b. Philip Persico Retirement Care c. Poinsettia Residential Care d. Persicona-Philips Mortuary
____/4	____/4	____/4	8. _____	a. Mcdonald, Calvin b. MacDonald, Carl, MD c. Macdonald, C. A. d. Dr. McDermott

JOB SKILL 8-3 *(continued)*

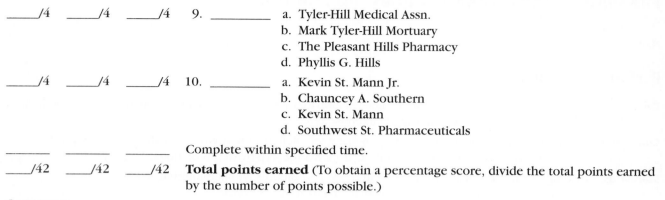

____/4   ____/4   ____/4   9. _____   a. Tyler-Hill Medical Assn.
                                                  b. Mark Tyler-Hill Mortuary
                                                  c. The Pleasant Hills Pharmacy
                                                  d. Phyllis G. Hills

____/4   ____/4   ____/4   10. _____   a. Kevin St. Mann Jr.
                                                  b. Chauncey A. Southern
                                                  c. Kevin St. Mann
                                                  d. Southwest St. Pharmaceuticals

_____   _____   _____   Complete within specified time.

____/42   ____/42   ___/42   **Total points earned** (To obtain a percentage score, divide the total points earned by the number of points possible.)

Comments:

Evaluator's Signature: _____   **Need to Repeat:** _____

National Curriculum Competency: CAAHEP: III.C.3.a(1)(d)   ABHES: VI.B.1.a.3(i)

JOB SKILL 8-4
Index Names on File Folder Labels and Arrange File Cards in Alphabetic Order

Name _____ Date _____ Score _____

Performance Objective

Task: Key names on file labels uniformly in correct indexing order. Affix labels to file cards or type names on file cards and alphabetize.

Conditions: Use Forms 17, 18, and 19, sixty file folder labels (optional), and sixty 3″ by 5″ index cards (or slips of paper). Refer in the textbook to alphabetic filing rules (Chapter 8) used for indexing and Procedure 8-5 for step-by-step directions.

Standards: Complete all steps listed in this skill in _____ minutes with a minimum score of _____. (Time element and accuracy criteria may be given by instructor.)

Time: **Start:** _____ **Completed:** _____ **Total:** _____ minutes

Scoring: One point for each step performed satisfactorily unless otherwise listed or weighted by instructor.

Directions with Performance Evaluation Checklist

Dr. Practon has asked you to key or type patient names appearing on Forms 17, 18, and 19 on file folder labels, as if they were to be attached to folder tabs, in proper indexing order. These can be printed neatly by hand using Forms 17, 18, and 19; typed using a typewriter; or keyed and printed from a computer on actual file folder labels. Affix labels to, or type names at the top right of index cards and arrange in alphabetic order. These may be spread out on your desk, or a small recipe box may be used for sorting. Note: There are several options for completing this job skill. Please read through all the steps prior to starting and determine if you will be using the worksheet (forms) provided for file labels or actual file folder labels and index cards.

1st Attempt	2nd Attempt	3rd Attempt	
_____	_____	_____	Gather materials (equipment and supplies) listed under "Conditions."
____/30	____/30	____/30	1. Use the labels on Forms 17, 18, and 19 as a worksheet and write (in pencil) each patient's name in the correct indexing order. Check with the instructor if you have problems determining units and indexing sequence. If you are not using actual file folder labels for this job skill, you may use a blank sheet of paper for the worksheet and these labels (which will be cut up into slips of paper for alphabetizing) for printing or typing patient names.
_____	_____	_____	2. Use blank labels marked "X" at the end of Form 19 for any names that need to be cross-referenced; these may vary per student.
____/30	____/30	____/30	3. Key or type names uniformly on file folder labels in indexing order starting at the left margin. At the right margin, key or type the reference number that appears by the patient's name as if it were an account number.

EXAMPLE—FILE LABEL

McDougall, Walter Louis	Acct. #1

1st	2nd	3rd	
____/30	____/30	____/30	4. Affix labels to index cards (top right), or key/type each name and number at the top of a card.
____/30	____/30	____/30	5. Alphabetize all cards or slips.

JOB SKILL 8-4 *(continued)*

____/10   ____/10   ____/10   6. Complete an answer sheet by either listing the account numbers in the order they were filed or keying each name in the sequence you have determined.

EXAMPLE—ANSWER SHEET

> 34. Albert, Frank
>
> 17. *Benjamin, Thomas
>
> 57. Bennett, C. Richard

_____   _____   _____   Complete within specified time.

___/133   ___/133   ___/133   **Total points earned** (To obtain a percentage score, divide the total points earned by the number of points possible.)

Comments:

Evaluator's Signature: _____   **Need to Repeat:** _____

National Curriculum Competency: CAAHEP: III.C.3.a(1)(d)   ABHES: VI.B.1.a.3(i)

JOB SKILL 8-5
Color-Code File Cards

Name _____ Date _____ Score _____

Performance Objective

Task: Color-code 60 file cards.

Conditions: Use file index cards from Job Skill 8-4 and highlight pens (orange, red, green, blue, violet).

Standards: Complete all steps listed in this skill in _____ minutes with a minimum score of _____.
(Time element and accuracy criteria may be given by instructor.)

Time: **Start:** _____ **Completed:** _____ **Total:** _____ minutes

Scoring: One point for each step performed satisfactorily unless otherwise listed or weighted by instructor.

Directions with Performance Evaluation Checklist

Dr. Practon may ask you to add color to the medical office filing system, or he may already use Remington's Varia-dex color-coding system. When a file is placed in a cabinet or drawer, or a card in a box, alphabetic dividers will indicate the first letter of the first filing unit. Then, the names are filed according to the color code of the *second* letter of the last name.

1st Attempt	2nd Attempt	3rd Attempt	
_____	_____	_____	Gather materials (equipment and supplies) listed under "Conditions."
___/60	___/60	___/60	1. Highlight the top edge of each 3″ by 5″ index card by color coding the *second* letter in the first unit of each name. Use the color guide in the following box. To help you remember the five divisions of the alphabetic system, notice that the first letter of each of the five groups is a vowel except for the last group, which begins with the letter "r."

If the second letter of the patient's surname is:	the tab guide color is:
a, b, c, or d	orange
e, f, g, or h	red
i, j, k, l, m, or n	green
o, p, or q	blue
r, s, t, u, v, w, x, y, or z	violet

_____	_____	_____	Complete within specified time.
___/62	___/62	___/62	**Total points earned** (To obtain a percentage score, divide the total points earned by the number of points possible.)

Comments:

Evaluator's Signature: _____ **Need to Repeat:** _____

CHAPTER 9

Medical Records

OBJECTIVES

After completing the exercises, the student will be able to:

1. Write meanings for chart note abbreviations.
2. Enhance spelling skills by learning new medical words.
3. Prepare a patient record and insert progress notes.
4. Prepare a patient record and format chart notes.
5. Correct a patient record.
6. Abstract from a medical record.
7. Prepare a history and physical report.

FOCUS ON CERTIFICATION*

CMA Content Summary

- Medical terminology
- Body systems
- Releasing patient information
- Living wills
- Medical records (types)
- Scanners
- Making corrections in records

RMA Content Summary

- A/P body systems
- Medical terminology
- Abbreviations
- Documentation of patient encounters
- Confidentiality
- Chart and records management
- Chart systems
- Transcription format
- Encryption and passwords

*This *Workbook* and accompanying textbook meet the entry-level administrative and general competencies for the CMA outlined by the AAMA Examination Content Outline and Role Delineation Study and for the RMA and CMAS outlined by the AMT Competencies and Examination Specifications (see Competency Grid in textbook Appendix B).

CMAS Content Summary

- Medical terminology
- Structure and function of body systems
- Diseases of body systems
- Chart patient information
- Patient record systems
- Documents and charts (paper and computerized)

- Chart contents
- Correct medical records
- Audits
- Confidentiality
- Confidentiality of computer-stored information

Abbreviation and Spelling Review

Read the following patient's chart note and write the meanings for the abbreviations listed below the note. To decode any abbreviations you do not understand or that appear unfamiliar to you, refer to the list of abbreviations in Part V of this *Workbook*. Step-by-step directions for this exercise are in Procedure 1-1 of Chapter 1 in the textbook. Medical terms in the chart note are italicized; study them for spelling. Use your medical dictionary to look up their definitions. Your instructor may give a spelling and definition test that includes these words and abbreviations.

Elizabeth A. Warner

November 16, 20XX CC: *constipation, rectal* bleeding & pain after BM. CPX reveals int & ext *hemorrhoids*. BP 150/95. *Sigmoidoscopy* to 15 cm. Rx: adv hospitalization for removal of hemorrhoids. Dg: bleeding hemorrhoids, int & ext; anal *fistula*; HBP.

Gerald Practon, MD
Gerald Practon, MD

CC	_____	cm	_____
BM	_____	Rx	_____
CPX	_____	adv	_____
int	_____	Dg	_____
ext	_____	HBP	_____
BP	_____		

Review Questions

Review the objectives, glossary, and chapter information before completing the following review questions.

1. List seven reasons for keeping medical records.

   a. _____

   b. _____

   c. _____

   d. _____

   e. _____

   f. _____

   g. _____

2. List some of the disadvantages of a paper-based medical record system.

   a. _____

   b. _____

   c. _____

   d. _____

   e. _____

3. What equipment is necessary to digitize medical records when converting from a paper-based system to

   an electronic-based system? _____

4. Why are flow sheets, charts, and graphs used in the medical record? _____

   _____

   _____

   _____

5. Name five advantages of using a medical record organizational system such as the problem-oriented medical record (POMR).

   a. _____

   b. _____

   c. _____

   d. _____

   e. _____

6. Match the physician titles in the left column with the definitions in the right column and insert the correct letter in the blank space.

   _____ attending physician

   _____ consulting physician

   _____ ordering physician

   _____ referring physician

   _____ treating or performing physician

   a. provider who sends the patient for testing

   b. provider whose opinion is requested

   c. medical staff member who is legally responsible for care of patient

   d. provider who renders service to patient

   e. provider directing selection, preparation or administration of tests, medication, or treatment

7. Since all documenters must sign their name to the portions of the medical record that they documented, when can initials legally be used? _____

   _____

   _____

8. List what the abbreviations stand for in the following chart format and briefly describe each term.

   a. S: _____

   b. O: _____

   c. A: _____

   d. P: _____

9. Using the documentation guidelines, state briefly what is said about the following.

   a. patient encounters: _____

   b. the assessment: _____

   c. abbreviations: _____

   d. diagnostic and ancillary services: _____

   e. risk factors: _____

   f. procedure and diagnostic codes: _____

   g. staff members assisting physician: _____

   h. patient education and instructions: _____

10. List items that should be documented in the medical record for skin lacerations and lesions.

   a. _____

   b. _____

   c. _____

   d. _____

   e. _____

11. List the four basic elements of a patient history and their abbreviations.

   a. _____

   b. _____

   c. _____

   d. _____

12. If a patient is seen in the office, a history and physical is dictated, and then the patient is admitted to the hospital, can the dictated history and physical be used for the hospital documentation? _____

   _____

   _____

13. Name ways in which the physician collects objective data.

   a. _____

   b. _____

   c. _____

   d. _____

14. Is there a difference between a chart note and a progress note? If yes, state the difference. _____

   _____

15. State types of patient encounters and common medical events that require charting on a medical record.

   a. _____

   b. _____

   c. _____

   d. _____

   e. _____

   f. _____

   g. _____

h. _____

i. _____

j. _____

Critical Thinking Exercise

1. The following phrases appeared on a history and physical. Place an *S* after those that are *subjective* and an *O* after those considered *objective*.

   a. Patient complains of feeling faint _____

   b. BP 120/80 _____

   c. Headache _____

   d. Skin shows no rashes _____

   e. Patient denies chest pain _____

   f. Mother L&W _____

   g. No inguinal hernia _____

   h. Heart tones normal _____

   i No masses palpable _____

   j. Patient had an episode of nausea _____

   k. Patient feels lethargic _____

   l. Temperature 101.1 F. _____

   m. Blood in stool _____

   n. Stomachache _____

   o. Leg cramping _____

   p. Blurred vision _____

   q. Vision 20/40 R. eye _____

   r. HCT 40% _____

   s. Pap smear class II _____

   t. Heel pain _____

   u. Lump in left breast _____

   v. Joint stiffness _____

   w. X-ray showed fracture R. ulna _____

   x. Urinalysis negative _____

   y. Acne _____

   z. Patient feels tired all the time _____

JOB SKILL 9-1
Prepare a Patient Record and Insert Progress Notes

Name _____ Date _____ Score _____

Performance Objective

Task: Key a patient record form with demographic information and progress notes; type a file card and file folder label.

Conditions: Computer, electronic typewriter, or word processor; one file folder, one file folder label, one patient record (Form 20), and one 3″ by 5″ file card.

Standards: Complete all steps listed in this skill in _____ minutes with a minimum score of _____. (Time element and accuracy criteria may be given by instructor.)

Time: Start: _____ Completed: _____ Total: _____ minutes

Scoring: One point for each step performed satisfactorily unless otherwise listed or weighted by instructor.

Directions with Performance Evaluation Checklist

Today is October 24, 20XX, and new patient Wayne G. Weather has come in as an emergency case; he was hurt on the job and has an injury to his lower back. He completed the patient information form (see Figure 7-1 in *Workbook* Job Skill 7-5). Complete the demographic information on the patient record form (20), file folder label, and file card. His wife, Nancy Weather, is a receptionist. His patient record number is 1180, which is keyed in the right corner of the record, file card, and file label. Use the detailed information listed in the directions to Job Skill 7-5 pertaining to Mr. Weather's condition, and enter the progress notes for today and the day of his hospital admit.

1st Attempt	2nd Attempt	3rd Attempt	
_____	_____	_____	Gather materials (equipment and supplies) listed under "Conditions."
____/2	____/2	____/2	1. Complete file folder label with patient name and medical record number; affix to file folder.
____/2	____/2	____/2	2. Complete file card with patient name and medical record number.
____/25	____/25	____/25	3. Key patient record number and demographic information on top portion of patient record.
____/15	____/15	____/15	4. Key progress note for 10/24/20XX noting emergency office visit, on-the-job injury, diagnosis, surgical scheduling information, and preadmission testing.
____/5	____/5	____/5	5. Key note for 10/28/20XX regarding hospital admit.
____/4	____/4	____/4	6. Proofread form, checking capitalization, punctuation, and spacing.
____/2	____/2	____/2	7. Finalize record for correct physician's signature.
_____	_____	_____	Complete within specified time.
____/57	____/57	____/57	**Total points earned** (To obtain a percentage score, divide the total points earned by the number of points possible.)

Comments:

Evaluator's Signature: _____ **Need to Repeat:** _____

National Curriculum Competency: CAAHEP: III.C.3.c(2)(c), III.C.3.c(2)(e) | ABHES: VI.B.1.a.3(b)

JOB SKILL 9-2
Prepare a Patient Record and Format Chart Notes

Name _____ Date _____ Score _____

Performance Objective

Task: Format and key a patient record, label a file folder, and type a file card.

Conditions: Computer, electronic typewriter or word processor; one file folder, one file label, one patient record (Form 21), and one 3″ by 5″ file card. Refer to Figure 9-7 in the textbook for chart note format example.

Standards: Complete all steps listed in this skill in _____ minutes with a minimum score of _____. (Time element and accuracy criteria may be given by instructor.)

Time: **Start:** _____ **Completed:** _____ **Total:** _____ minutes

Scoring: One point for each step performed satisfactorily unless otherwise listed or weighted by instructor.

Directions with Performance Evaluation Checklist

You will be preparing a patient record, filling in the top portion with demographic information and the bottom portion with progress notes. Refer to Figure 9-7 in the textbook for an example of the charting format using the chief complaint (CC), physical examination (PE), diagnosis (DX), and "Plan" as headings for the appropriate lines.

1st Attempt	2nd Attempt	3rd Attempt	
_____	_____	_____	Gather materials (equipment and supplies) listed under "Conditions."
_____/2	_____/2	_____/2	1. Use the name Krista Lee Carlisle and medical record number 1181. Complete a file folder label; affix to file folder.
_____/2	_____/2	_____/2	2. Type a 3″ by 5″ file card with patient name and medical record number at top right.
_____/25	_____/25	_____/25	3. Complete the top portion of medical record form (#21) using your own personal information, or interview a person in class or someone at home to obtain this information (address, telephone number, insurance name, and so forth).
_____/5	_____/5	_____/5	4. Complete the bottom portion of the medical record using the data found in *Workbook* Figure 9-1. Use a format similar to that found in textbook Figure 9-7 and abbreviate medical terms when appropriate.
_____/10	_____/10	_____/10	5. Make a separate entry for Dr. Fran Practon's examination on October 25, 20XX.
_____/10	_____/10	_____/10	6. Make a separate entry for the follow-up visit on October 28, 20XX.
_____/10	_____/10	_____/10	7. Make a separate entry for the follow-up visit on November 15, 20XX.
_____/2	_____/2	_____/2	8. Make a separate entry for the canceled appointment.
_____	_____	_____	Complete within specified time.
_____/68	_____/68	_____/68	**Total points earned** (To obtain a percentage score, divide the total points earned by the number of points possible.)

JOB SKILL 9-2 (*continued*)

10/25/XX   Height 5′10″ Weight 222 pounds. Blood pressure 140/60. Chief complaint: Patient complained of several weeks' history of fatigue, lack of appetite, and headache; has lost approximately 8 pounds since October 1, 20XX. Denies smoking. Averages three beers a day. On examination liver appears somewhat enlarged, tender on palpitation. All other systems appear normal. No apparent jaundice. Urinalysis findings: dark amber urine, bilirubinemia and proteinuria 2+. Patient sent to laboratory for blood workup; complete blood count, chemistry panel, liver panel, hepatitis panel. Diagnosis: hepatomegaly, rule out hepatitis. Patient instructed to adhere to strict bed rest, low-fat, high-carbohydrate diet. Disability for 2 weeks; instructions given. Return to the office in three days. Call sooner if symptoms increase. Tylenol tablets every 4 to 6 hours for headache.

10/28/XX   Weight: 220 pounds. Blood pressure 128/64. Chief complaint: Follow-up visit for laboratory results. Definitive diagnosis: hepatitis A. All other laboratory results normal. Patient to increase disability to 8 weeks, mild activity as tolerated. Instructions to use no alcohol, continue same diet, fluids as tolerated. Tylenol as needed. Call office immediately if unable to tolerate fluids or diet. Return to office in one week.

11/15/XX   Weight: 224 pounds. Blood pressure 130/66. Chief complaint: Follow-up visit. Patient states "is feeling much better," tolerating diet and fluids, good weight gain; urinalysis: clear yellow urine, protein-trace. Vital signs normal. On examination, no tenderness on palpitation of abdomen. Patient to follow up in two weeks. Continue modified activity as tolerated. Call if symptoms increase.

12/03/XX   Pt called to cancel appointment (3:00 p.m.); did not reschedule.

Figure 9-1

Comments:

Evaluator's Signature: _____   **Need to Repeat:** _____

National Curriculum Competency: CAAHEP: III.C.3.b(4)(c), III.C.3.c(2)(c), III.C.3.c(2)(e)   ABHES: VI.B.1.a.3(b), VI.B.1.a.4(a)

JOB SKILL 9-3
Correct a Patient Record

Name _____ Date _____ Score _____

Performance Objective

Task: Make a correction on a patient record.

Conditions: Use the medical record for Krista Lee Carlisle (Record No. 1181 from Job Skill 92). Refer to Procedure 9-2 in the textbook for step-by-step directions.

Standards: Complete all steps listed in this skill in _____ minutes with a minimum score of _____.
                     (Time element and accuracy criteria may be given by instructor.)

Time: **Start:** _____ **Completed:** _____ **Total:** _____ minutes

Scoring: One point for each step performed satisfactorily unless otherwise listed or weighted by instructor.

Directions with Performance Evaluation Checklist

On October 28, 20XX, Dr. Fran Practon indicated the patient would be disabled for eight weeks. On November 15, she realized she should have indicated the disability for six weeks. Correct the medical record.

1st Attempt	2nd Attempt	3rd Attempt	
_____	_____	_____	Gather materials (equipment and supplies) listed under "Conditions."
_____	_____	_____	1. Make the necessary change on the patient record by crossing out the incorrect entry ("~~X 8 weeks~~").
_____	_____	_____	2. Handwrite, in ink, the correct entry above the words "~~X 8 weeks~~."
____/3	____/3	____/3	3. In the margin, write the word "correction," your initials, and the date you are making the correction.
_____	_____	_____	Complete within specified time.
____/7	____/7	____/7	**Total points earned** (To obtain a percentage score, divide the total points earned by the number of points possible.)

Comments:

Evaluator's Signature: _____ **Need to Repeat:** _____

National Curriculum Competency: CAAHEP: III.C.3.c(2)(b), III.C.3.c(2)(c), III.C.3.c(2)(e)	ABHES: VI.B.1.a.3(b), VI.B.1.a.5(b)

JOB SKILL 9-4
Abstract from a Medical Record

Name _____ Date _____ Score _____

Performance Objective

Task: Abstract information from a patient record to answer questions and fill in a Medical Record Abstract Form.

Conditions: Use Patient Record No. 1181 for Krista Lee Carlisle from Job Skill 9-2, pen or pencil, and Medical Record Abstract Form (22). Refer to Procedure 9-3 in the textbook for step-by-step directions.

Standards: Complete all steps listed in this skill in _____ minutes with a minimum score of _____. (Time element and accuracy criteria may be given by instructor.)

Time: **Start:** _____ **Completed:** _____ **Total:** _____ minutes

Scoring: One point for each step performed satisfactorily unless otherwise listed or weighted by instructor.

Directions with Performance Evaluation Checklist

1st Attempt	2nd Attempt	3rd Attempt	
_____	_____	_____	Gather materials (equipment and supplies) listed under "Conditions."
____/25	____/25	____/25	1. Abstract information from the medical record (1181) and answer each question on the abstract form; complete the form.
_____	_____	_____	Complete within specified time.
____/27	____/27	____/27	**Total points earned** (To obtain a percentage score, divide the total points earned by the number of points possible.)

Comments:

Evaluator's Signature: _____ **Need to Repeat:** _____

National Curriculum Competency: CAAHEP: III.C.3.c(2)(e)   ABHES: VI.B.1.a.5(b)

JOB SKILL 9-5
Prepare a History and Physical (H & P) Report

Name _____ Date _____ Score _____

Performance Objective

Task: Complete a patient record with demographic information, key a history and physical report, prepare a file folder with file label, type a 3″ by 5″ file card, and make a photocopy of the H & P report.

Conditions: Computer, electronic typewriter, or word processor; photocopy machine; patient record (Form 23), patient information form for Sun Low Chung (Figure 9-2); history and physical data (Figure 9-3); one file folder, one file folder label, one file card (3″ by 5″), and two sheets of 8½″ by 11″ white paper. Refer to textbook Figures 9-6A and B for history and physical format examples.

Standards: Complete all steps listed in this skill in _____ minutes with a minimum score of _____. (Time element and accuracy criteria may be given by instructor.)

Time: Start: _____ **Completed:** _____ **Total:** _____ minutes

Scoring: One point for each step performed satisfactorily unless otherwise listed or weighted by instructor.

Directions with Performance Evaluation Checklist

You will be completing the demographic information on a patient record for Sun Low Chung and keying the history and physical examination in report form on separate paper.

1st Attempt	2nd Attempt	3rd Attempt	
_____	_____	_____	Gather materials (equipment and supplies) listed under "Conditions."
_____	_____	_____	1. Prepare a file folder label for Sun Low Chung with medical record number 1182; affix to file folder.
_____	_____	_____	2. Prepare a 3″ by 5″ file card for Sun Low Chung.
____/20	____/20	____/20	3. Use Sun Low Chung's patient information form (*Workbook* Figure 9-2) to key her patient record number and demographic information on the top portion of patient record (Form 23).
_____	_____	_____	4. Read the H & P in *Workbook* Figure 9-3.
____/20	____/20	____/20	5. Highlight the proper headings that will be used when keying the data in a History and Physical Examination format (see textbook Figures 9-6A and B for examples).
____/20	____/20	____/20	6. Key data in *Workbook* Figure 9-3 using proper history and physical format. Note: You will not be using the bottom portion of the patient record (Form 23) for this patient because a complete H & P report is being prepared for the medical record; reference it in the area of the progress notes.
_____	_____	_____	7. Date report using current dates as dictated and transcribed dates.
_____	_____	_____	8. Key in full block style.
_____	_____	_____	9. Set margins so they are even, equal, and of correct size.
____/15	____/15	____/15	10. Insert main topic headings and correct paragraphing.
____/7	____/7	____/7	11. Insert subtopic headings.
____/4	____/4	____/4	12. Insert capitalization, punctuation, tab stops, and correct spacing.
_____	_____	_____	13. Insert page 2 heading.
_____	_____	_____	14. Place a signature line at end of H & P; Dr. Gerald Practon is the physician.
_____	_____	_____	15. Insert typist's identifying signoff data for the H & P.
_____	_____	_____	16. Proofread report for spelling and typographical errors on screen or while H & P remains in word processor or typewriter.

JOB SKILL 9-5 *(continued)*

_____ _____ _____   17. Finalize document for physician to review and sign.

_____ _____ _____   18. Make a photocopy of the completed H & P report.

_____ _____ _____   Complete within specified time.

___/100 ___/100 ___/100   **Total points earned** (To obtain a percentage score, divide the total points earned by the number of points possible.)

Comments:

Evaluator's Signature: _____ **Need to Repeat:** _____

National Curriculum Competency: CAAHEP: III.C.3.c(2)(c), III.C.3.c(2)(e)	ABHES: VI.B.1.a.2(i), VI.B.1.a.2(n), VI.B.1.a.3(b), VI.B.1.a.3(e), VI.B.1.a.5(b)

JOB SKILL 9-5 (*continued*)

PATIENT INFORMATION FOR MEDICAL RECORDS (*Please Print*)		DATE: 10/25/XX

PATIENT ⬤MR. ○MRS. ○MISS

LAST NAME	FIRST NAME	MIDDLE
Chung	Sun	Low

PATIENT ADDRESS

STREET	CITY	STATE	ZIP	HOME PHONE
→ 2375 Laney Street	Woodland Hills, XY 12345		555/278-6135	

SOCIAL SECURITY NUMBER	DATE OF BIRTH	AGE	DRIVER'S LICENSE NO.
→ 738-XX-6712	5-20-45		6-0065-178

PATIENT EMPLOYER	OCCUPATION
→ Civil Service Maintenance	Mechanic

EMPLOYER'S ADDRESS

STREET	CITY	STATE	ZIP	BUS PHONE
→ 742 Redwood Highway,	Port Davis,	XY	12346	555/271-4811

SPOUSE'S NAME	MARITAL STATUS	REFERRED BY
→ Song Su Chung ⬤M ○S ○D ○W ○SEP.		Employer

SPOUSE'S EMPLOYER

STREET	CITY	STATE	ZIP	BUS. PHONE
Best Market 214 Main Street,	Woodland Hills,	XY	12345	555/279-4827

IN CASE OF EMERGENCY CONTACT:

NAME	ADDRESS	CITY	STATE	ZIP	TELEPHONE
Pat Chung (brother)	2851 Laney St,	Woodland Hills,	XY	12345	555/278-7812

▼ MEDICAL INSURANCE INFORMATION

COMPANY	POLICY NUMBER
Blue Shield 2751 Courntney St., Woodland Hills, XY 12345	
COMPANY	POLICY NUMBER
	27894B
COMPANY	POLICY NUMBER

▼ IF SOMEONE OTHER THAN PATIENT IS RESPONSIBLE FOR PAYMENT PLEASE COMPLETE THIS SECTION

RESPONSIBLE PARTY ○MR. ○MRS. ○MISS

LAST NAME	FIRST NAME	MIDDLE	RELATION

ADDRESS

STREET	CITY	STATE	ZIP	TELEPHONE
→				

OCCUPATION	EMPLOYED BY
→	

EMPLOYER'S ADDRESS

STREET	CITY	STATE	ZIP	BUS. PHONE
→				

I hereby authorize Dr. *Gerald Praxton* to furnish to the above insurance company(s) or to a designated attorney, all information which said insurance company(s) or attorney may request. I hereby assign to Dr. *Gerald Praxton* all money to which I am entitled for medical and/or surgical expense relative to the service rendered by him, but not to exceed my indebtedness to said physician and/or surgeon. It is understood that any money received from the above named insurance company, over and above my indebtedness will be refunded to me when my bill is paid in full. I understand I am financially responsible to said doctor(s) for charges not covered by this assignment. I further agree in the event of non-payment, to bear the cost of collection, and/or Court cost and reasonable legal fees should this be required.

Sun Low Chung
INSURED OR GUARDIAN SIGNATURE

Sun Low Chung
PATIENT'S SIGNATURE

58-8409   © 1976 BIBBERO SYSTEMS, INC., SAN FRANCISCO

Figure 9-2

JOB SKILL 9-5 (*continued*)

Sun Low Chung

History. Chief complaint. Palpitations for 1 week. Present illness. This patient has had known hypertension for 4 years. He has been taking Serpasil 0.25 mg daily. About 1 month ago, the medication was changed to Dyazide 250 mg, one tablet per day. Since that time, the patient has felt more nervous and anxious, with occasional chest tightness. One week ago the patient noted some skipped heartbeats occurring in the evening. There were no other associated symptoms and no history of paroxysmal nocturnal dyspnea, orthopnea, or ankle edema. Palpitation subsided spontaneously but recurred the following night, with a fast throbbing sensation in his right ear. He was seen by Dr. Chan 2 weeks later and had a chest x-ray and cardiac enzymes done. These were normal values. An electrocardiogram showed normal sinus rhythm, with nonspecific ST abnormalities. He experiences palpitations in the evening. The patient has been asked to avoid any strenuous exercise and to stay at home until he is seen by the undersigned physician. Past history. The patient was born in Hankow, China, but has lived in the United States since 1952. He has worked in the Air Force and airplane industry but lately is working for civil service at Port Davis. He has been subjected to some work pressure recently. There was no history of coronary artery disease, heart murmurs, rheumatic fever, or joint problems in childhood. Malaria in his youth in China. Hypothyroidism diagnosed about 10 years ago, and he has been on thyroid 1 grain q.d. Operations none. Allergies none. Medication as stated above, and Valium 5 milligrams one b.i.d. to t.i.d. p.r.n., Thyroid 1 grain q.d. Social history. The patient smoked one pack of cigarettes per day for 10 years but has discontinued for about 15 years. He does not drink. He consumes about two cups of coffee per day and very little tea. The family history. Most of the family members were separated during the war, and their health conditions are not known. Mother died from an unknown illness at the age of 35. The patient has two children, 36 and 27, both in good health. No known diabetes, hypertension, or heart problems in the family. The review of systems. General. No recent weight gain or weight loss. No unusual fatigue. No recent fevers. The patient has myopia in both eyes. Glasses have not been checked for the past 5 years, and distant vision is not good. EENT. Negative. CR. As in PI. No history of hemoptysis or chronic cough. GI. Negative. GU. Nocturia once a night for many years. NP. No history of headache, syncope, or light-headedness. No history of paralysis. MS. No history of joint problems. Physical examination. General. This patient is an elderly Asian male in no acute distress. Blood pressure is right arm 148 over 80 and left arm 138 over 88. Pulse 80 and regular. Respirations 18. Height 5 feet, 7 inches. Weight 176 1/4 pounds. The patient is afebrile. HEENT. Not pale or cyanotic. Tympanic membranes intact. Fundus normal in the left; right cannot be visualized because of question of early cataract or marked refractive error. Neck. Supple. No jugular venous pulse, thyromegaly, or lymphadenopathy. Carotid upstrokes normal. Chest. Point of maximum, impulse in the fifth intercostal space in the midclavicular line. S1, S2 normal. A soft S4 was heard. No S3. No murmurs. Lungs clear. Abdomen. Soft, nontender. No hepatosplenomegaly. No masses felt. No abdominal bruits. Musculoskeletal. Bilateral hallux valgus. No edema or clubbing. All peripheral pulses normal and equal. Neurological. No gross abnormalities. Diagnosis. 1. Palpitations, probably premature ventricular contractions. Rule out coronary artery disease. Rule out malignant arrhythmias. 2. History of hypertension. 3. History of hypothyroidism. Therapeutic Plan. 1. Review old records. 2. Tumor skin test. 3. EKG with 12-hour Holter monitor. 4. Measure blood pressure once a week x 3 weeks. Decide whether long-term hypertensive medication is necessary. 5. Ophthalmology consult.

Figure 9-3

CHAPTER 10

Drug and Prescription Records

OBJECTIVES

After completing the exercises, the student will be able to:

1. Enhance knowledge of medical terminology, interpret abbreviations, and accurately spell medical words.

2. Spell drug names.

3. Use a *Physicians' Desk Reference* (*PDR*).

4. Translate prescriptions.

5. Record prescription refills in medical records.

6. Write a prescription.

7. Interpret a medication log.

8. Record on a medication schedule.

FOCUS ON CERTIFICATION*

CMA Content Summary

- Medical abbreviations
- Facility accreditation
- Controlled substances
- Drug enforcement administration
- Computer database
- Restocking supplies
- Classes of drugs

- Drug forms
- Drug action/uses
- Side effects/adverse effects
- Substance abuse
- Prescriptions
- Maintaining medication records
- Medication disposal

*This *Workbook* and accompanying textbook meet the entry-level administrative and general competencies for the CMA outlined by the AAMA Examination Content Outline and Role Delineation Study and for the RMA and CMAS outlined by the AMT Competencies and Examination Specifications (see Competency Grid in textbook Appendix B).

RMA Content Summary

- Medical terms and abbreviations
- Patient instruction
- Documentation of medications
- Chart medication information
- Maintain inventory

- Prescriptions
- Drug Enforcement Administration
- Drug categories
- Routes of administration
- *Physicians' Desk Reference*

CMAS Content Summary

- Medical terminology
- Chart information (paper/computerized)

- Pharmacology concepts

Abbreviation and Spelling Review

Read the following patient's chart note and write the meanings for the abbreviations listed below the note. To decode any abbreviations you do not understand or that appear unfamiliar to you, refer to the list of abbreviations in Part V of this *Workbook*. Step-by-step directions for this exercise are in Procedure 1-1 of Chapter 1 in the textbook. Medical terms in the chart note are italicized; study them for spelling. Use your medical dictionary to look up their definitions. Your instructor may give a spelling and definition test that includes these words and abbreviations.

Lillian M. Chan

February 17, 20XX OB case. LMP 12-14-20XX. Pt had D & C in 1989 following *spontaneous abortion*. First child delivered by *C-section*. Ordered CBC, UR, and WR. Pt to ret in 1 mo.

Fran Practon, MD

Fran Practon, MD

OB	_____	CBC	_____
LMP	_____	UR	_____
Pt	_____	WR	_____
D & C	_____	ret	_____
C-section	_____	mo	_____

Review Questions

Review the objectives, glossary, and chapter information before completing the following review questions.

1. Match the law or agency in the right column with the description in the left column and insert the correct letter in the blank space.

   _____ Law requiring transfer tax for those who sold marijuana.

   _____ Federal law that requires the pharmaceutical industry to maintain physical security and strict record keeping for scheduled drugs.

   _____ First law to control the prescription, sale, and possession of narcotic drugs.

   _____ Organization that regulates the manufacturing and dispensing of dangerous and potentially abused drugs.

   a. Harrison Narcotic Act

   b. Volstead Act

   c. Marijuana Tax Act

   d. Food, Drug, and Cosmetic Act

   e. Controlled Substance Act

   f. Food and Drug Administration

   g. Drug Enforcement Administration

_____ Law that prohibited the manufacture, transportation, and sale of beverages containing more than 0.5% alcohol.

_____ Agency that determines the safety of drugs before it permits them to be marketed.

_____ First law that required the labeling of drugs with directions for safe use.

2. Where must the physician register for a narcotic license and when must the license be renewed?

_____

3. Refer to textbook Table 10-1, Five Schedules of Controlled Substances, and answer the following questions:

a. On which schedule(s) may prescriptions be written by the health care worker?

_____

b. On which schedule(s) will the medical assistant most likely be handling triplicate forms for the doctor?

_____

c. On which schedule(s) do drugs have the most potential for abuse?

_____

4. Name and define the three types of drug names.

a. _____

b. _____

c. _____

5. Define *generic drug*. _____

_____

6. In the *Physicians' Desk Reference (PDR)*, which section is used most frequently by the medical assistant? _____

_____

7. Name and define the four components of a prescription.

a. _____

b. _____

c. _____

d. _____

8. Match the drug route in the right column with the correct definition in the left column and insert the letter in the blank space.

_____ Medication administered into a joint   a. ophthalmic

_____ Medication administered through the ear   b. otic

_____ Medication absorbed through the skin using a patch c. endotracheal

_____ Medication placed between the cheek and gum   d. intra-articular

_____ Medication administered to the eye   e. buccal

_____ Medication placed under the tongue   f. sublingual

_____ Medication administered through the trachea   g. transdermal

9. Write the abbreviation or symbol for the following pharmaceutical terms.

   a. after meals _____

   b. drops _____

   c. every morning _____

   d. every two hours _____

   e. intramuscular _____

   f. when necessary _____

10. Name several ways the medical assistant can instruct the patient about drug dosages to be sure the patient understands the directions.

    a. _____

    b. _____

    c. _____

    d. _____

    e. _____

11. Name three important items to include when instructions are given to patients taking antibiotics.

    a. _____

    b. _____

    c. _____

12. Match the drug categories in the right column with the definitions in the left column by writing letters in the blanks.

    _____ Drug that causes general or local loss of sensation to pain and touch   a. narcotic

    _____ Drug that decreases congestion   b. antiemetic

    _____ Drug that exerts a tranquilizing effect   c. stimulant

    _____ Drug that increases excretion of urine   d. diuretic

    _____ Drug that relieves pain and produces sleep   e. coagulant

    _____ Drug that causes blood to clot   f. sedative

    _____ Drug that relieves vomiting   g. hemostatic

    _____ Drug that increases activity in the body or any of its organs   h. anesthetic

    _____ Drug used to check bleeding   i. antitussive

    _____ Drug used to relieve cough   j. decongestant

13. Name two ways a medical assistant can track a patient's drug use habits.

    a. _____

    b. _____

14. Name five ways to protect prescription pads from being misused.

    a. _____

    b. _____

    c. _____

    d. _____

    e. _____

15. Name some common side effects associated with medications.

a. _____   g. _____

b. _____   h. _____

c. _____   i. _____

d. _____   j. _____

e. _____   k. _____

f. _____   l. _____

16. If the patient does not have any known allergies, what is the abbreviation listed on the "alert tag" on the front of the patient's chart? _____

_____

Critical Thinking Exercises

1. If a pharmacist calls the office and the physician approves a refill on Mr. Hamilton's prescription, what administrative task should the medical assistant then perform (list details)?

_____

_____

_____

_____

2. Mrs. Schwartz telephones and says that the doctor prescribed Hytrin, but she cannot remember why. With the physician's permission, you would tell her that the medication is being prescribed for her _____.

a. headaches   c. nerves

b. hypertension   d. hypotension

(Find the answer in the *Physicians' Desk Reference* or other drug reference book.)

3. Rewrite the following statements as they would appear on a prescription, using Latin abbreviations.

a. Proventil (albuterol) inhaler, one hundred milligrams per five milliliters, one or two inhalations every four ours whenever necessary.

_____

b. Cardizem CD (diltiazem HCl) capsules, 180 milligrams, number one hundred, once a day before meals, and one before bedtime.

_____

c. Lanoxin (digoxin) tablets, zero point one hundred and twenty-five milligrams, number sixty, one every day.

_____

d. Vantin (cefpodoxime proxetil) tablets, two hundred milligrams, number twenty-eight, one by mouth, every twelve hours for fourteen days.

_____

JOB SKILL 10-1
Spell Drug Names

Name _____ Date _____ Score _____

Performance Objective

Task: Correctly spell brand or generic drug names.

Conditions: Use the 10 drug names listed next to each step; a computer, typewriter, or word processor; and a drug reference book such as the *Physicians' Desk Reference (PDR)*, *Instant Drug Index*, *Hospital Formulary*, or *Pharmaceutical Terminology*. Refer to Procedure 10-1 in the textbook for step-by-step directions.

Standards: Complete all steps listed in this skill in _____ minutes with a minimum score of _____.
(Time element and accuracy criteria may be given by instructor.)

Time: **Start:** _____ **Completed:** _____ **Total:** _____ minutes

Scoring: One point for each step performed satisfactorily unless otherwise listed or weighted by instructor.

Directions with Performance Evaluation Checklist

Dr. Practon has dictated ten drug names for several patients, and you have written them phonetically. Find the correct spelling for each drug. Be sure to begin all brand names with a capital letter and all generic names with a lowercase letter.

1st Attempt	2nd Attempt	3rd Attempt	
_____	_____	_____	Gather materials (equipment and supplies) listed under "Conditions."
_____/3	_____/3	_____/3	1. Spell **Car-de-zem** _____
_____/3	_____/3	_____/3	2. Spell **di-ah-BEN-eze** _____
_____/3	_____/3	_____/3	3. Spell **FEE-a-sol** _____
_____/3	_____/3	_____/3	4. Spell **NAP-ro-sin** _____
_____/3	_____/3	_____/3	5. Spell **LIP-a-tour** _____
_____/3	_____/3	_____/3	6. Spell **LAY-six** _____
_____/3	_____/3	_____/3	7. Spell **eye-bu-PRO-fen** _____
_____/3	_____/3	_____/3	8. Spell **die-AS-a-pam** _____
_____/3	_____/3	_____/3	9. Spell **TEN-or-min** _____
_____/3	_____/3	_____/3	10. Spell **aug-MEN-tin** _____
_____	_____	_____	Complete within specified time.
_____/32	_____/32	_____/32	**Total points earned** (To obtain a percentage score, divide the total points earned by the number of points possible.)

Comments:

Evaluator's Signature: _____ **Need to Repeat:** _____

National Curriculum Competency: CAAHEP: III.C.3.c(2)(e)   ABHES: VI.B.1.a.2(j), VI.B.1.a.5(b)

JOB SKILL 10-2
Determine the Correct Spellings of Drug Names

Name _____ Date _____ Score _____

Performance Objective

Task: Determine the correct spellings for brand, generic, or over-the-counter drug names.

Conditions: Use the 10 sentences in the steps below, which each have two spellings of a medication; a pen or pencil; and a drug reference book such as the *Physicians' Desk Reference (PDR)*, *Instant Drug Index*, *Hospital Formulary*, or *Pharmaceutical Terminology*. Refer to Procedure 10-1 in the textbook for step-by-step directions. For over-the-counter drugs, use your common knowledge, an over-the-counter drug book, or visit a local drug store to locate the medication on the shelf.

Standards: Complete all steps listed in this skill in _____ minutes with a minimum score of _____. (Time element and accuracy criteria may be given by instructor.)

Time: Start: _____ **Completed:** _____ **Total:** _____ minutes

Scoring: One point for each step performed satisfactorily unless otherwise listed or weighted by instructor.

Directions with Performance Evaluation Checklist

Read the following sentences and circle the correct spelling from each pair of generic or brand-name medications. These sentences contain some frequently misspelled drug names.

1st Attempt	2nd Attempt	3rd Attempt	
_____	_____	_____	Gather materials (equipment and supplies) listed under "Conditions."
____/3	____/3	____/3	1. Dr. Practon's last chart note on Mr. Hoy Cho states, "advised the patient to take (a) Aspirin, (b) aspirin, 1 tab b.i.d."
____/3	____/3	____/3	2. After Ray Nunez suffered a mild heart attack, the physician prescribed a (a) nitroglycerin, (b) nitroglycerine patch daily.
____/3	____/3	____/3	3. Maria Sanchez telephoned stating she had a cold and wanted to know if it was all right to take (a) Contac, (b) Contact, an over-the-counter drug.
____/3	____/3	____/3	4. Mrs. Hatakeyama's allergy was easily treated with (a) Actafed, (b) Actifed.
____/3	____/3	____/3	5. Rosaria LaMaccia suffered a mild respiratory infection and Dr. Practon gave her a prescription for (a) Ceclor, (b) Seklor.
____/3	____/3	____/3	6. The patient came in complaining of muscle spasms in the lumbar region, so a prescription for (a) Flexeril, (b) Flexoril was given.
____/3	____/3	____/3	7. Fayetta Brown's diagnosis was duodenal ulcer, and she was given a prescription for (a) Bentil, (b) Bentyl.
____/3	____/3	____/3	8. A year ago Mae James had a urinary tract infection and was prescribed (a) Ceptra, (b) Septra.
____/3	____/3	____/3	9. Ventricular arrhythmias were diagnosed in Cameron Lesser's case, so (a) Quiniglute, (b) Quinaglute was given.
____/3	____/3	____/3	10. After the death of her spouse, Danielle La Fleur became depressed and Dr. Practon prescribed (a) Amatriptyline, (b) Amitriptyline.
_____	_____	_____	Complete within specified time.
____/32	____/32	____/32	**Total points earned** (To obtain a percentage score, divide the total points earned by the number of points possible.)

JOB SKILL 10-2 *(continued)*

Comments:

Evaluator's Signature: _____ **Need to Repeat:** _____

National Curriculum Competency: CAAHEP: III.C.3.c(2)(e)   ABHES: VI.B.1.a.2(j), VI.B.1.a.5(b)

JOB SKILL 10-3
Use the *Physicians' Desk Reference (PDR)*

Name _____ Date _____ Score _____

Performance Objective

Task: Identify medication in the correct section of the *Physicians' Desk Reference (PDR)*.

Conditions: *Physician's Desk Reference* (or Figure 10-3 in textbook); pen or pencil. Refer to Procedure 10-1 in the textbook for step-by-step directions.

Standards: Complete all steps listed in this skill in _____ minutes with a minimum score of _____.
(Time element and accuracy criteria may be given by instructor.)

Time: **Start:** _____ **Completed:** _____ **Total:** _____ minutes

Scoring: One point for each step performed satisfactorily unless otherwise listed or weighted by instructor.

Directions with Performance Evaluation Checklist

Dr. Practon has just received a prothrombin time report on Mrs. Darcuiel. He asks you to call the patient and verify her present dosage of Coumadin before he makes an adjustment. When you call the patient, she states she put all the pills in a medication container and no longer remembers her dosage. She says it is the only medication she is taking and it is *yellow*. Refer to the *PDR* or Figure 10-3 in the textbook to determine how many milligrams she is taking.

1st Attempt	2nd Attempt	3rd Attempt	
_____	_____	_____	Gather materials (equipment and supplies) listed under "Conditions."
____/5	____/5	____/5	1. Dosage Mrs. Darcuiel is taking: _____
____/3	____/3	____/3	2. In which section of the PDR did you find the information? _____
_____	_____	_____	Complete within specified time.
___/10	___/10	___/10	**Total points earned** (To obtain a percentage score, divide the total points earned by the number of points possible.)

Comments:

Evaluator's Signature: _____   **Need to Repeat:** _____

National Curriculum Competency: CAAHEP: III.C.3.a(1)(h)	ABHES: VI.B.1.a.3(e)

JOB SKILL 10-4
Translate Prescriptions

Name _____ Date _____ Score _____

Performance Objective

Task: Translate prescriptions from Latin into common English.

Conditions: Nine written prescriptions, one sheet of plain paper, and pen or pencil. Refer to Procedure 10-2 in the textbook for step-by-step directions.

Standards: Complete all steps listed in this skill in _____ minutes with a minimum score of _____. (Time element and accuracy criteria may be given by instructor.)

Time: **Start:** _____ **Completed:** _____ **Total:** _____ minutes

Scoring: One point for each step performed satisfactorily unless otherwise listed or weighted by instructor.

Directions with Performance Evaluation Checklist

Translate the nine prescriptions in Figure 10-1 into common English by referring to textbook Table 10-3, Common Prescription Abbreviations and Symbols. Refer to Procedure 10-2 in the textbook for step-by-step instructions.

EXAMPLE:

Valium 10 mg
#21
Sig.: ī p.o. t.i.d.

Translation: Valium, ten milligrams, number twenty-one, one by mouth three times a day.

1st Attempt	2nd Attempt	3rd Attempt	
_____	_____	_____	Gather materials (equipment and supplies) listed under "Conditions."
_____/5	_____/5	_____/5	1. Translate prescription for Tagamet.
_____/5	_____/5	_____/5	2. Translate prescription for Darvocet.
_____/5	_____/5	_____/5	3. Translate prescription for Diovan.
_____/5	_____/5	_____/5	4. Translate prescription for Tenormin.
_____/5	_____/5	_____/5	5. Translate prescription for Robitussin.
_____/5	_____/5	_____/5	6. Translate prescription for Isordil.
_____/5	_____/5	_____/5	7. Translate prescription for Compazine.
_____/5	_____/5	_____/5	8. Translate prescription for Vanceril.
_____/5	_____/5	_____/5	9. Translate prescription for Timoptic Solution.
_____	_____	_____	Complete within specified time.
____/47	____/47	____/47	**Total points earned** (To obtain a percentage score, divide the total points earned by the number of points possible.)

Comments:

Evaluator's Signature: _____ **Need to Repeat:** _____

National Curriculum Competency: CAAHEP: III.C.3.c(2)(e)   ABHES: VI.B.1.a.4(n)

JOB SKILL 10-4 (continued)

1
Tagamet 400 mg
#30
Sig.: ī p.o. h.s.

6
Isordil
(isosorbide dinitrate)
20 mg
30
ī p.o. q.12°

2
Darvocet N-100
#60 Tabs
Sig.: īī q.4h.
p.r.n. pain

7
Compazine
25 mg suppositories
#14
ī rectally b.i.d.
p.r.n. vomiting

3
Diovan HCT
160mg/12.5mg
#100
Sig.: ī p.o. every day

8
Vanceril Inhalation Aerosol
42 mcg
#1 bottle
2 inhalations q.i.d.
p.r.n. asthma

4
Tenormin 50 mg
#100
ī every day

9
Timoptic Solution
0.25%
1 bottle
ī gt. each eye b.i.d.

5
Robitussin DAC
4 oz. bottle
2 tsp. q. 4 h. p.r.n.
cough

Figure 10-1

JOB SKILL 10-5
Record Prescription Refills in Medical Records

Name _____ Date _____ Score _____

Performance Objective

Task: Record four prescription refills in patient medical records.

Conditions: Four large file folder labels (Form 24) and pen. Use (1) medical record for Wayne G. Weather completed in Job Skill 7-5 (*Workbook* Figure 7-1) and Job Skill 9-1; (2) medical record for Krista Lee Carlisle completed in Job Skill 9-2; and (3) medical record for Sun Low Chung completed in Job Skill 9-5 (*Workbook* Figures 9-2 and 9-3). Refer to Procedure 10-3 in the textbook for step-by-step directions. Use pharmaceutical abbreviations and symbols found in the textbook Table 10-3 or Part V of the *Workbook*.

Standards: Complete all steps listed in this skill in _____ minutes with a minimum score of _____. (Time element and accuracy criteria may be given by instructor.)

Time: Start: _____ Completed: _____ Total: _____ minutes

Scoring: One point for each step performed satisfactorily unless otherwise listed or weighted by instructor.

Directions with Performance Evaluation Checklist

Read the following scenarios and abstract the prescription information. Record each transaction on a label, use the current date, initial it, and then secure the label in the patient's medical record.

1st Attempt	2nd Attempt	3rd Attempt	
_____	_____	_____	Gather materials (equipment and supplies) listed under "Conditions."
___/10	___/10	___/10	1. Record: The ABC Pharmacy calls about a prescription for Wayne G. Weather. Dr. Practon approves a refill for Darvocet N-100, number twenty, one tablet every four hours whenever necessary for pain.
___/10	___/10	___/10	2. Record: The Dalton Pharmacy calls about Krista Lee Carlisle. The pharmacist asks if a refill on Sonata, ten milligram capsules, number ten, one by mouth at bedtime, can be approved. Dr. Practon approves.
___/10	___/10	___/10	3. Record: The Georgetown Pharmacy calls regarding Sun Low Chung. He has a urinary tract infection again and would like a refill on his Bactrim, double strength, number twenty-eight, one by mouth two times a day for fourteen days. Dr. Practon approves.
___/10	___/10	___/10	4. Record: Two days later, Sun Low Chung calls Dr. Practon reporting an adverse reaction to the Bactrim. Dr. Practon calls the Main Street Pharmacy to order Macrodantin, one-hundred milligram capsules, number forty, one by mouth four times a day with milk or meals for ten days.
___/4	___/4	___/4	5. Secure prescription documentation (on labels) in correct medical records.
_____	_____	_____	Complete within specified time.
___/46	___/46	___/46	**Total points earned** (To obtain a percentage score, divide the total points earned by the number of points possible.)

JOB SKILL 10-5 *(continued)*

Comments:

Evaluator's Signature: _____ **Need to Repeat:** _____

National Curriculum Competency: CAAHEP: III.C.3.c(2)(e)   ABHES: VI.B.1.a.4(n)

JOB SKILL 10-6
Write a Prescription

Name _____ Date _____ Score _____

Performance Objective

Task: Write a prescription.

Conditions: In some regions, medical assistants may be allowed to write prescriptions for patients; the physician must sign all originals. This exercise is designed to help understand the different components of a prescription form and the abbreviations used. Use one prescription (Form 25) and refer to textbook Figure 10-5 for a visual example. Refer to Table 10-3, Common Prescription Abbreviations and Symbols, or the list of abbreviations in Part V of this *Workbook*.

Standards: Complete all steps listed in this skill in _____ minutes with a minimum score of _____. (Time element and accuracy criteria may be given by instructor.)

Time: **Start:** _____ **Completed:** _____ **Total:** _____ minutes

Scoring: One point for each step performed satisfactorily unless otherwise listed or weighted by instructor.

Directions with Performance Evaluation Checklist

Read the following scenario and write a prescription using today's date:

Felisha Weiss, 456 Los Angeles Avenue, Woodland Hills, XY 12345, needs prophylactic treatment for migraine headache syndrome. She will be given verapamil, one hundred eighty milligrams, sustained release, number one-hundred and twenty tablets. Directions are to take one by mouth every morning; she may have two refills.

1st Attempt	2nd Attempt	3rd Attempt	
_____	_____	_____	Gather materials (equipment and supplies) listed under "Conditions."
____/5	____/5	____/5	1. Complete patient demographic information and enter today's date.
____/4	____/4	____/4	2. Complete inscription.
____/2	____/2	____/2	3. Complete subscription.
____/4	____/4	____/4	4. Complete signature.
_____	_____	_____	5. Indicate number of refills.
_____	_____	_____	6. Proofread form prior to physician's signature.
_____	_____	_____	Complete within specified time.
____/19	____/19	____/19	**Total points earned** (To obtain a percentage score, divide the total points earned by the number of points possible.)

Comments:

Evaluator's Signature: _____ **Need to Repeat:** _____

National Curriculum Competency: CAAHEP: III.C.3.c(2)(e)	ABHES: VI.B.1.a.2(j), VI.B.1.a.4(n)

JOB SKILL 10-7
Interpret a Medication Log

Name _____ Date _____ Score _____

Performance Objective

Task:　　　　Study the medication log and determine the drug use habits of a patient.

Conditions:　Refer to the medication log (*Workbook* Figure 10-2) and use a pen or pencil. See Procedure 10-3 in the textbook for step-by-step directions.

Standards:　Complete all steps listed in this skill in _____ minutes with a minimum score of _____. (Time element and accuracy criteria may be given by instructor.)

Time:　　　　**Start:** _____ **Completed:** _____ **Total:** _____ minutes

Scoring:　　One point for each step performed satisfactorily unless otherwise listed or weighted by instructor.

Directions with Performance Evaluation Checklist

It is November 17, current year, and Mary Beth Foley calls wanting a refill on her Glucotrol. Study the medication log and answer the following questions.

1st Attempt	2nd Attempt	3rd Attempt	
_____	_____	_____	Gather materials (equipment and supplies) listed under "Conditions."
_____/2	_____/2	_____/2	1. Has Mary Beth Foley been prescribed the medication? YES NO
_____/2	_____/2	_____/2	2. How many days has it been since she got her last refill? _____ days
_____/2	_____/2	_____/2	3. Is it time to refill the medication? YES NO
_____/2	_____/2	_____/2	4. When may she call for the next refill? _____
_____	_____	_____	Complete within specified time.
____/10	____/10	____/10	**Total points earned** (To obtain a percentage score, divide the total points earned by the number of points possible.)

Comments:

Evaluator's Signature: _____ **Need to Repeat:** _____

National Curriculum Competency: CAAHEP: III.C.3.c(3)(b)　　　　　　　　　ABHES: VI.B.1.a.3(b)

JOB SKILL 10-7 *(continued)*

MEDICATION LOG

PATIENT NAME: FOLEY, Mary Beth   **DATE OF BIRTH:** 9-30-52

ALLERGIES: NKA

DATE	MEDICATIONS	DOSE	#	INSTRUCTIONS (SIG)	PRN REG	TEL WRIT	PHARMACY	DR. SIG.
8/5/XX	Amitriptyline	100 mg	90	i p.o. h.s.	R	T	ABC Pharm	GMP
10/28/XX	Amitriptyline	100 mg	90	i p.o. h.s.	R	T	ABC Pharm	GMP
9/23/XX	Glucotrol	10 mg	30	i p.o. a.c./a.m.	R	T	ABC Pharm	GMP
9/23/XX	Verapamil SR	240 mg	30	i p.o. q.a.m.	R	T	ABC Pharm	GMP
10/7/XX	Glucotrol	10 mg	90	i p.o. a.c./a.m.	R	W	mail order pharmacy	GMP
10/7/XX	Tetracycline	250 mg	30	i p.o. T.I.D. p.r.n. yellow sputum	P	T	ABC Pharm	GMP
10/16/XX	Verapamil SR	240 mg	90	i p.o. q.a.m.	R	W	mail order pharmacy	GMP

Figure 10-2

JOB SKILL 10-8
Record on a Medication Schedule

Name _____ Date _____ Score _____

Performance Objective

Task: Record medication name, dosage, and instructions on a medication schedule.

Conditions: Medication schedule (Form 26) and a pen or pencil. Refer to textbook Figure 10-7 for a visual example.

Standards: Complete all steps listed in this skill in _____ minutes with a minimum score of _____. (Time element and accuracy criteria may be given by instructor.)

Time: Start: _____ Completed: _____ Total: _____ minutes

Scoring: One point for each step performed satisfactorily unless otherwise listed or weighted by instructor.

Directions with Performance Evaluation Checklist

Mr. Delbert Silva has just seen Dr. Fran Practon. She has prescribed Paxil for his depression. The dosage is 20 milligrams every morning. He is very confused, and Dr. Practon would like you to record all of his prescription information on a medication schedule for him. There is information in his chart indicating he is also taking Sinemet 20/250 milligrams for his Parkinson's disease. He takes two tablets four times a day. He is also on Lopressor, 100 milligrams twice a day, for his hypertension. You have verified that Mr. Silva is still on these medications. Please set up and fill out the medication schedule for Mr. Silva.

1st Attempt	2nd Attempt	3rd Attempt	
_____	_____	_____	Gather materials (equipment and supplies) listed under "Conditions."
____/2	____/2	____/2	1. Fill in patient name and physician name.
____/4	____/4	____/4	2. Set up schedule for "a.m.," "NOON," "p.m.," and "BED."
____/4	____/4	____/4	3. Record information for Paxil medication.
____/8	____/8	____/8	4. Record information for Sinemet medication.
____/5	____/5	____/5	5. Record information for Lopressor medication.
_____	_____	_____	6. Proofread schedule prior to giving it to the patient.
_____	_____	_____	Complete within specified time.
___/26	___/26	___/26	**Total points earned** (To obtain a percentage score, divide the total points earned by the number of points possible.)

Comments:

Evaluator's Signature: _____ **Need to Repeat:** _____

National Curriculum Competency: CAAHEP: III.C.3.c(2)(e), III.C.3.c(3)(b) | ABHES: VI.B.1.a.3(b), VI.B.1.a.4(n), VI.B.1.a.5(b)

Written Correspondence

OBJECTIVES

After completing the exercises, the student will be able to:

1. Enhance knowledge of medical terminology, interpret abbreviations, and accurately spell medical words.
2. Identify spelling errors and select correctly spelled terms.
3. Key a letter of withdrawal.
4. Edit written communication.
5. Compose and key a letter for a failed appointment.
6. Compose and key a letter for an initial visit.
7. Compose and key a letter to another physician.
8. Compose and key a letter requesting payment.
9. Abstract information and key interoffice memorandums.
10. Abstract information from a medical record, and compose and key a letter.
11. Key a two-page letter.

FOCUS ON CERTIFICATION*

CMA Content Summary

- Medical terminology
- Spelling, correspondence, letters, memos
- Data entry; keyboard fundamentals
- Letter and memo formats
- Envelopes
- Computer and printer usage
- Computer storage devices
- Word processing
- Databases

*This *Workbook* and accompanying textbook meet the entry-level administrative and general competencies for the CMA outlined by the AAMA Examination Content Outline and Role Delineation Study and for the RMA and CMAS outlined by the AMT Competencies and Examination Specifications (see Competency Grid in textbook Appendix B).

RMA Content Summary

- Medical terminology
- Spelling
- Written communication skills

- Compose correspondence
- Transcription and dictation
- Word processing computer applications

CMAS Content Summary

- Spell medical terms
- Written communication
- Format business documents
- Basic computer operations

- Fundamental knowledge of a PC-based environment
- Word processing and databases
- Medical office software applications

Abbreviation and Spelling Review

Read the following patient's chart note and write the meanings for the abbreviations listed below the note. To decode any abbreviations you do not understand or that appear unfamiliar to you, refer to the list of abbreviations in Part V of this *Workbook*. Step-by-step directions for this exercise are in Procedure 1-1 of Chapter 1 in the textbook. Medical terms in the chart note are italicized; study them for spelling. Use your medical dictionary to look up their definitions. Your instructor may give a spelling and definition test that includes these words and abbreviations.

DATE	PROGRESS
1-3-20XX	Maria K Morgan CC: Pt complains of back pain, *nausea, dysuria,* & *oliguria* of 1 wk.
	PH: *Congenital stricture* rt. *ureter* at *ureterovesical junction.* UA: Occ WBC, occ epith. pH
	7, alb 1, sugar O. Dr. Woodman's summary rev. Dilat to K35 c̄ Brev ordered IVP. *Unilateral*
	nephrectomy may be indicated. Dx possible *urinary calculi* RTO 1 wk. for UA &
	possible Dilat. Ḡ Practon MD

CC	_____	alb	_____
Pt	_____	rev	_____
WK	_____	dilat	_____
PH	_____	K35	_____
UA	_____	c̄	_____
Occ	_____	Brev	_____
WBC	_____	IVP	_____
epith.	_____	Dx	_____
pH	_____	RTO	_____

Review Questions

Review the objectives, glossary, and chapter information before completing the following review questions.

1. How should a letter of an official or legal nature be sent when there is a need to expedite it? _____
   _____

2. Define the term *ergonomics*. _____
   _____

3. Why would a computerized medical office have a typewriter? _____
   _____

4. When keying a letter on a computer, what type of software would you use? _____

5. List three flaws that would make a letter unmailable.

    a. _____

    b. _____

    c. _____

6. Which style is the least personal of the various letter formats? _____

7. Which two punctuation styles are most commonly used? Briefly describe each.

    a. _____

    b. _____

8. What are the typical default settings for right and left margins? _____

9. Name three devices you could use to arouse the reader's interest in the first paragraph of a letter you are writing for the physician.

    a. _____

    b. _____

    c. _____

10. Explain the following text-editing features of electronic word processors.

    a. Directional keys _____

    b. Function keys _____

    c. Memory functions _____

    d. Tool features _____

    e. Edit features _____

    f. Printing feature _____

    g. Format functions _____

11. When checking for layout or format prior to printing, what software program option would you use to view an entire page of a document? _____

12. Transcription needs in the physician's office will be based on the following factors:

    a. _____

    b. _____

    c. _____

    d. _____

13. What procedure should be followed when the transcriptionist cannot understand a word or phrase of a physician's dictation? _____

14. Below are three methods the physician may use to create letters. Briefly describe the physician's and medical transcriber's roles when using these methods.

a. Dictation equipment: _____

_____

_____

b. Voice-activated software: _____

_____

_____

c. Remote device (PDA): _____

_____

_____

15. List five ways to increase the productivity of photocopy machines.

a. _____

b. _____

c. _____

d. _____

e. _____

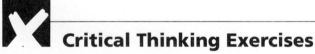

Critical Thinking Exercises

1. The following examples are parts of a letter. Read each example, and then identify and name the part of the letter.

a. Attn: Philip Kellogg, MD

_____

b. Re: Administrative Medical Assisting, 6th edition

_____

c. P.S. Please call me if you need directions.

_____

d. Sincerely,

_____

e. Arthur Miller, MD
   2300 Broad Avenue
   Woodland Hills, XY 12345-4700

_____

f. Dear Dr. Rogers:

_____

g. CC: Bernice Brantley, MD

_____

h. Enc. (3)

_____

MO
SS
MEDICAL OFFICE SIMULATION SOFTWARE

Computer Competency

Go to the Online Companion for this book at www.delmarlearning.com/companions to complete Medical Office Simulation Software activities for this chapter.

JOB SKILL 11-1
Spell Medical Words

Name _____ Date _____ Score _____

Performance Objective

Task: Identify correctly spelled medical terms.

Conditions: Pen or pencil.

Standards: Complete all steps listed in this skill in _____ minutes with a minimum score of _____.
(Time element and accuracy criteria may be given by instructor.)

Time: Start: _____ Completed: _____ Total: _____ minutes

Scoring: One point for each step performed satisfactorily unless otherwise listed or weighted by instructor.

Directions with Performance Evaluation Checklist

Select and circle the correctly spelled medical word from the choices given.

1st Attempt	2nd Attempt	3rd Attempt			
_____	_____	_____	Gather materials (equipment and supplies) listed under "Conditions."		
_____	_____	_____	1. conchiousness	consciousness	consceousness
_____	_____	_____	2. exhaustion	exsaustion	exhausion
_____	_____	_____	3. theraputic	therapuetic	therapeutic
_____	_____	_____	4. antidiarretic	antidiarrhetic	antidiarhetic
_____	_____	_____	5. neurolysis	nuerolysis	neurolosis
_____	_____	_____	6. medisinal	medicinal	medicenal
_____	_____	_____	7. roentegenogram	rentegenogram	roentgenogram
_____	_____	_____	8. kinesiology	kenesiology	kenisiology
_____	_____	_____	9. pharmasuetical	pharmacuetical	pharmaceutical
_____	_____	_____	10. humeris	humerus	humerous
_____	_____	_____	11. esophaglagia	esophagalgia	esopagalgia
_____	_____	_____	12. critereon	criterion	creiterion
_____	_____	_____	13. cauterisation	caterization	cauterization
_____	_____	_____	14. methastasize	metastasize	metasthasize
_____	_____	_____	15. spontaneous	spontenous	spontaneus
_____	_____	_____	16. capitation	captation	capitasion
_____	_____	_____	17. pancretectomy	pancraetectomy	pancreatectomy
_____	_____	_____	18. indemity	endemnity	indemnity
_____	_____	_____	19. negoteable	negotiable	negotable
_____	_____	_____	20. intemperance	intemperence	intemparance
_____	_____	_____	21. ajudicate	adjudicate	adgudicate
_____	_____	_____	22. cursor	curser	courser
_____	_____	_____	23. stethoscope	steathescope	stethescrope
_____	_____	_____	24. purelent	purulent	peurulent
_____	_____	_____	25. ausculation	auscultation	auscultasion
_____	_____	_____	Complete within specified time.		
____/27	____/27	____/27	**Total points earned** (To obtain a percentage score, divide the total points earned by the number of points possible.)		

JOB SKILL 11-1 *(continued)*

Comments:

Evaluator's Signature: _____ **Need to Repeat:** _____

| National Curriculum Competency: CAAHEP: III.C.3.c(1)(a) | ABHES: VI.B.1.a(2)(j) |

JOB SKILL 11-2
Key a Letter of Withdrawal

Name _____ Date _____ Score _____

Performance Objective

Task: Key a letter of withdrawal for the physician's signature.

Conditions: Letterhead for Practon Medical Group, Inc., formatted in a word processing program, or one sheet of letterhead (Form 27). Refer to textbook Figures 11-7 and 11-8 for format. Refer to Figure 3-11 in textbook Chapter 3 for an example and Procedure 11-2 in the textbook for step-by-step directions.

Standards: Complete all steps listed in this skill in _____ minutes with a minimum score of _____. (Time element and accuracy criteria may be given by instructor.)

Time: Start: _____ **Completed:** _____ **Total:** _____ minutes

Scoring: One point for each step performed satisfactorily unless otherwise listed or weighted by instructor.

Directions with Performance Evaluation Checklist

Mrs. Stanfield refused to follow the treatment prescribed by Dr. Gerald Practon and he has asked you to type a letter of withdrawal on his letterhead. Follow the steps below to complete this job skill.

1st Attempt	2nd Attempt	3rd Attempt	
_____	_____	_____	Gather materials (equipment and supplies) listed under "Conditions."
_____	_____	_____	1. Format letterhead or use Form 27.
_____	_____	_____	2. Use current date.
_____	_____	_____	3. Address letter to Constance M. Stanfield, 2090 Hope Street, Woodland Hills, XY 12345.
_____	_____	_____	4. Use correct salutation.
_____	_____	_____	5. Key in full block style.
_____	_____	_____	6. Use open punctuation.
_____	_____	_____	7. Use even and equal left and right margins.
_____	_____	_____	8. Place letter on stationery with correct spacing.
___/10	___/10	___/10	9. Write appropriate letter with wording that is legally correct.
_____	_____	_____	10. Check paragraphing and punctuation.
___/2	___/2	___/2	11. Place complimentary close and signature line in appropriate place.
_____	_____	_____	12. Key reference initials.
_____	_____	_____	13. Key enclosure notation.
_____	_____	_____	14. Proofread for spelling and typographical errors while on screen or in typewriter.
_____	_____	_____	15. Correct, print, and proofread again.
_____	_____	_____	16. Correct all errors and ready for physician's signature.
_____	_____	_____	Complete within specified time.
___/28	___/28	___/28	**Total points earned** (To obtain a percentage score, divide the total points earned by the number of points possible.)

JOB SKILL 11-2 *(continued)*

Comments:

Evaluator's Signature: _____ Need to Repeat: _____

National Curriculum Competency: CAAHEP: III.C.3.c(1)(a)	ABHES: VI.B.1.a.2(g), VI.B.1.a.2(j),
	VI.B.1.a.2(o), VI.B.1.a.3(a)

JOB SKILL 11-3
Edit Written Communication

Name _____ Date _____ Score _____

Performance Objective

Task:　　　　Edit sentences for improvement.

Conditions:　Assemble 20 sentences and pen or pencil.

Standards:　Complete all steps listed in this skill in _____ minutes with a minimum score of _____.
　　　　　　　(Time element and accuracy criteria may be given by instructor.)

Time:　　　Start: _____ **Completed:** _____ **Total:** _____ minutes

Scoring:　　One point for each step performed satisfactorily unless otherwise listed or weighted by instructor.

Directions with Performance Evaluation Checklist

Read each sentence below and edit to eliminate words, change the sequence of words, and eliminate redundant phrases.

1st Attempt	2nd Attempt	3rd Attempt	
_____	_____	_____	Gather materials (equipment and supplies) listed under "Conditions."
_____	_____	_____	1. Mrs. Benson just recovered from an attack of pneumonia.
_____	_____	_____	2. The letter arrived at a time when we were busy.
_____	_____	_____	3. During the year of 19XX the unpaid accounts were numerous.
_____	_____	_____	4. If the population, as in the general case, increases, we'll plan on expanding our practice.
_____	_____	_____	5. The water is for drinking purposes only.
_____	_____	_____	6. The close proximity of the police department scared the thief.
_____	_____	_____	7. It costs the sum of 20 dollars.
_____	_____	_____	8. The young secretary has a beautiful future before her.
_____	_____	_____	9. The wreck occurred at the corner of Fourth and Rampart Streets.
_____	_____	_____	10. The color of the prize rose was dark red.
_____	_____	_____	11. We are now engaged in building a new medical office.
_____	_____	_____	12. Somebody or other must assume the responsibility.
_____	_____	_____	13. The file is made out of steel.
_____	_____	_____	14. There is much construction in the city of Ventura.
_____	_____	_____	15. It happened at the hour of midnight.
_____	_____	_____	16. The package should be there in three weeks' time.
_____	_____	_____	17. We will ship the office supplies at a later date.
_____	_____	_____	18. The character of the road was smooth.
_____	_____	_____	19. The physician spoke at a meeting held in Miami Beach.
_____	_____	_____	20. The patient appeared for her appointment at the hour of 2:30 p.m.
_____	_____	_____	Complete within specified time.
____/22	____/22	____/22	**Total points earned** (To obtain a percentage score, divide the total points earned by the number of points possible.)

JOB SKILL 11-3 *(continued)*

Comments:

Evaluator's Signature: _____ **Need to Repeat:** _____

National Curriculum Competency: CAAHEP: III.C.3.c(1)(a)   ABHES: VI.B.1.a.2(g), VI.B.1.a.2(j),
                                                                         VI.B.1.a.2(o), VI.B.1.a.3(a)

JOB SKILL 11-4
Compose and Key a Letter for a Failed Appointment

Name _____ Date _____ Score _____

Performance Objective

Task: Compose and key an original letter dealing with a failed appointment.

Conditions: Letterhead for Practon Medical Group, Inc., formatted in a word processing program, or one sheet of letterhead (Form 28) and dictionary. Refer to textbook Figures 11-7 and 11-8 for format. Refer to Procedure 11-2 in the textbook for step-by-step directions.

Standards: Complete all steps listed in this skill in _____ minutes with a minimum score of _____. (Time element and accuracy criteria may be given by instructor.)

Time: **Start:** _____ **Completed:** _____ **Total:** _____ minutes

Scoring: One point for each step performed satisfactorily unless otherwise listed or weighted by instructor.

Directions with Performance Evaluation Checklist

Margaret B. Hanson (Mrs. C. L.) of 2319 Warren Street, Woodland Hills, XY 12345 calls on September 20 to make a 4 p.m. appointment for her 18-year-old son, James P. Hanson, on September 25. The patient does not show (DNS) for the appointment. Write a letter with a reference line to Mrs. Hanson notifying her about her son's failure to keep his appointment. Remember that this is a legal document that must be prepared for Dr. Fran Practon's signature. Key this letter in full-block style with mixed punctuation; assume a file copy will be made.

1st Attempt	2nd Attempt	3rd Attempt	
_____	_____	_____	Gather materials (equipment and supplies) listed under "Conditions."
_____	_____	_____	1. Design letterhead or use Form 28.
_____	_____	_____	2. Date letter using current date.
_____	_____	_____	3. Key inside address.
_____	_____	_____	4. Key appropriate salutation.
_____	_____	_____	5. Key reference or subject line.
_____	_____	_____	6. Use full-block style.
_____	_____	_____	7. Use mixed punctuation.
_____	_____	_____	8. Center letter with even margins.
____/5	____/5	____/5	9. Mention failed appointment with date and time in body of letter in a clear, concise manner.
_____	_____	_____	10. Insert proper paragraphing.
____/2	____/2	____/2	11. Key appropriate complimentary close and signature line.
_____	_____	_____	12. Insert proper reference initials.
_____	_____	_____	13. Proofread while document is on screen or in typewriter for spelling, punctuation, capitalization, and typing errors.
_____	_____	_____	14. Correct, print, and proofread again.
_____	_____	_____	15. Make corrections and ready for physician's signature.
_____	_____	_____	Complete within specified time.
____/22	____/22	____/22	**Total points earned** (To obtain a percentage score, divide the total points earned by the number of points possible.)

JOB SKILL 11-4 *(continued)*

Comments:

Evaluator's Signature: _____ **Need to Repeat:** _____

National Curriculum Competency: CAAHEP: III.C.3.c(1)(a)	ABHES: VI.B.1.a.2(g), VI.B.1.a.2(j), VI.B.1.a.2(o), VI.B.1.a.3(a)

JOB SKILL 11-5
Compose and Key a Letter for an Initial Visit

Name _____ Date _____ Score _____

Performance Objective

Task:　　Compose and key an original letter to a new patient explaining procedures for the initial visit and requesting insurance information.

Conditions:　Letterhead for Practon Medical Group, Inc., formatted in a word processing program, or one sheet of letterhead (Form 29) and dictionary. Refer to textbook Figures 11-7 and 11-8 for format. Refer to Procedure 11-2 in the textbook for step-by-step directions.

Standards:　Complete all steps listed in this skill in _____ minutes with a minimum score of _____. (Time element and accuracy criteria may be given by instructor.)

Time:　　**Start:** _____ **Completed:** _____ **Total:** _____ minutes

Scoring:　One point for each step performed satisfactorily unless otherwise listed or weighted by instructor.

Directions with Performance Evaluation Checklist

Write a letter over your own signature to Raymond E. Stokes Jr., 4053 Magnolia Boulevard, Woodland Hills, XY 12345. Remind him of his appointment at 2:30 p.m. on Thursday, October 2, (current year). Inform him that the fee for an initial office visit is approximately $70.92. Suggest that he bring all insurance information if he has insurance coverage. Use full-block style with mixed punctuation.

1st Attempt	2nd Attempt	3rd Attempt	
_____	_____	_____	Gather materials (equipment and supplies) listed under "Conditions."
_____	_____	_____	1. Design letterhead or use Form 29.
_____	_____	_____	2. Date letter using current date.
_____	_____	_____	3. Key inside address.
_____	_____	_____	4. Key appropriate salutation.
_____	_____	_____	5. Key reference or subject line.
_____	_____	_____	6. Use full-block style.
_____	_____	_____	7. Use mixed punctuation.
_____	_____	_____	8. Center letter with even margins.
____/5	____/5	____/5	9. Mention appointment time, date, fee, and insurance coverage information in body of letter.
_____	_____	_____	10. Insert proper paragraphing.
____/2	____/2	____/2	11. Key appropriate complimentary close and signature line.
_____	_____	_____	12. Insert proper reference initials.
_____	_____	_____	13. Proofread while document is on screen or in typewriter for spelling, punctuation, capitalization, and typing errors.
_____	_____	_____	14. Correct, print, and proofread again.
_____	_____	_____	15. Make corrections and sign.
_____	_____	_____	Complete within specified time.
____/22	____/22	____/22	**Total points earned** (To obtain a percentage score, divide the total points earned by the number of points possible.)

JOB SKILL 11-5 *(continued)*

Comments:

Evaluator's Signature: _____ **Need to Repeat:** _____

National Curriculum Competency: CAAHEP: III.C.3.c(1)(a)	ABHES: VI.B.1.a.2(g), VI.B.1.a.2(j), VI.B.1.a.2(o), VI.B.1.a.3(a)

JOB SKILL 11-6
Compose and Key a Letter to Another Physician

Name _____ Date _____ Score _____

Performance Objective

Task: Compose and key an original letter referring a patient to another physician.

Conditions: Letterhead for Practon Medical Group, Inc., formatted in a word processing program, or one sheet of letterhead (Form 30) and dictionary. Refer to textbook Figures 11-7 and 11-8 for format. Refer to Procedure 11-2 in textbook for step-by-step directions.

Standards: Complete all steps listed in this skill in _____ minutes with a minimum score of _____. (Time element and accuracy criteria may be given by instructor.)

Time: Start: _____ Completed: _____ Total: _____ minutes

Scoring: One point for each step performed satisfactorily unless otherwise listed or weighted by instructor.

Directions with Performance Evaluation Checklist

Write a letter to Dr. Manuel Madero-Gonzales, Av. Mexico 131, Parque San Andraes, Mexico 21, D.F., referring Dr. Fran Practon's patient, Mr. Hector Gutierrez, who may need medical attention while vacationing in Mexico from September 30 through October 21, 20XX. He has been treated for infectious hepatitis, and his recent laboratory studies and clinical evaluations were within normal limits; assume you are enclosing copies of the most recent laboratory report and clinical evaluation. Tell Dr. Madero-Gonzales that you have instructed Mr. Gutierrez to contact him if any medical problems develop during his three-week stay. Use modified block-style and open punctuation; make a copy to mail to the patient.

1st Attempt	2nd Attempt	3rd Attempt	
_____	_____	_____	Gather materials (equipment and supplies) listed under "Conditions."
_____	_____	_____	1. Design letterhead or use Form 30.
_____	_____	_____	2. Date letter using current date.
_____	_____	_____	3. Key inside address.
_____	_____	_____	4. Key appropriate salutation.
_____	_____	_____	5. Key reference or subject line.
_____	_____	_____	6. Use modified block style.
_____	_____	_____	7. Use open punctuation.
_____	_____	_____	8. Center letter with even margins.
____/5	____/5	____/5	9. Mention enclosed clinical evaluation in body of letter.
_____	_____	_____	10. Insert proper paragraphing.
____/2	____/2	____/2	11. Key appropriate complimentary close and signature line.
_____	_____	_____	12. Key enclosure notation.
_____	_____	_____	13. Key copy notation.
_____	_____	_____	14. Insert proper reference initials.
_____	_____	_____	15. Proofread while document is on screen or in typewriter for spelling, punctuation, capitalization, and typing errors.
_____	_____	_____	16. Correct, print, and proofread again.
_____	_____	_____	17. Make corrections and prepare for physician's signature.
_____	_____	_____	18. Make a copy to mail to patient.
_____	_____	_____	Complete within specified time.
____/25	____/25	____/25	**Total points earned** (To obtain a percentage score, divide the total points earned by the number of points possible.)

JOB SKILL 11-6 (*continued*)

Comments:

Evaluator's Signature: _____ **Need to Repeat:** _____

National Curriculum Competency: CAAHEP: III.C.3.c(1)(a)   ABHES: VI.B.1.a.2(g), VI.B.1.a.2(j),
                                                                          VI.B.1.a.2(o), VI.B.1.a.3(a)

JOB SKILL 11-7
Compose and Key a Letter Requesting Payment

Name _____ Date _____ Score _____

Performance Objective

Task: Compose and key a letter requesting payment on an overdue bill.

Conditions: Letterhead for Practon Medical Group, Inc., formatted in a word processing program, or one sheet of letterhead (Form 31) and dictionary. Refer to textbook Figures 11-7 and 11-8 for format. Refer to Procedure 11-2 in the textbook for step-by-step directions.

Standards: Complete all steps listed in this skill in _____ minutes with a minimum score of _____. (Time element and accuracy criteria may be given by instructor.)

Time: Start: _____ **Completed:** _____ **Total:** _____ minutes

Scoring: One point for each step performed satisfactorily unless otherwise listed or weighted by instructor.

Directions with Performance Evaluation Checklist

When checking the financial records, you find that Christine LaMairre (Mrs. C. J.), 247 South Lincoln Boulevard, Apartment 5, Topanga, XY 12345, has not paid her bill for three months. She was seen for a consultation and complete physical examination; the fee was $70.92. She has no insurance coverage. Write a firm letter requesting payment by a specific date so it is not necessary to turn her account over to a collection agency. Enclose a copy of the current statement. Compose and key an original letter over Dr. Gerald Practon's signature in modified block style with open punctuation; assume a file copy of the letter will be made.

1st Attempt	2nd Attempt	3rd Attempt	
_____	_____	_____	Gather materials (equipment and supplies) listed under "Conditions."
_____	_____	_____	1. Design letterhead or use Form 31.
_____	_____	_____	2. Date letter using current date.
_____	_____	_____	3. Key inside address.
_____	_____	_____	4. Key appropriate salutation.
_____	_____	_____	5. Key reference or subject line.
_____	_____	_____	6. Use modified block style.
_____	_____	_____	7. Use open punctuation.
_____	_____	_____	8. Center letter with even margins.
____/5	____/5	____/5	9. Request payment, stating amount owed in body of letter using firm language.
_____	_____	_____	10. Insert proper paragraphing.
____/2	____/2	____/2	11. Key appropriate complimentary close and signature line.
_____	_____	_____	12. Key enclosure notation.
_____	_____	_____	13. Insert proper reference initials.
_____	_____	_____	14. Proofread while document is on screen or in typewriter for spelling, punctuation, capitalization, and typing errors.
_____	_____	_____	15. Correct, print, and proofread again.
_____	_____	_____	16. Make corrections and prepare for physician's signature.
_____	_____	_____	17. Make a file copy.
_____	_____	_____	Complete within specified time.
____/24	____/24	____/24	**Total points earned** (To obtain a percentage score, divide the total points earned by the number of points possible.)

JOB SKILL 11-7 *(continued)*

Comments:

Evaluator's Signature: _____ **Need to Repeat:** _____

| National Curriculum Competency: CAAHEP: III.C.3.c(1)(a) | ABHES: VI.B.1.a.2(g), VI.B.1.a.2(j), VI.B.1.a.2(o), VI.B.1.a.3(a) |

JOB SKILL 11-8
Key an Interoffice Memoranda

Name _____ Date _____ Score _____

Performance Objective

Task: Key an interoffice memorandum.

Conditions: Use interoffice memo (Form 32) and handwritten note (*Workbook* Figure 11-1). See textbook Figure 11-10 for an example.

Standards: Complete all steps listed in this skill in _____ minutes with a minimum score of _____. (Time element and accuracy criteria may be given by instructor.)

Time: **Start:** _____ **Completed:** _____ **Total:** _____ minutes

Scoring: One point for each step performed satisfactorily unless otherwise listed or weighted by instructor.

Directions with Performance Evaluation Checklist

Dr. Practon has written a note and asked you to key a memorandum to Dr. Yong Hall. Abstract information from his handwritten note and key the message accurately on an interoffice memo. Use guide words such as those found on Form 32.

1st Attempt	2nd Attempt	3rd Attempt	
_____	_____	_____	Gather materials (equipment and supplies) listed under "Conditions."
_____	_____	_____	1. Read the note before beginning to compose the memo.
_____	_____	_____	2. Prepare a rough draft of the memo.
_____	_____	_____	3. Align and key memo headings (or use those on Form 32).
_____	_____	_____	4. Fill in spaces after each guide word with appropriate data.
_____	_____	_____	5. Choose appropriate information for the subject heading.
____/5	____/5	____/5	6. Write a concise message using appropriate sentence structure.
_____	_____	_____	7. Include all relevant information.
_____	_____	_____	8. Proofread memo while document is on screen or in typewriter for spelling, punctuation, capitalization, and typing errors.
_____	_____	_____	9. Print hard copy.
_____	_____	_____	Complete within specified time.
____/15	____/15	____/15	**Total points earned** (To obtain a percentage score, divide the total points earned by the number of points possible.)

Comments:

Evaluator's Signature: _____   **Need to Repeat:** _____

National Curriculum Competency: CAAHEP: III.C.3.c(1)(a)	ABHES: VI.B.1.a.2(g), VI.B.1.a.2(j), VI.B.1.a.2(o), VI.B.1.a.3(a)

JOB SKILL 11-8 *(continued)*

From the Desk of... *G. P.*

3-22

Jean:

Ask Dr. Hall if he saw article "Evaluation of Biofeedback Training + Its Effects Upon Pt's with Tension Headaches" - Jan, 20XX. AMA Journal by Dr. Hugh James, pgs 21-25 - relevant to his research; very informative!

G. P.

P.S. Does he need a reprint?

Figure 11-1

JOB SKILL 11-9
Key a Memoranda from Handwritten Notes

Name _____ Date _____ Score _____

Performance Objective

Task: Key an interoffice memorandum from a handwritten note.

Conditions: Use interoffice memo (Form 33) and handwritten note (*Workbook* Figure 11-2). See textbook Figure 11-10 for an example.

Standards: Complete all steps listed in this skill in _____ minutes with a minimum score of _____. (Time element and accuracy criteria may be given by instructor.)

Time: **Start:** _____ **Completed:** _____ **Total:** _____ minutes

Scoring: One point for each step performed satisfactorily unless otherwise listed or weighted by instructor.

Directions with Performance Evaluation Checklist

Dr. Fran Practon has written you a note (Figure 11-2) asking you to key a memorandum to Cathy Crowe, RPT. Dr. Practon will take it to the hospital and place it in Cathy's box. Key the appropriate memo.

1st Attempt	2nd Attempt	3rd Attempt	
_____	_____	_____	Gather materials (equipment and supplies) listed under "Conditions."
_____	_____	_____	1. Read the note before beginning to compose the memo.
_____	_____	_____	2. Prepare a rough draft of the memo.
_____	_____	_____	3. Align and key memo headings (or use those on Form 32).
_____	_____	_____	4. Fill in spaces after each guide word with appropriate data.
_____	_____	_____	5. Choose appropriate information for the subject heading.
____/5	____/5	____/5	6. Write a concise message using appropriate sentence structure.
_____	_____	_____	7. Include all relevant information.
_____	_____	_____	8. Proofread memo while document is on screen or in typewriter for spelling, punctuation, capitalization, and typing errors.
_____	_____	_____	9. Print hard copy.
_____	_____	_____	Complete within specified time.
____/15	____/15	____/15	**Total points earned** (To obtain a percentage score, divide the total points earned by the number of points possible.)

Comments:

Evaluator's Signature: _____ **Need to Repeat:** _____

National Curriculum Competency: CAAHEP: III.C.3.c(1)(a)	ABHES: VI.B.1.a.2(g), VI.B.1.a.2(j), VI.B.1.a.2(o), VI.B.1.a.3(a)

JOB SKILL 11-9 *(continued)*

From the Desk of... *Fran*
                                    3-22

J.-

Please type a memo so I can take it to the hospital today to Cathy Crowe, RPT. Tell her we haven't rec'd copy of muscle strength Evaluation form for pt. Eric Willard. I desperately need it by 24th before I see Eric.

                    Thanks!

                    F.P.

Figure 11-2

JOB SKILL 11-10
Abstract Information from a Medical Record, Compose, and Key a Letter

Name _____ Date _____ Score _____

Performance Objective

Task:　　　　Abstract patient information from a chart note, then key a letter to a referring physician.

Conditions:　Letterhead for Practon Medical Group, Inc., formatted in a word processing program, or one sheet of letterhead (Form 34) and dictionary. Refer to textbook Figures 11-7 and 11-8 for format. Refer to textbook Procedure 11-2 for step-by-step directions.

Standards:　Complete all steps listed in this skill in _____ minutes with a minimum score of _____. (Time element and accuracy criteria may be given by instructor.)

Time:　　　 **Start:** _____ **Completed:** _____ **Total:** _____ minutes

Scoring:　　One point for each step performed satisfactorily unless otherwise listed or weighted by instructor.

Directions with Performance Evaluation Checklist

Dr. Fran Practon has asked you to review the chart notes of Ben Olman (*Workbook* Figure 11-3) and send a letter, dated March 22, 20XX, to the referring physician outlining the treatment since the last letter. Use full block style with mixed punctuation and key the letter for the physician's signature.

1st Attempt	2nd Attempt	3rd Attempt	
_____	_____	_____	Gather materials (equipment and supplies) listed under "Conditions."
_____	_____	_____	1. Design letterhead or use Form 34.
_____	_____	_____	2. Date letter.
_____	_____	_____	3. Key inside address.
_____	_____	_____	4. Key appropriate salutation.
_____	_____	_____	5. Key reference or subject line.
_____	_____	_____	6. Use full block style.
_____	_____	_____	7. Use mixed punctuation.
_____	_____	_____	8. Center letter with even margins.
____/3	____/3	____/3	9. Include patient's name and purpose of letter at the beginning of letter.
____/10	____/10	____/10	10. Include all dates and medical information since previous letter.
_____	_____	_____	11. Insert proper paragraphing.
____/2	____/2	____/2	12. Key appropriate closing sentence.
____/2	____/2	____/2	13. Key appropriate complimentary close and signature line.
_____	_____	_____	14. Insert proper reference initials.
_____	_____	_____	15. Proofread while document is on screen or in typewriter for spelling, punctuation, capitalization, and typing errors.
_____	_____	_____	16. Correct, print, and proofread again.
_____	_____	_____	17. Make corrections and prepare for physician's signature.
_____	_____	_____	Complete within specified time.
____/32	____/32	____/32	**Total points earned** (To obtain a percentage score, divide the total points earned by the number of points possible.)

JOB SKILL 11-10 *(continued)*

DATE	PROGRESS
2/3/XX	Pt moved recently to area and was referred to me by Dr. Ann Coleman, 4021 Indiana Ave, Ste 2, Pacific Palisades, CA 90272. **Olman, Ben A.** States he has a long HX of tonsillitis. Pt seen in ofc complaining of chills, sore throat since January 26. Temp. 102.6° F. CPX shows tonsils that appear enlarged & red. Throat culture taken. llf *Fran Practon, MD*
2/5/XX	Pt improved. Tonsils appear less swollen. Throat culture neg. for strep. Continue penicillin Rx for 10 days p.o. t.i.d. Call if not improved. llf *Fran Practon, MD*
2/20/XX	Pt comes in again with severe sore throat. Began 3 days after penicillin was dc. Malaise. Temp 101.4° F. Tonsil culture taken and await results before prescribing antibiotic. Ret 3 days. llf *Fran Practon, MD*
2/23/XX	Pt presents with acute sore throat, red & inflamed. Temp 102.4° F. Adv tonsillectomy after acute phase subsides. Rx antibiotic, Suprax, 20 mg q. 12 h. llf *Fran Practon, MD*
2/23/XX	Letter mailed to Dr. Coleman.
3/2/XX	Pt RTO. Throat improved. Scheduled T & A at College Hospital for 3/15/XX. llf *Fran Practon, MD*
3/15/XX	Pt adm to outpatient surgery at College Hospital. T & A with disc. same day. llf
3/21/XX	PO; no complaints. Temp 98.4° F. To retn p.r.n. llf *Fran Practon, MD*

Figure 11-3

Comments:

Evaluator's Signature: _____ **Need to Repeat:** _____

National Curriculum Competency: CAAHEP: III.C.3.c(1)(a)	ABHES: VI.B.1.a.2(g), VI.B.1.a.2(j), VI.B.1.a.2(o), VI.B.1.a.3(a)

JOB SKILL 11-11
Key a Two-Page Letter

Name _____ Date _____ Score _____

Performance Objective

Task: Key a two-page letter using appropriate second-page heading.

Conditions: Letterhead for Practon Medical Group, Inc., formatted in a word processing program, or one sheet of letterhead (Form 35) and dictionary. Refer to textbook Figures 11-7 and 11-8 for format and Example 11-20 for second-page heading. Refer to Procedure 11-2 in the textbook for step-by-step directions.

Standards: Complete all steps listed in this skill in _____ minutes with a minimum score of _____. (Time element and accuracy criteria may be given by instructor.)

Time: **Start:** _____ **Completed:** _____ **Total:** _____ minutes

Scoring: One point for each step performed satisfactorily unless otherwise listed or weighted by instructor.

Directions with Performance Evaluation Checklist

Using the current date, format and key a two-page letter to the attention of the education chair of your local county medical society; use their address. The subject for the letter is "Work Experience for the Medical Office Student," and the text, written by Dr. Gerald Practon, is found in *Workbook* Figure 11-4. Set 1½" margins, use full block style with open punctuation, determine paragraphing, and make capitalization corrections as required.

1st Attempt	2nd Attempt	3rd Attempt	
_____	_____	_____	Gather materials (equipment and supplies) listed under "Conditions."
_____	_____	_____	1. Design letterhead or use Form 35 and one sheet of plain paper for second page.
_____	_____	_____	2. Date letter using current date.
_____	_____	_____	3. Key inside address.
_____	_____	_____	4. Include attention line.
_____	_____	_____	5. Key appropriate salutation.
_____	_____	_____	6. Key reference or subject line.
_____	_____	_____	7. Use full block style.
_____	_____	_____	8. Use open punctuation.
_____	_____	_____	9. Center letter using 1½" margins.
____/6	____/6	____/6	10. Insert proper paragraphing.
_____	_____	_____	11. Make necessary capitalization corrections.
_____	_____	_____	12. Choose appropriate line to end page 1.
____/3	____/3	____/3	13. Insert second-page heading.
____/5	____/5	____/5	14. Key all information accurately.
_____	_____	_____	15. Key appropriate concluding sentence.
____/2	____/2	____/2	16. Key appropriate complimentary close and signature line.
_____	_____	_____	17. Insert proper reference initials.
_____	_____	_____	18. Proofread while document is on screen or in typewriter for spelling, punctuation, capitalization, and typing errors.
_____	_____	_____	19. Correct, print, and proofread again.
_____	_____	_____	20. Make corrections and prepare for physician's signature.
_____	_____	_____	Complete within specified time.
____/34	____/34	____/34	**Total points earned** (To obtain a percentage score, divide the total points earned by the number of points possible.)

JOB SKILL 11-11 (*continued*)

In reply to your request for information on work experience, I am enclosing a summary of the material I have found for your group, and I hope it answers some of your questions. Physicians, administrators, educational and medical associations, and officials of school districts have expressed increased interest in the value of on-the-job training and career-related work-study programs for their medical office students. Some colleges have instituted major curriculum changes to provide for internships and hospital work-study assignments. As a result of this interest, employers, including medical agencies, as well as federal agencies, are being asked to support the objectives of this new educational concept by providing new training opportunities for medical office students. Many agencies have inquired as to the role that they may play in making medical facilities available and in providing training to support these work-study medical programs. These inquiries have requested clarification in three general program areas: (1) programs established through legislation; (2) part-time, intermittent, or temporary employment; and (3) the selective exposure of students, in a nonpaid status, to learning projects related to educational objectives. Agencies are now providing and are encouraged to expand work-study opportunities for students and enrollees in programs authorized by legislation. Such legislation includes the Higher Education, Vocational Education Training, economic opportunity, and Social Security acts. Under these programs, students receive stipends from financial grants provided by statute. Similar support is urged for part-time, intermittent, and cyclic employment programs for students. Hospital programs such as cooperative work-study, summer and vacation employment, and part-time employment during the school year offer agencies an excellent opportunity to make significant contributions through medical-related assignments. These programs are also in keeping with federal long-range recruitment objectives. I hope this summarizes for your group the information you requested. If I can be of any further assistance in setting up the program in your area, please feel free to contact me.

Figure 11-4

Comments:

Evaluator's Signature: _____   **Need to Repeat:** _____

National Curriculum Competency: CAAHEP: III.C.3.c(1)(a)   ABHES: VI.B.1.a.2(g), VI.B.1.a.2(j),
VI.B.1.a.2(o), VI.B.1.a.3(a)

CHAPTER 12

Processing Mail and Telecommunications

OBJECTIVES

After completing the exercises, the student will be able to:

1. Enhance knowledge of medical terminology, interpret abbreviations, and accurately spell medical words.

2. Process incoming mail.

3. Annotate mail.

4. Classify outgoing mail.

5. Address envelopes for optical character reader (OCR) scanning.

6. Complete a mail-order form for postal supplies.

7. Compose letters and prepare envelopes for certified mailing.

8. Prepare a cover sheet for fax transmission.

9. Key and fold original letters, address small and large envelopes for certified mail, return-receipt requested.

FOCUS ON CERTIFICATION*

CMA Content Summary

- Medical terminology and abbreviations
- Receive, organize, prioritize, and transmit information
- Format envelopes
- Operate photocopy machine
- Operate fax machine
- Send electronic mail
- Security/passwords
- Screen and process incoming and outgoing mail
- Classify mail
- OCR guidelines
- Postal meter

*This *Workbook* and accompanying textbook meet the entry-level administrative and general competencies for the CMA outlined by the AAMA Examination Content Outline and Role Delineation Study and for the RMA and CMAS outlined by the AMT Competencies and Examination Specifications (see Competency Grid in textbook Appendix B).

RMA Content Summary

- Medical terminology
- Common abbreviations
- Written communication

- Encryption and personal passwords
- Understand firewall software
- Compose correspondence

CMAS Content Summary

- Medical terminology
- Written communication
- Process incoming and outgoing mail
- Confidentiality

- Ensure confidentiality of computer-stored information
- Software and e-mail applications
- Manage office mailing and shipping services

Abbreviation and Spelling Review

Read the following patient's chart note and write the meanings for the abbreviations listed below the note. To decode any abbreviations you do not understand or that appear unfamiliar to you, refer to the list of abbreviations in Part V of this *Workbook*. Step-by-step directions for this exercise are in Procedure 1-1 of Chapter 1 in the textbook. Medical terms in the chart note are italicized; study them for spelling. Use your medical dictionary to look up their definitions. Your instructor may give a spelling and definition test that includes these words and abbreviations.

Stephen L. Boasberg

January 17, 20XX OC: Biopsy report pos. for CA of *prostate*. TURP & *bilateral orchiectomy, scrotal*. Adm to hosp in 2 days. Est. TD: 6 wks. Adv dc pain medication in 3 days.

Fran Practon, MD

Fran Practon, MD

OC	_____	est.	_____
pos.	_____	TD	_____
CA	_____	wks	_____
TURP	_____	adv	_____
adm	_____	dc	_____
hosp	_____		

Terence O. Williams

January 17, 20XX Sunday, 4 a.m. pt seen in ER complaining of pain, R ear, abt 3 days, PX revealed fluid & pus. Temp. 100°F.

Fran Practon, MD

Fran Practon, MD

AM	_____	abt	_____
pt	_____	PX	_____
ER	_____	temp.	_____
R	_____	F	_____

Review Questions

Review the objectives, glossary, and chapter information before completing the following review questions.

1. According to the U.S. Postal Service, the *domestic mail* zone includes _____

   _____ .

2. OCR stands for _____ .

3. List three advantages for using a postage meter.

   a. _____

   b. _____

   c. _____

4. Name three ways in which postage stamps can be obtained.

   a. _____

   b. _____

   c. _____

5. List the items that should be available when opening mail.

   a. _____

   b. _____

   c. _____

   d. _____

   e. _____

   f. _____

6. Why should all incoming correspondence be dated? _____

   _____

7. Generally, a letter marked _____ or _____
   is not opened by the medical assistant.

8. Parcel Post is also known as _____ mail.

9. The most expedient way to send letters that weigh under 13 ounces is _____ ,

   and the most expedient way to send letters that weigh over 13 ounces is _____ .

10. The fastest and most reliable delivery service offered by the U.S. Postal Service, which guarantees overnight

    delivery, is called _____ .

11. OCR envelope guidelines require keying the attention line _____

    _____ .

12. Name four service endorsements that can be placed on envelopes to notify the U.S. Postal Service of action to
    take when a piece of mail is undeliverable-as-addressed.

    a. _____

    b. _____

    c. _____

    d. _____

13. A type of mail service that electronically sends, receives, stores, and forwards messages in digital form over telecommunication lines is known as _____ .

14. An e-mail business communication should follow the format of a/an _____ .

15. Answer "True" or "False" to the following statements.

    a. _____ Informal salutations may be used with e-mail.

    b. _____ Informal complimentary closings may be used with e-mail.

    c. _____ Pronouns are recommended in the composition of all e-mails.

    d. _____ It is all right to forward chain letters via office e-mail as long as it is done quickly.

    e. _____ E-mail attachments should never be sent with office e-mail.

    f. _____ Even though HIPAA does not directly address e-mail in its standards, both the privacy and security rules apply.

    g. _____ A secure messaging service allows e-mail to be encrypted.

    h. _____ It is recommended that you check your e-mail box at work every hour.

16. Describe five situations in which the physician might use facsimile (fax) transmission from the office.

    a. _____

    b. _____

    c. _____

    d. _____

    e. _____

17. What method of mailing should be used to send a patient chart to a lawyer for use in a malpractice court hearing?

    _____

18. List six legal requirements that apply when faxing confidential medical records.

    a. _____

    b. _____

    c. _____

    d. _____

    e. _____

    f. _____

Critical Thinking Exercises

1. Respond to the following statements regarding composing e-mail messages.

    a. There is no need to worry about typographical or spelling errors. _____

    _____

    b. It is *more important* to proofread for spelling and accuracy. _____

    _____

    c. It is permissible to use abbreviations because the recipient will understand what you mean. _____

    _____

2. Respond to the following statements regarding receiving e-mail messages.

    a. Respond as soon as possible, but after you finish the task you are doing. _____

    _____

    b. Answer immediately. _____

    _____

    c. Print the message, put it in your inbox with other fax and telephone requests, and answer when convenient.

    _____

    d. Always acknowledge that the message has been received. _____

3. Respond to the following statements regarding the insertion of your telephone number on e-mail messages.

    a. It is not necessary because you reply directly to the sender of the message. _____

    _____

    b. Always include it. _____

    c. It depends on the preference of the employer or individual sending the message. _____

    _____

4. Respond to the following statements regarding printing e-mail messages.

    a. If the message is important or if a hard copy record is needed, then print the message. _____

    _____

    b. Always print the message. _____

    c. Never print the message. _____

JOB SKILL 12-1
Process Incoming Mail

Name _____ Date _____ Score _____

Performance Objective

Task: Sort and process incoming mail; determine the disbursement and action for each communication.

Conditions: List of incoming mail; pen or pencil.

Standards: Complete all steps listed in this skill in _____ minutes with a minimum score of _____.
(Time element and accuracy criteria may be given by instructor.)

Time: **Start:** _____ **Completed:** _____ **Total:** _____ minutes

Scoring: One point for each step performed satisfactorily unless otherwise listed or weighted by instructor.

Directions with Performance Evaluation Checklist

You will be opening today's mail and determining what action needs to take place for each piece. Some of the mail will be placed on the physician's desk; please designate its importance by indicating "top," "middle," or "bottom" of mail stack. You may need to route mail to other office workers, pull a patient's chart, record items on a calendar (physician or medical assistant), or set up a file folder. All money received needs to be posted or recorded on the patient's ledger or account, the daysheet or journal, and the bank deposit (you can simply put "record payment") and then put in a safe place (locked drawer or safe). You will need to check the address on the check against the office records to verify that the address is current. You have the ability to write checks if an invoice needs to be paid.

Study the following list of mail items. Use critical thinking skills to give a written explanation in the designated space of what you would do with each piece of mail.

1st Attempt	2nd Attempt	3rd Attempt		
_____	_____	_____	Gather materials (equipment and supplies) listed under "Conditions."	
_____	_____	_____	1. Letter and check from a patient:	_____
_____	_____	_____	2. Announcement of a medical society meeting:	_____
_____	_____	_____	3. Advertisement for an x-ray machine:	_____
_____	_____	_____	4. Mail-order gardening catalog:	_____
_____	_____	_____	5. Letter from Mr. C. J. Conway:	_____
_____	_____	_____	6. Check from Mr. Bill Owen:	_____
_____	_____	_____	7. Advertisement of a new tranquilizer drug:	_____
_____	_____	_____	8. *Journal of the American Medical Association* (current issue):	_____
_____	_____	_____	9. A request for a reprint of an article written by Dr. Practon:	_____
_____	_____	_____	10. Letter marked "Personal" to Dr. Fran Practon:	_____
_____	_____	_____	11. A drug sample:	_____
_____	_____	_____	12. Letter referring a patient to Dr. Gerald Practon:	_____
_____	_____	_____	13. A piece of pornographic literature:	_____
_____	_____	_____	14. Letter announcing an evening professional meeting in two months:	_____
_____	_____	_____	15. License tax-due notice:	_____
_____	_____	_____	16. Charity solicitation letter:	_____
_____	_____	_____	17. Insurance query about Mrs. Dorothy Ranger:	_____

JOB SKILL 12-1 (*continued*)

_____ _____ _____ 18. Medicare payment for Beth Cook: _____

_____ _____ _____ 19. Lab test results on Mrs. Murdock: _____

_____ _____ _____ 20. Consultant report on Mr. Bill McKean: _____

_____ _____ _____ 21. Check from Aetna Insurance Company for service
rendered to Samantha Boatman: _____

_____ _____ _____ 22. Prudential insurance form on Mr. Tom Patten: _____

_____ _____ _____ 23. Invoice from V. Mueller Supply Company: _____

_____ _____ _____ 24. Letter from Mrs. Todd Stark without date or address
(these do appear on the envelope):   _____

_____ _____ _____ 25. Letter from Dr. Lees concerning a research project: _____

_____ _____ _____ 26. Letter about cancellation of appointment by patient
who is on vacation: _____

_____ _____ _____ 27. *Time* magazine: _____

_____ _____ _____ 28. Mutual funds investment letter: _____

_____ _____ _____ 29. Local medical society agenda for monthly meeting: _____

_____ _____ _____ 30. Ad for new filing equipment: _____

_____ _____ _____ 31. Mail-order medical instrument catalog: _____

_____ _____ _____ 32. Gift parcel from Mrs. Gaspar Whelan (patient):   _____

_____ _____ _____ 33. Letter notifying Dr. Fran Practon of the death of a
colleague: _____

_____ _____ _____ 34. Telegram from Dr. Perry Cardi congratulating
Dr. Gerald Practon on his election as vice president
of local medical society: _____

_____ _____ _____ 35. Personal letter, opened by mistake: _____

_____ _____ _____ Complete within specified time.

___/37 ___/37 ___/37 **Total points earned** (To obtain a percentage score, divide the total points earned
by the number of points possible.)

Comments:

Evaluator's Signature: _____ **Need to Repeat:** _____

National Curriculum Competency: CAAHEP: III.C.3.a(1)   ABHES: VI.B.1.a.3(a)

JOB SKILL 12-2
Annotate Mail

Name _____ Date _____ Score _____

Performance Objective

Task: Read a letter, annotate significant words or phrases, and make comments in the margin concerning the action to be taken.

Conditions: Use the letter in *Workbook* Figure 12-1 for reference and a highlighter or colored pen. Refer to textbook Procedure 12-2 for step-by-step directions.

Standards: Complete all steps listed in this skill in _____ minutes with a minimum score of _____. (Time element and accuracy criteria may be given by instructor.)

Time: Start: _____ **Completed:** _____ **Total:** _____ minutes

Scoring: One point for each step performed satisfactorily unless otherwise listed or weighted by instructor.

Directions with Performance Evaluation Checklist

Read the letter from Mr. Glen Marchall (Figure 12-1) that arrived today. Note significant words or phrases by highlighting them or by underlining with colored pen. Annotate any action requirements in the right margin using colored pen.

1st Attempt	2nd Attempt	3rd Attempt	
_____	_____	_____	Gather materials (equipment and supplies) listed under "Conditions."
____/10	____/10	____/10	1. Underline important words or phrases.
____/5	____/5	____/5	2. Annotate action areas of letter.
_____	_____	_____	Complete within specified time.
____/17	____/17	____/17	**Total points earned** (To obtain a percentage score, divide the total points earned by the number of points possible.)

Comments:

Evaluator's Signature: _____ **Need to Repeat:** _____

National Curriculum Competency: CAAHEP: III.C.3.a(1)   ABHES: VI.B.1.a.3(a)

JOB SKILL 12-2 *(continued)*

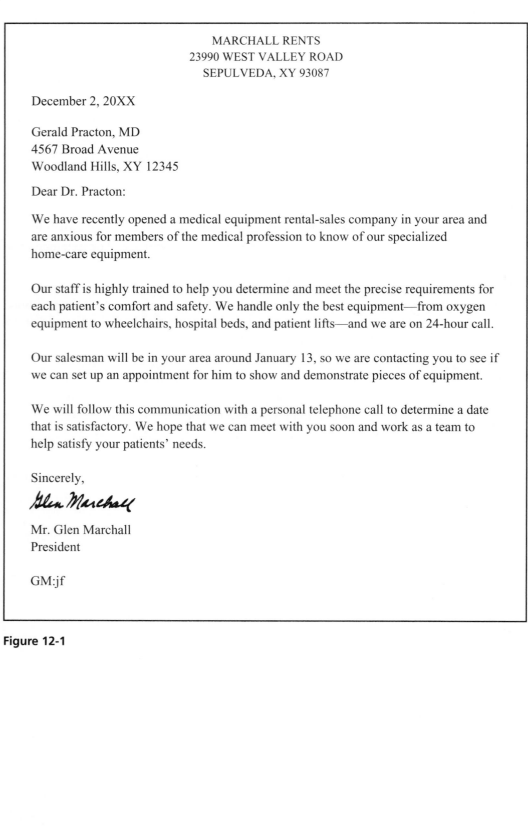

MARCHALL RENTS
23990 WEST VALLEY ROAD
SEPULVEDA, XY 93087

December 2, 20XX

Gerald Practon, MD
4567 Broad Avenue
Woodland Hills, XY 12345

Dear Dr. Practon:

We have recently opened a medical equipment rental-sales company in your area and are anxious for members of the medical profession to know of our specialized home-care equipment.

Our staff is highly trained to help you determine and meet the precise requirements for each patient's comfort and safety. We handle only the best equipment—from oxygen equipment to wheelchairs, hospital beds, and patient lifts—and we are on 24-hour call.

Our salesman will be in your area around January 13, so we are contacting you to see if we can set up an appointment for him to show and demonstrate pieces of equipment.

We will follow this communication with a personal telephone call to determine a date that is satisfactory. We hope that we can meet with you soon and work as a team to help satisfy your patients' needs.

Sincerely,

Glen Marchall

Mr. Glen Marchall
President

GM:jf

Figure 12-1

JOB SKILL 12-3
Classify Outgoing Mail

Name _____ Date _____ Score _____

Performance Objective

Task: Identify classes of mail.

Conditions: Use list of outgoing mail and pen or pencil. Refer to "Mail Classifications" under the section titled "Handling Outgoing Mail" and Procedure 12-3 in the textbook for help.

Standards: Complete all steps listed in this skill in _____ minutes with a minimum score of _____. (Time element and accuracy criteria may be given by instructor.)

Time: Start: _____ Completed: _____ Total: _____ minutes

Scoring: One point for each step performed satisfactorily unless otherwise listed or weighted by instructor.

Directions with Performance Evaluation Checklist

You will be mailing various pieces and types of mail for the physicians, and it will be helpful if you can determine classifications before going to the post office. After each piece of mail, indicate the appropriate classification or special services used.

1st Attempt	2nd Attempt	3rd Attempt		
_____	_____	_____	Gather materials (equipment and supplies) listed under "Conditions."	
_____	_____	_____	1. Income tax forms mailed on deadline date	_____
_____	_____	_____	2. Proof that estimated income tax form was mailed by deadline	_____
_____	_____	_____	3. Prescription	_____
_____	_____	_____	4. Postal card	_____
_____	_____	_____	5. Photograph	_____
_____	_____	_____	6. Medical pamphlet	_____
_____	_____	_____	7. Newspaper	_____
_____	_____	_____	8. Bound 28-page manuscript	_____
_____	_____	_____	9. Unsealed circular weighing 12 ounces	_____
_____	_____	_____	10. Green diamond border envelope to enclose an item weighing more than 2 pounds	_____
_____	_____	_____	11. U.S. treasury bond	_____
_____	_____	_____	12. X-rays with letter	_____
_____	_____	_____	13. Cultured pearl necklace	_____
_____	_____	_____	14. Sealed dental catalog	_____
_____	_____	_____	15. Monthly statement	_____
_____	_____	_____	16. Letter with check enclosed	_____
_____	_____	_____	17. Laboratory report	_____
_____	_____	_____	18. Package weighing 36 pounds	_____
_____	_____	_____	19. Fastest delivery for a medical tape	_____
_____	_____	_____	20. Important item to be delivered within 24 hours; it is Saturday noon	_____
_____	_____	_____	21. A final collection letter from medical office	_____
_____	_____	_____	22. 30-page book with advertising	_____
_____	_____	_____	23. Medical society journal	_____

JOB SKILL 12-3 *(continued)*

_____ _____ _____   Complete within specified time.

____/25 ____/25 ____/25 **Total points earned** (To obtain a percentage score, divide the total points earned by the number of points possible.)

Comments:

Evaluator's Signature: _____ **Need to Repeat:** _____

National Curriculum Competency: CAAHEP: III.C.3.a(1)   ABHES: VI.B.1.a.3(a)

JOB SKILL 12-4
Address Envelopes for OCR Scanning

Name _____ Date _____ Score _____

Performance Objective

Task: Address small envelopes for OCR scanning using acceptable abbreviations and correct ZIP codes.

Conditions: Three number 6 envelopes or Forms 36 and 37. Use the format recommended for OCR processing found in textbook Table 12-2 and Figure 12-6. See textbook Table 12-3 for address abbreviations, and refer to *Workbook* Figure 12-2 for those that cannot be abbreviated to 13 positions. Refer to textbook Table 12-4 for two-letter state abbreviations and *Workbook* Figure 12-2 for ZIP codes from the National ZIP Code directory.

Standards: Complete all steps listed in this skill in _____ minutes with a minimum score of _____. (Time element and accuracy criteria may be given by instructor.)

Time: Start: _____ Completed: _____ Total: _____ minutes

Scoring: One point for each step performed satisfactorily unless otherwise listed or weighted by instructor.

Directions with Performance Evaluation Checklist

Dr. Fran Practon has three letters that need to be mailed immediately. Key the three addresses listed below on number 6 envelopes using standard abbreviations and ZIP codes. If using real envelopes, key Dr. Practon's office address (see *Workbook* Part IV) in the upper left corner of each envelope.

1. Mr. and Mrs. Arthur L. Duncally
   Post Office Box 286
   West Boothbay Harbor, Maine

2. Coastal Community Hospital
   8900 West Elvingston Drive
   Brooklyn-Curtis Bay, Maryland
   Attn: Elizabeth Collingswood, MD

3. Mr. Randolph G. Greenworthy Jr.
   49021 67th Avenue North
   Apartment 8
   Washington Grove, Maryland

1st Attempt	2nd Attempt	3rd Attempt	
_____	_____	_____	Gather materials (equipment and supplies) listed under "Conditions."
____/9	____/9	____/9	1. Key return address if not using Forms 36 and 37.
____/9	____/9	____/9	2. Key addresses for three envelopes.
____/9	____/9	____/9	3. Use OCR format.
____/9	____/9	____/9	4. Look up and use abbreviations.
____/3	____/3	____/3	5. Look up and key correct ZIP codes.
_____	_____	_____	6. Place attention line in correct position.
_____	_____	_____	7. Proofread for typographical, spelling, and spacing errors.
_____	_____	_____	Complete within specified time.
____/43	____/43	____/43	**Total points earned** (To obtain a percentage score, divide the total points earned by the number of points possible.)

JOB SKILL 12-4 *(continued)*

```
                              MAINE
04006-0000  Biddeford Pool .............................. BIDDEFRD POOL
04625-0000  Cranberry Isles.................................. CRANBERRY IS
04021-0000  Cumberland Center ........................... CUMBRLND CTR
04426-0000  Dover-Foxcroft .............................. DOVR FOXCROFT
04940-0000  Farmington Falls............................. FARMINGTN FLS
04575-0000  West Boothbay Harbor ........................ W BOOTHBY HBR

                             MARYLAND
21005-0000  Aberdeen Proving Ground ...................... ABRDN PRV GRD
20331-0000  Andrews Air Force Hospital ..................... ANDRS AF HOSP
21225-0000  Brooklyn-Curtis Bay ........................... BKLYN CTS BAY
20622-0000  Charlotte Hall ................................ CHARLOTE HALL
20732-0000  Chesapeake Beach............................... CHESAPKE BCH
20904-0000  Ednor Cloverly ............................. EDNR CLOVERLY
21713-0000  Fahrney Keedy Memorial Home ................. FHRN MEM HOME
20755-0000  Fort George G. Meade ............................ FT MEADE
21240-0000  Friendship Airport ........................... FRNDSHP ARPRT
21078-0000  Havre de Grace ............................. HVRE DE GRACE
20014-0000  National Naval Medical Center .................. NAVAL MED CTR
20390-0000  Naval Air Facility................................ NAV AIR FACIL
20678-0000  Prince Frederick............................. PRNC FREDERCK
20788-0000  Prince Georges Plaza........................... PRNC GEO PLZ
21152-0000  Sparks Glencoe ............................... SPRKS GLENCOE
21784-0000  Springfield State Hospital ........................ SPRINFLD HOSP
20390-0000  U.S. Naval Communications Center .............. NAV COMMS CTR
20880-0000  Washington Grove ........................... WASHINGTN GRV
```

Figure 12-2

Comments:

Evaluator's Signature: _____ **Need to Repeat:** _____

JOB SKILL 12-5
Complete a Mail-Order Form for Postal Supplies

Name _____ Date _____ Score _____

Performance Objective

Task: Complete a mail-order form for postal supplies and compute the total amount owed.

Conditions: Use Form 38 and pen.

Standards: Complete all steps listed in this skill in _____ minutes with a minimum score of _____.
(Time element and accuracy criteria may be given by instructor.)

Time: Start: _____ **Completed:** _____ **Total:** _____ minutes

Scoring: One point for each step performed satisfactorily unless otherwise listed or weighted by instructor.

Directions with Performance Evaluation Checklist

Complete in ink the mail-order form for stamps. For each item ordered, list the quantity and multiply it by the price to obtain the cost, and then add all figures in the "cost" column to determine the total cost of the order. A check would ordinarily be made out to the U.S. Postmaster and enclosed with the order; however, since check writing is discussed in a future chapter, a check will not be written for this exercise.

1st Attempt	2nd Attempt	3rd Attempt	
_____	_____	_____	Gather materials (equipment and supplies) listed under "Conditions."
____/5	____/5	____/5	1. Print the medical practice's telephone number, name, and complete address.
____/3	____/3	____/3	2. Order five roles of 41-cent stamps; 100 in each roll.
____/3	____/3	____/3	3. Order three sets of 80-cent stamps (5 stamps per set) for first ounce of flat mail.
____/2	____/2	____/2	4. Order one book of "Forever Stamps," which can be used for First Class mail regardless of future postal rate increases.
____/3	____/3	____/3	5. Order forty 2-cent stamps for extra postage.
____/3	____/3	____/3	6. Order two-hundred 17-cent additional ounce stamps for First Class postage (10 stamps per set).
_____	_____	_____	7. Compute the total cost and insert.
_____	_____	_____	Complete within specified time.
____/22	____/22	____/22	**Total points earned** (To obtain a percentage score, divide the total points earned by the number of points possible.)

Comments:

Evaluator's Signature: _____ **Need to Repeat:** _____

National Curriculum Competency: CAAHEP: III.C.3.a(1)   ABHES: VI.B.1.a.3(a)

JOB SKILL 12-6
Compose a Letter and Prepare an Envelope for Ceritified Mail

Name _____ Date _____ Score _____

Performance Objective

Task: Compose and key a letter in a specified format; address and prepare a large envelope for OCR processing as Certified Mail.

Conditions: One letterhead (create on a word-processing program or use Form 39), one number 10 envelope or Form 40 (see textbook Figure 12-6), a Certified Mail form or Form 41 (see textbook Figures 12-4 and 12-5), and pen. Refer to textbook Procedures 12-3 and 12-4 for step-by-step directions.

Standards: Complete all steps listed in this skill in _____ minutes with a minimum score of _____. (Time element and accuracy criteria may be given by instructor.)

Time: **Start:** _____ **Completed:** _____ **Total:** _____ minutes

Scoring: One point for each step performed satisfactorily unless otherwise listed or weighted by instructor.

Directions with Performance Evaluation Checklist

Mrs. Jane K. Call of 199 Eisenhower Boulevard, Apartment 17-J, Canoga Park, XY 12345-0001 telephoned yesterday stating that she wanted no further treatment from Dr. Gerald Practon. Write a letter to confirm this discharge by the patient stating that Dr. Practon feels further treatment is necessary and recommends that she contact the Valley Medical Society at (555) 659-2234 to obtain the name of another physician. See Chapter 3, Figure 3-12, for help with letter composition. Read through and follow the format specifications listed below for the letter, envelope, and certification form.

1st Attempt	2nd Attempt	3rd Attempt	
_____	_____	_____	Gather materials (equipment and supplies) listed under "Conditions."

LETTER

1st	2nd	3rd	
_____	_____	_____	1. Use Practon letterhead.
_____	_____	_____	2. Use modified block style.
_____	_____	_____	3. Use mixed punctuation.
_____	_____	_____	4. Use current date.
_____	_____	_____	5. Center letter with even margins.
_____	_____	_____	6. Key inside address.
_____	_____	_____	7. Key appropriate salutation.
_____	_____	_____	8. Mention patient name and purpose of letter at beginning.
_____	_____	_____	9. Compose appropriate letter with wording that is legally correct.
_____	_____	_____	10. Insert proper paragraphing.
_____	_____	_____	11. Key complimentary closing line in correct position.
_____	_____	_____	12. Key signature line.
_____	_____	_____	13. Key reference initials.
_____	_____	_____	14. Proofread letter while the document is on screen or in typewriter for typographical, spelling, punctuation, and capitalization errors.
_____	_____	_____	15. Correct errors.
_____	_____	_____	16. Print letter and proofread again.
_____	_____	_____	17. Present letter ready for physician to read and sign.

JOB SKILL 12-6 *(continued)*

ENVELOPE

____/8 ____/8 ____/8   18. Key large envelope in OCR format with no errors.

_____ _____ _____   19. Determine the correct postage via the Internet or by calling your local Post Office and write the amount where the stamp would be placed on the envelope.

CERTIFICATION FORM

____/5 ____/5 ____/5   20. Complete data on front of certification form.

____/5 ____/5 ____/5   21. Complete data on back of certification form.

____/5 ____/5 ____/5   22. Complete Receipt for Certified Mail.

_____ _____ _____   23. Fold letter correctly and insert in envelope; do not seal.

_____ _____ _____   Complete within specified time.

____/44 ____/44 ____/44   **Total points earned** (To obtain a percentage score, divide the total points earned by the number of points possible.)

Comments:

Evaluator's Signature: _____ **Need to Repeat:** _____

National Curriculum Competency: CAAHEP: III.C.3.a(1), III.C.3.c(1)(a)   ABHES: VI.B.1.a.2(j), VI.B.1.a.2(o), VI.B.1.a.3(a)

JOB SKILL 12-7
Prepare a Cover Sheet for Fax Transmission

Name _____ Date _____ Score _____

Performance Objective

Task: Prepare a transmission slip to accompany a message for fax communication.

Conditions: Fax transmittal (Form 42) and computer or typewriter. Refer to textbook Procedure 12-7 for step-by-step directions and Figure 12-12 for a visual example of a cover sheet.

Standards: Complete all steps listed in this skill in _____ minutes with a minimum score of _____. (Time element and accuracy criteria may be given by instructor.)

Time: **Start:** _____ **Completed:** _____ **Total:** _____ minutes

Scoring: One point for each step performed satisfactorily unless otherwise listed or weighted by instructor.

Directions with Performance Evaluation Checklist

Dr. Fran Practon is scheduled to speak at the Massachusetts American Women's Medical Association convention on November 20 in Boston. She asks you to prepare a fax cover sheet to accompany a two-page letter she will write for fax transmission. The fax will be directed to Dr. Elmo Reardon, 891 So. Revere Way, Boston, MA 02100; fax number: (555) 326-9923; phone number: (555) 326-9921. Abstract the necessary information and complete the fax cover sheet dated November 13, current year.

1st Attempt	2nd Attempt	3rd Attempt	
_____	_____	_____	Gather materials (equipment and supplies) listed under "Conditions."
____/8	____/8	____/8	1. Complete the top portion of the fax cover sheet.
_____	_____	_____	2. Indicate number of pages sent.
____/3	____/3	____/3	3. Request prompt confirmation of fax receipt by fax or telephone.
_____	_____	_____	4. List student name as contact.
_____	_____	_____	Complete within specified time.
____/15	____/15	____/15	**Total points earned** (To obtain a percentage score, divide the total points earned by the number of points possible.)

Comments:

JOB SKILL 12-8

Key and Fold an Original Letter; Address a Small Envelope for Certified Mail, Return-Receipt Requested

Name _____ Date _____ Score _____

Performance Objective

Task: Key a letter using specified format, prepare an envelope for OCR processing, fold and insert the letter into the envelope, and attach special mailing forms.

Conditions: One letterhead (create on a word-processing program or use Form 43), one number 6 envelope or Form 44 (see textbook Figure 12-6), a Certified Mail form or Form 45 (see textbook Figures 12-4 and 12-5), and pen. Refer to textbook Procedures 12-3 and 12-4 for step-by-step directions.

Standards: Complete all steps listed in this skill in _____ minutes with a minimum score of _____. (Time element and accuracy criteria may be given by instructor.)

Time: **Start:** _____ **Completed:** _____ **Total:** _____ minutes

Scoring: One point for each step performed satisfactorily unless otherwise listed or weighted by instructor.

Directions with Performance Evaluation Checklist

Mr. Henry J. Stone, One April Circle, Pacoima, XY 91331-0000, has had surgery and is negligent about following Dr. Gerald Practon's advice; he is at risk of having further injury. Compose an appropriate letter to Mr. Stone advising him of Dr. Practon's withdrawal from the case as of 30 days from the date of this notice. Refer to Chapter 3, Figure 3-11 for help with letter composition. Read and follow the format specifications listed below for the letter, envelope, and certification form.

1st Attempt	2nd Attempt	3rd Attempt	
_____	_____	_____	Gather materials (equipment and supplies) listed under "Conditions."

LETTER

1st Attempt	2nd Attempt	3rd Attempt	
_____	_____	_____	1. Use Practon letterhead.
_____	_____	_____	2. Use full block style.
_____	_____	_____	3. Use mixed punctuation.
_____	_____	_____	4. Use current date.
_____	_____	_____	5. Center letter with even margins.
_____	_____	_____	6. Key inside address.
_____	_____	_____	7. Key appropriate salutation.
_____	_____	_____	8. Compose letter of withdrawal with wording that is legally correct.
_____	_____	_____	9. Insert proper paragraphing.
_____	_____	_____	10. Key complimentary closing line in correct position.
_____	_____	_____	11. Key signature line.
_____	_____	_____	12. Key reference initials.
_____	_____	_____	13. Proofread letter while the document is on screen or in typewriter for typographical, spelling, punctuation, and capitalization errors.
_____	_____	_____	14. Correct errors.
_____	_____	_____	15. Print letter and proofread again.
_____	_____	_____	16. Present letter ready for physician to read and sign.

JOB SKILL 12-8 (*continued*)

ENVELOPE

____/8   ____/8   ____/8   17. Key small envelope in OCR format with no errors.

_____   _____   _____   18. Determine the correct postage via the Internet or by calling your local Post Office and write the amount where the stamp would be placed on the envelope.

CERTIFICATION FORM

____/5   ____/5   ____/5   19. Complete data on front of certification form.

____/5   ____/5   ____/5   20. Complete data on back of certification form.

____/5   ____/5   ____/5   21. Complete Receipt for Certified Mail.

_____   _____   _____   22. Fold letter correctly and insert in envelope; do not seal.

_____   _____   _____   Complete within specified time.

____/43   ____/43   ____/43   **Total points earned** (To obtain a percentage score, divide the total points earned by the number of points possible.)

Comments:

Evaluator's Signature: _____   **Need to Repeat:** _____

National Curriculum Competency: CAAHEP: III.C.3.a(1), III.C.3.c(1)(a)	ABHES: VI.B.1.a.2(o), VI.B.1.a.3(a)

JOB SKILL 12-9
Key and Fold an Original Letter; Address a Large Envelope for Certified Mail, Return-Receipt Requested

Name _____ Date _____ Score _____

Performance Objective

Task: Key a letter, prepare a large envelope for OCR processing, fold and insert the letter into the envelope, and attach special mailing forms.

Conditions: One letterhead (create on a word-processing program or use Form 46), one number 10 envelope or Form 47 (see textbook Figure 12-6), a Certified Mail form or Form 48 (see textbook Figures 12-4 and 12-5), and pen. Refer to textbook Procedures 12-3 and 12-4 for step-by-step directions.

Standards: Complete all steps listed in this skill in _____ minutes with a minimum score of _____. (Time element and accuracy criteria may be given by instructor.)

Time: Start: _____ Completed: _____ Total: _____ minutes

Scoring: One point for each step performed satisfactorily unless otherwise listed or weighted by instructor.

Directions with Performance Evaluation Checklist

Miss Henrietta M. Marskovskie of 4311 Eberly Street, Woodland Hills, XY 12345-4700 was referred to Practon Medical Group by Dr. Ambrose Kistler, 698 Madison Way, Gretna, NE 54321-0009, when she relocated in Woodland Hills. Dr. Gerald Practon went to medical school at the University of Omaha, Nebraska, with Dr. Kistler. Dr. Kistler and his wife, Julie, share the Practon's love for the game of golf; they have played many rounds together. Dr. Practon would like you to write a letter acknowledging this kind referral, and he will edit it prior to its finalization. He saw the patient yesterday and will be taking over her care. She is being treated for renal disease, which is now under control; the patient is doing well and looks very healthy. She is thrilled to be in her new home and close to her grandchildren. Write a friendly referral thank you letter under Dr. Gerald Practon's signature.

1st Attempt	2nd Attempt	3rd Attempt	
_____	_____	_____	Gather materials (equipment and supplies) listed under "Conditions."

LETTER

1st	2nd	3rd	
_____	_____	_____	1. Use Practon letterhead.
_____	_____	_____	2. Use modified block style.
_____	_____	_____	3. Use mixed punctuation.
_____	_____	_____	4. Use current date.
_____	_____	_____	5. Center letter with even margins.
_____	_____	_____	6. Key inside address.
_____	_____	_____	7. Key appropriate salutation.
_____	_____	_____	8. Compose a friendly letter thanking Dr. Kistler for the referral.
_____	_____	_____	9. Insert proper paragraphing.
_____	_____	_____	10. Key complimentary closing line in correct position.
_____	_____	_____	11. Key signature line.
_____	_____	_____	12. Key reference initials.
_____	_____	_____	13. Proofread letter while the document is on screen or in typewriter for typographical, spelling, punctuation, and capitalization errors.
_____	_____	_____	14. Correct errors.
_____	_____	_____	15. Print letter and proofread again.
_____	_____	_____	16. Present letter ready for physician to read and edit.
_____	_____	_____	17. Incorporate any changes into the letter, print, and present for signature.

JOB SKILL 12-9 (*continued*)

ENVELOPE

_____/8 _____/8 _____/8   18. Key large envelope in OCR format with no errors.

_____ _____ _____   19. Determine the correct postage via the Internet or by calling your local Post Office and write the amount where the stamp would be placed on the envelope.

CERTIFICATION FORM

_____/5 _____/5 _____/5   20. Complete data on front of certification form.

_____/5 _____/5 _____/5   21. Complete data on back of certification form.

_____/5 _____/5 _____/5   22. Complete Receipt for Certified Mail.

_____ _____ _____   23. Fold letter correctly and insert in envelope; do not seal.

_____ _____ _____   Complete within specified time.

____/44 ____/44 ____/44   **Total points earned** (To obtain a percentage score, divide the total points earned by the number of points possible.)

Comments:

C H A P T E R **13**

Fees, Credit, and Collection

OBJECTIVES

After completing the exercises, the student will be able to:

1. Enhance knowledge of medical terminology, interpret abbreviations, and accurately spell medical words.

2. Role-play and discuss how to handle fee collection in various situations.

3. Use a calculator to compute figures on a ledger card.

4. Complete and post on a ledger card.

5. Complete receipts for cash-paying patients.

6. Compose a collection letter, prepare an envelope and ledger, and post transactions.

7. Complete a credit card authorization form.

8. Complete a financial agreement.

FOCUS ON CERTIFICATION*

CMA Content Summary
- Medical abbreviations
- Telephone technique
- Ledgers
- Charges, payments, adjustments
- Collecting and updating demographic data
- Itemized and cycle billing
- Aging accounts receivable
- Collection procedures

RMA Content Summary
- Medical terminology and abbreviations
- Payments and write-off amounts
- Aging reports
- Fee schedules
- Calculate and post payments
- Ledgers and accounts
- Truth in Lending Statements
- Itemized statements and billing methods
- Skip tracing
- Fair Debt Collection Practices Act
- Bankruptcy and small claims procedures
- Collection procedures

*This *Workbook* and accompanying textbook meet the entry-level administrative and general competencies for the CMA outlined by the AAMA Examination Content Outline and Role Delineation Study and for the RMA and CMAS outlined by the AMT Competencies and Examination Specifications (see Competency Grid in textbook Appendix B).

CMAS Content Summary

- Spell medical terms
- Accounts receivable
- Fee structure
- Credit arrangements
- Patient accounts/ledgers
- Billing methods
- Collections

Abbreviation and Spelling Review

Read the following patient's chart note and write the meanings for the abbreviations listed below the note. To decode any abbreviations you do not understand or that appear unfamiliar to you, refer to the list of abbreviations in Part V of this *Workbook*. Step-by-step directions for this exercise are found in Procedure 1-1 of Chapter 1 in the textbook. Medical terms in the chart note are italicized; study them for spelling. Use your medical dictionary to look up their definitions. Your instructor may give a spelling and definition test that includes these words and abbreviations.

3-4-20XX	Robert M Feldman–Pt seen for *bronchial asthma*, ASHD, HBP & *sebaceous cyst*. ECG ordered stat. Lab & x-rays ordered. Comp PX to be done on Friday. PTR next wk. for I & D of *sebaceous cyst* of Ⓡ *axilla*.
	Fran Practon, MD

Pt   _____   Comp   _____

ASHD   _____   PX   _____

HBP   _____   PTR   _____

ECG   _____   wk.   _____

stat.   _____   I&D   _____

lab   _____   Ⓡ   _____

Review Questions

Review the objectives, glossary, and chapter information before completing the following review questions.

1. Match the terms in the right column with the definitions in the left column by writing the letters in the blanks.

   _____ Analysis of accounts receivable showing 30, 60, 90, and 120 days' delinquency   a. garnishment

   _____ A legal proceeding in which money (salary) and property are attached so   b. credit
               they can be used to pay a debt   c. open accounts

   _____ A list of the physician's procedures, services, and fees   d. dun

   _____ A message to remind a patient about delinquent payment   e. skip

   _____ Record of business transactions on the books that represents an unsecured   f. aging account
               accounts receivable where credit has been extended without a formal
               written contract   g. fee schedule

   _____ To trust in an individual's integrity to meet financial obligations

   _____ A debtor who moves and does not leave a forwarding address

2. Name three reasons why a patient registration (information) form is valuable for the collection process.

   a. _____

   b. _____

   c. _____

3. How often should a patient information form be updated? _____

4. The job of discussing and collecting fees is usually relegated to the _____ .

5. Name four factors involved in establishing fees for a physician.

   a. _____

   b. _____

   c. _____

   d. _____

6. For states that allow multiple fee schedules, a medical practice may have separate fee schedules for what type of programs or plans?

   a. _____

   b. _____

   c. _____

   d. _____

7. To increase the percentage of patients who pay their bills and for good public relations, how should a person handle himself or herself when approaching a patient?

   a. _____

   b. _____

   c. _____

   d. _____

   e. _____

8. When is a managed care copayment usually collected? _____

   _____

9. Name several things to look for in a deadbeat patient.

   a. _____

   b. _____

   c. _____

   d. _____

   e. _____

   f. _____

   g. _____

   h. _____

10. When is the best time to collect for an office visit and why? _____

   _____

   _____

11. What are some names used for the form that serves as a combination bill, insurance form, and routing document?

   a. _____

   b. _____

   c. _____

   d. _____

   e. _____

   f. _____

   g. _____

   h. _____

   i. _____

12. Explain cycle billing. _____

   _____

   _____

13. Name four advantages of using a billing service.

   a. _____

   b. _____

   c. _____

   d. _____

14. If a patient is called about a delinquent bill at 10 p.m., what federal law is being violated? _____

   _____

15. If credit is refused to a patient, what federal legislation must be complied with? _____

   _____

16. If, in an obstetrical case, a patient is asked for monthly payments before delivery of the baby, what form must

   be completed, signed, and given to the patient? _____

   If there are fewer than _____ payment installments, this form is not necessary.

17. If interest is charged on a monthly billing statement, what law requires the disclosure of these costs before

   the time of service? _____

   _____

18. Which law states the requirements and limitations for the patient and the medical practice when a complaint

   is registered about a billing statement error? _____

   _____

19. Name the time limit for collection on an open account in your state. _____

20. Explain aging an account and state why it is necessary. _____

   _____

   _____

21. An itemized billing statement is usually sent every _____ days, and when an account becomes delinquent

   a _____ message is sent to prompt payment.

22. What is the average time frame for turning an account over to a collection agency? _____

_____

23. If a physician asks you to file a claim in small-claims court, where would you go to get the form and detailed information about the process? _____

_____

_____

24. Define wage garnishment. _____

_____

25. State where you would file an estate claim and how long you have to file it in your state. _____

_____

27. Name two types of bankruptcy.

    a. _____

    b. _____

✗ Critical Thinking Exercises

1. Mr. Hernandez starts an argument with you about the physician's fee. What would be your response?

_____

_____

_____

_____

2. Dr. Practon expects you to ask patients to pay at the time of their office visits. Mr. Owen passes your desk without stopping after seeing the doctor. What would you say? _____

_____

_____

_____

_____

3. What do you feel are the most important precautions to take in case a patient becomes a *skip* and you have to conduct a *trace*? _____

_____

_____

_____

_____

JOB SKILL 13-1
Role-Play Collection Scenarios

Name _____ Date _____ Score _____

Performance Objective

Task: State how you would handle fee collection in 20 scenarios illustrated in this exercise.

Conditions: Practon Medical Group, Inc., office policy and fee schedule (Part IV of this *Workbook*), two sheets of plain bond paper, pencil or pen, and computer or typewriter.

Standards: Complete all steps listed in this skill in _____ minutes with a minimum score of _____. (Time element and accuracy criteria may be given by instructor.)

Time: **Start:** _____ **Completed:** _____ **Total:** _____ minutes

Scoring: One point for each step performed satisfactorily unless otherwise listed or weighted by instructor.

Directions with Performance Evaluation Checklist

Write how you would handle each of the following collection situations, keeping in mind Practon Medical Group office policies.

1st Attempt	2nd Attempt	3rd Attempt	
_____	_____	_____	Gather materials (equipment and supplies) listed under "Conditions."
____/5	____/5	____/5	1. A new patient, Anne Rule, called for an appointment for Monday morning. It is your office policy to collect the physician's fee at the time of the first visit. Convey this information during your conversation.
____/5	____/5	____/5	2. An established patient, Sylvia Cone, came in on Wednesday for a level IV examination. She calls today and says she is not going to pay the bill because she is not satisfied with the treatment. She says, "Go ahead and send my account to a collection agency. I'll call my attorney. I can make trouble for you and Dr. Practon, too." Prepare your response.
____/5	____/5	____/5	3. Mrs. Katrina Frenzel calls to ask you about the bill she just received for her son, Paul, who recently made his first visit to the office. She thinks the bill for $70.92 is "very high" and wonders if there is a mistake because the fee seems out of line. She says she has recently moved into this area. Prepare your response and state what action you would take.
____/5	____/5	____/5	4. Today you call Miss Wendy Snow about her account, which is overdue. You have sent her two statements, telephoned her, and finally sent a letter asking her to call the office about the $80 she owes. She has not responded. According to your records, she was seen on November 2, she lives at home with her parents, and she has health insurance but has not paid the deductible. Prepare questions you would ask her.
____/5	____/5	____/5	5. Recently, Dr. Gerald Practon performed a two-hour operation and billed the patient his standard fee, which is what physicians generally charge in your region. However, the patient's husband considers the fee exorbitant and has paid only part of it. What action would you take, and how would you collect the outstanding amount?
____/5	____/5	____/5	6. Last week, Dr. Fran Practon made a lengthy long-distance telephone call to check on a postoperative patient who had complicated major surgery. Should you bill the patient for the telephone charges? Explain your answer.
____/5	____/5	____/5	7. Recently, a patient whose account you have turned over to a collection agency meets you in the supermarket and mentions that she will be telephoning for an appointment soon. Before making the appointment, you notify Dr. Practon of this circumstance. He insists she pay what she owes, and requires any future bills be paid in cash. Is this ethical? Explain your answer.

JOB SKILL 13-1 (*continued*)

_____/5 _____/5 _____/5   8. You routinely bill Dr. Practon's patients the amount that appears on the fee schedule he approved. In reviewing a ledger, Dr. Practon finds that a certain patient has been charged more than was intended. The patient makes no complaint and pays the bill in full. What action would you take?

_____/5 _____/5 _____/5   9. Sister Mary Benedict Ramer, a new patient, is seen in consultation. She gives you her insurance card and asks whether she will be given a discount because she is a member of the clergy. How would you respond?

_____/5 _____/5 _____/5   10. Dr. Practon's fee for an appendectomy is $568.36 (*CPT* code 44950). Mr. Jefferson's hospital stay for his appendectomy is unusually troublesome. His first symptoms appeared after midnight, and he was admitted to the hospital as a emergency patient. A decision to operate immediately was postponed by Dr. Practon when the patient began to improve; however, he had several abnormal laboratory results. During the following night, the patient's condition worsened, and the appendectomy was performed, thereby interrupting Dr. Practon's sleep for a second night. After the operation, the patient had a bad case of postanesthesia nausea and was quite demanding while in the hospital. Would Dr. Practon be justified in charging him extra because he was a "lot of trouble?" Explain.

_____/5 _____/5 _____/5   11. You send a bill for $1,500 to Mrs. Jamison for major surgery. She tells you that the physician had told her in a presurgery conversation that the charge would be "about $1,300." Dr. Practon says he does not remember quoting the figure to her. If the usual charge is $1,500 for this procedure, what should you do about the bill? Explain.

_____/5 _____/5 _____/5   12. Mr. French calls in complaining about an overdue refund. He, as well as the insurance company, paid for a procedure, and he is owed a return of his payment. You have been swamped with billing and reply that the statements come first and when you can "get to it" you will mail the refund. What is the proper procedure in this instance? Describe.

_____/5 _____/5 _____/5   13. Patient Joanie Franklin comes in to see Dr. Practon for an initial visit. When asked about insurance coverage, she states, "According to our divorce settlement, my husband's insurance should be billed first." How would you respond?

_____/5 _____/5 _____/5   14. An established patient telephones and says, "The letter I received from the insurance company said you charged too much." How would you respond?

_____/5 _____/5 _____/5   15. New patient Bill Songer comes in to see Dr. Gerald Practon. He says, "My wife handles all the bills, so you will have to call her." How would you reply?

_____/5 _____/5 _____/5   16. An established patient was seen by Dr. Fran Practon and returned the following week to have a treadmill. His insurance was billed; however, the explanation of benefits was sent to the patient denying payment for the treadmill. The patient came in and stated, "My insurance should have covered that service." What questions would you ask and what action would you take?

_____/5 _____/5 _____/5   17. You call patient Mary Edwards regarding an overdue account and reach an answering machine—the patient is not home. What will you do?

_____/5 _____/5 _____/5   18. A patient who has not seen Dr. Practon in a long time comes in for an office visit. Upon leaving, the patient states, "My attorney told me not to pay the bill." What would you say and what question(s) would you ask?

_____/5 _____/5 _____/5   19. A longstanding patient owes over $500, which is now past due. She calls stating, "I have just declared bankruptcy." How would you respond?

_____/5 _____/5 _____/5   20. You are calling Jana Lynn Rose about an overdue account. Her spouse answers the phone and states that the patient is deceased. How would you respond?

JOB SKILL 13-1 *(continued)*

_____ _____ _____   Complete within specified time.

___/102   ___/102   ___/102   **Total points earned** (To obtain a percentage score, divide the total points earned by the number of points possible.)

Comments:

Evaluator's Signature: _____   **Need to Repeat:** _____

National Curriculum Competency: CAAHEP: III.C.3.a(2)(d),	ABHES: VI.B.1.a.2(a), VI.B.1.a.2(b), VI.B.1.a.2(d)
III.C.3.c(1)(b)	VI.B.1.a.2(i), VI.B.1.a.2(k), VI.B.1.a.3(m), VI.B.1.a.7(a),

JOB SKILL 13-2
Use a Calculator

Name _____ Date _____ Score _____

Performance Objective

Task: Compute charges, payments, and adjustments on a ledger card using a calculator and determine a running balance.

Conditions: Use calculator, adding machine, or computer calculator; pen or pencil; and ledger card (Form 49). Refer to Procedure 13-2 and 13-3 in the textbook for step-by-step directions.

Standards: Complete all steps listed in this skill in _____ minutes with a minimum score of _____. (Time element and accuracy criteria may be given by instructor.)

Time: **Start:** _____ **Completed:** _____ **Total:** _____ minutes

Scoring: One point for each step performed satisfactorily unless otherwise listed or weighted by instructor.

Directions with Performance Evaluation Checklist

Using a calculator, practice touch operation by moving your fingers correctly from the home row to other numbered keys as shown in the illustration. Set up a ledger card for the patient, and add charges and subtract payments and adjustments line by line to determine a running balance.

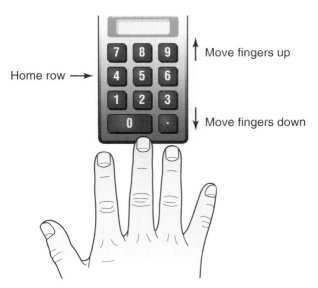

1st Attempt	2nd Attempt	3rd Attempt	
_____	_____	_____	Gather materials (equipment and supplies) listed under "Conditions."
_____/8	_____/8	_____/8	1. Set up ledger card for patient John Dearborn (DOB 9/30/50), 112 South Fifth Street, Woodland Hills, XY 12345; home telephone number: (555) 486-0943; work telephone number: (555) 486-5098; insured with Aetna Casualty, policy no. 12345 AET.
_____/2	_____/2	_____/2	2. Starting from top of ledger card, add the balance forward and the charge from Line 1, and insert the total in the balance column on the right.
_____/2	_____/2	_____/2	3. Add the charge from Line 2, and insert the total in the balance column.
_____/2	_____/2	_____/2	4. Add the charge from Line 3, and insert the total in the balance column.
_____/2	_____/2	_____/2	5. Add the charge from Line 4, and insert the total in the balance column.
_____/2	_____/2	_____/2	6. Add the charge from Line 5, and insert the total in the balance column.

JOB SKILL 13-2 *(continued)*

_____ _____ _____			7. Bring down the balance from Line 5 to Line 6 in the balance column. Rationale: When a line is used for notations only, the balance should always be brought forward to the next line.
____/2 ____/2 ____/2			8. Add the charge from Line 7, and insert the total in the balance column.
____/2 ____/2 ____/2			9. Add the charge from Line 8, and insert the total in the balance column.
____/2 ____/2 ____/2			10. Subtract the payment from Line 9, and insert the total in the balance column.
____/2 ____/2 ____/2			11. Subtract the payment from Line 10, and insert the total in the balance column.
____/2 ____/2 ____/2			12. Subtract the adjustment from Line 11, and insert the total in the balance column.
_____ _____ _____			13. Bring down the balance from Line 11 to Line 12 in the balance column.
____/2 ____/2 ____/2			14. Subtract the payment from Line 13, and insert the total in the balance column.
____/2 ____/2 ____/2			15. Subtract the payment from Line 14, and insert the total in the balance column.
____/2 ____/2 ____/2			16. Subtract the adjustment from Line 15, and insert the total in the balance column.
_____ _____ _____			17. Circle the running balance on the ledger that appears in Line 15 (keep calculator tape when applicable).
_____ _____ _____			Complete within specified time.
___/39 ___/39 ___/39			**Total points earned** (To obtain a percentage score, divide the total points earned by the number of points possible.)

Comments:

Evaluator's Signature: _____   **Need to Repeat:** _____

National Curriculum Competency: CAAHEP: III.C.3.a(2)   ABHES: VI.B.1.a(3)

JOB SKILL 13-3

Complete and Post on a Ledger Card: Charges, Payments, a Returned Check, and a Check from a Collection Agency

Name _____ Date _____ Score _____

Performance Objective

Task: Prepare a ledger card: post charges, payments, a returned check for NSF, and a check from a collection agency, making correct notations and calculating a running balance.

Conditions: Use calculator, adding machine, or computer calculator; pen or pencil; and ledger card (Form 50). Refer to Procedure 13-2 and 13-3 in the textbook for step-by-step directions. See textbook Example 13-3 and Figure 13-4 for posting illustrations. Refer to fee schedule for procedure (*CPT*) codes and mock fees.

Standards: Complete all steps listed in this skill in _____ minutes with a minimum score of _____. (Time element and accuracy criteria may be given by instructor.)

Time: Start: _____ **Completed:** _____ **Total:** _____ minutes

Scoring: One point for each step performed satisfactorily unless otherwise listed or weighted by instructor.

Directions with Performance Evaluation Checklist

Set up a ledger card for the patient. Post entries line by line, adding all charges and subtracting all payments and adjustments to determine a running balance.

1st Attempt	2nd Attempt	3rd Attempt	
			Gather materials (equipment and supplies) listed under "Conditions."
____8	____/8	____/8	1. Set up ledger card for established patient Helen Rice (DOB 1/17/58), 212 Hemmingway Road, Woodland Hills, XY 12345; home telephone number: (555) 486-7721; work telephone number: (555) 486-3333; insured with QRS Insurance Company, policy no. QRS 212345-678.
_____	_____	_____	2. Enter balance forward of $360.00.
____/5	____/5	____/5	3. Enter charge for a Level IV office visit on 3/16/XX with proper reference and description; compute a running balance.
____/4	____/4	____/4	4. Enter notation that the insurance company was billed on 3/17/XX for these services.
____/5	____/5	____/5	5. Post patient payment (check #987) on 3/20/XX in the amount of $360 for amount owed.
____/5	____/5	____/5	6. The bank called stating check #987 is being returned for non-sufficient funds (NSF). Post a reversal of the payment and calculate a new running balance. Patient was called and asked to bring in cash or money order within 3 days.
____/5	____/5	____/5	7. On 3/30/XX, you received notification from insurance company that the patient no longer has insurance coverage. Bill patient for entire balance and make notation on ledger; bring down running balance.
____/5	____/5	____/5	8. On 4/30/XX, you sent second statement to patient indicating "Account is overdue, please play balance." Make entry on ledger and bring down running balance.
____/5	____/5	____/5	9. On 5/30/XX, you sent third statement to patient indicating, "If payment is not received in five days, your account will be sent to a collection agency."
____/3	____/3	____/3	10. On 6/5/XX, you sent account to Collect 4U Agency. Make notation on ledger; adjust entire balance (subtract it from the running balance), circle it, and post a zero balance.

JOB SKILL 13-3 *(continued)*

_____/6   _____/6   _____/6   12. On 7/15/XX, patient paid collection agency $200. Agency sent check #9876543 to the office. Post agency check on patient's ledger, reverse the adjustment by $200, and indicate account closed.

_____   _____   _____   Complete within specified time.

_____/54   _____/54   _____/54   **Total points earned** (To obtain a percentage score, divide the total points earned by the number of points possible.)

Comments:

Evaluator's Signature: _____ **Need to Repeat:** _____

National Curriculum Competency: CAAHEP: III.C.3.a(2)(e), III.C.3.a(2)(h), III.C.3.a(2)(i)	ABHES: VI.B.1.a.3(p), VI.B.1.a.3(s), VI.B.1.a.3(t)

JOB SKILL 13-4
Complete Cash Receipts

Name _____ Date _____ Score _____

Performance Objective

Task: Complete four cash receipt forms.

Conditions: Use one sheet of cash receipts (Form 51), photocopy machine, and pen. Refer to the Fee Schedule in Part IV and Abbreviations (Tables 7-1 and 15-2) in Part V of this *Workbook*.

Standards: Complete all steps listed in this skill in _____ minutes with a minimum score of _____. (Time element and accuracy criteria may be given by instructor.)

Time: Start: _____ Completed: _____ Total: _____ minutes

Scoring: One point for each step performed satisfactorily unless otherwise listed or weighted by instructor.

Directions with Performance Evaluation Checklist

The following patients have paid in full for professional services. Post all entries and make a copy of each receipt for Dr. Practon's file (which you can keep for your records). Give the original receipts to the instructor for grading; these originals in a real situation would be given to the patient for his or her records.

1st Attempt	2nd Attempt	3rd Attempt	
_____	_____	_____	Gather materials (equipment and supplies) listed under "Conditions."
_____	_____	_____	1. Use February 16 of the current year as the date of service and posting date.
_____	_____	_____	2. Refer to the number in the bottom right corner of the receipt to use for the "reference" column.
____/3	____/3	____/3	3. The first patient is established and had a Level I office visit and therapeutic estrogen injection. Charge separately for the administration of the injection (intramuscular) and the drug (supply). Use correct abbreviations to list the description.
____/2	____/2	____/2	4. Post the charges and add to the previous balance, list payments or adjustments and subtract from the previous balance, then calculate and post current balance. The first patient had no previous balance.
_____	_____	_____	5. The first patient is Ms. Beth T. Hobson; record the last name first.
_____	_____	_____	6. Indicate in "Other" area if the payment is by cash, or list check and check number.
____/10	____/10	____/10	7. Follow steps 2 through 7, post and produce a cash receipt for new patient Henry P. Morgan. He had a Level IV examination and paid in cash.
____/10	____/10	____/10	8. Follow steps 2 through 7 to post and produce a cash receipt for a Level II office consultation for Mrs. Harriet F. Garber. She paid in cash.
____/10	____/10	____/10	9. Follow steps 2 through 7 to post and produce a cash receipt for established patient Miss Carole V. Putnam. She had a Level III office visit and a 2-view x-ray of her right wrist. Previous balance $50; paid for services with check no. 4706.
_____	_____	_____	Complete within specified time.
____/41	____/41	____/41	**Total points earned** (To obtain a percentage score, divide the total points earned by the number of points possible.)

JOB SKILL 13-4 *(continued)*

Comments:

JOB SKILL 13-5
Compose a Collection Letter, Prepare an Envelope and Ledger; Post Transactions

Name _____ Date _____ Score _____

Performance Objective

Task: Compose a collection letter, address an envelope, and complete a ledger card. Make notations on the ledger and make a photocopy of the letter and ledger.

Conditions: One letterhead (Form 52), one number 10 envelope (Form 53), and one ledger card (Form 54). Refer to step-by-step directions in Chapter 11 of the textbook (Procedure 11-2) for written correspondence and Chapter 13 (Procedure 13-3) for ledger card posting. Refer to Chapter 12 in the textbook (Figure 12-6) for illustration of a business envelope.

Standards: Complete all steps listed in this skill in _____ minutes with a minimum score of _____. (Time element and accuracy criteria may be given by instructor.)

Time: Start: _____ **Completed:** _____ **Total:** _____ minutes

Scoring: One point for each step performed satisfactorily unless otherwise listed or weighted by instructor.

Directions with Performance Evaluation Checklist

1st Attempt	2nd Attempt	3rd Attempt	
_____	_____	_____	Gather materials (equipment and supplies) listed under "Conditions."

Ledger

1st Attempt	2nd Attempt	3rd Attempt	
____/8	____/8	____/8	1. Prepare a ledger card for Mrs. Mae Van Alystine (DOB 4/12/56) of 2381 Maple Street, Woodland Hills, XY 12345; home telephone (555) 421-8700. She is insured with Mutual Insurance Company, policy number J148, and employed by TBC Import Company, work telephone number (555) 421-0707.
____/10	____/10	____/10	2. On July 10, current year, she was a new patient and had a 30-minute office visit (Level III) and an intrauterine device inserted (58300). Post both charges, listing *CPT* code numbers in the "reference" column, and calculate a running balance.
____/4	____/4	____/4	3. Indicate on the ledger that the insurance company was billed on the same day services were rendered; bring forward the balance owed.
____/4	____/4	____/4	4. On July 25 the insurance company denied payment because the visit was for a contraceptive device. Indicate that the patient was billed on the ledger card.
____/4	____/4	____/4	5. The patient was billed a second time on August 25; indicate this on the ledger card and bring forward the balance owed.
____/4	____/4	____/4	6. The patient was billed a third time on September 25; indicate this on the ledger card and bring forward the balance owed.
____/4	____/4	____/4	7. Compose a rough draft of a collection letter (letter #1) to be sent on October 25 with a copy of the ledger (statement); indicate this on the ledger card, and bring forward the balance owed.

Letter

1st Attempt	2nd Attempt	3rd Attempt	
____/8	____/8	____/8	8. Use letterhead to produce a collection letter, centered on page with full block style; even and equal margins; consistent punctuation; and appropriate paragraphing, capitalization, and abbreviations.
_____	_____	_____	9. Date letter October 25 of current year.
____/3	____/3	____/3	10. Use proper address format for inside address.

JOB SKILL 13-5 (continued)

_____	_____	_____	11. Place salutation identifying person to whom the letter is being written.
_____	_____	_____	12. Include reference line indicating date of service and charges.
____/5	____/5	____/5	13. In body of letter, state reason for letter and indicate expected response.
____/2	____/2	____/2	14. Place complimentary close and signature line.
_____	_____	_____	15. Insert proper enclosure notation.
_____	_____	_____	16. Proofread for spelling and typographical errors while letter remains on computer screen or in typewriter.
_____	_____	_____	17. Make corrections, proof again, and prepare final copy for signature.

Envelope

____/5	____/5	____/5	18. Prepare envelope using the U.S. Postal Service's approved format.
_____	_____	_____	19. Copy letter, ledger card, and envelope.
_____	_____	_____	20. Attach original letter and ledger card to envelope.
_____	_____	_____	Complete within specified time.
___/71	___/71	___/71	**Total points earned** (To obtain a percentage score, divide the total points earned by the number of points possible.)

Comments:

Evaluator's Signature: _____ **Need to Repeat:** _____

National Curriculum Competency: CAAHEP: III.C.3.a(1), III.C.3.c(1)(a)	ABHES: VI.B.1.a.2(j), VI.B.1.a.2(o), VI.B.1.a.3(a)

JOB SKILL 13-6
Complete a Credit Card Authorization Form

Name _____ Date _____ Score _____

Performance Objective

Task: Fill in authorization form with correct information to charge credit card.

Conditions: Authorization to charge credit card (Form 55) and pen or pencil. Refer to textbook Figure 13-7 for a visual example.

Standards: Complete all steps listed in this skill in _____ minutes with a minimum score of _____. (Time element and accuracy criteria may be given by instructor.)

Time: Start: _____ Completed: _____ Total: _____ minutes

Scoring: One point for each step performed satisfactorily unless otherwise listed or weighted by instructor.

Directions with Performance Evaluation Checklist

It is May 15 of the current year, and you are called to the reception area of Dr. Fran Practon's office because a patient has come in and has a large unpaid balance. It is up to you to discuss the situation with him and come to an agreement on how the account can be paid. After having a discussion, the patient agrees to use his credit card and make monthly payments until the account is paid in full.

1st Attempt	2nd Attempt	3rd Attempt	
_____	_____	_____	Gather materials (equipment and supplies) listed under "Conditions."
_____/2	_____/2	_____/2	1. Fill in the patient's name, Mr. Stewart T. Wilson; he is the cardholder.
_____/2	_____/2	_____/2	2. Mr. Wilson will be using his Visa credit card, account number 4444-2222-8888-777, expiration date August, 2011.
_____/3	_____/3	_____/3	3. Mr. Wilson agrees to make monthly payments of $100 on the 15th of each month; his balance is $800.
_____/2	_____/2	_____/2	4. Have the patient sign and date the form.
_____	_____	_____	Complete within specified time.
_____/11	_____/11	_____/11	**Total points earned** (To obtain a percentage score, divide the total points earned by the number of points possible.)

Comments:

Evaluator's Signature: _____ **Need to Repeat:** _____

National Curriculum Competency: CAAHEP: III.C.3.a(2)(d)   ABHES: VI.B.1.a.3(m)

JOB SKILL 13-7
Complete a Financial Agreement

Name _____ Date _____ Score _____

Performance Objective

Task: Fill in a financial agreement with a schedule of payments.

Conditions: Financial Agreement (Form 56), calculator, and pen or pencil. Refer in the textbook to Figure 13-8 for a visual example and Procedure 13-5 for step-by-step directions.

Standards: Complete all steps listed in this skill in _____ minutes with a minimum score of _____. (Time element and accuracy criteria may be given by instructor.)

Time: Start: _____ Completed: _____ Total: _____ minutes

Scoring: One point for each step performed satisfactorily unless otherwise listed or weighted by instructor.

Directions with Performance Evaluation Checklist

Mr. Biederman has received an itemization of all charges that are now overdue. He has no insurance and has agreed to a payment plan; there will be no financial charge.

1st Attempt	2nd Attempt	3rd Attempt	
_____	_____	_____	Gather materials (equipment and supplies) listed under "Conditions."
_____/2	_____/2	_____/2	1. Enter patient's name, Alan Biederman, and telephone number, (555) 486-9093, on the financial agreement form.
_____/9	_____/9	_____/9	2. Mr. Biederman has incurred $3,000 for medical services with Dr. Gerald Practon and has agreed to pay $600 as a down payment. Determine the unpaid balance and fill in Sections 1 through 9 on the agreement form.
_____/8	_____/8	_____/8	3. Mr. Biederman agrees to pay $200 on the first of every month starting August 1 (current year). Calculate the amount and number of monthly payments and fill in the lower section of the form.
_____	_____	_____	4. Have Mr. Biederman sign and date the form; it is July 1 (current year).
_____/3	_____/3	_____/3	5. On the Schedule of Payment, fill in the total amount owed, the down payment (DP), and the balance owed in the top right portion of the form.
_____/24	_____/24	_____/24	6. Complete the Schedule of Payment by filling in all dates and the amount of each installment payment.
_____	_____	_____	7. Present the form to Dr. Practon for his signature.
_____	_____	_____	Complete within specified time.
_____/50	_____/50	_____/50	**Total points earned** (To obtain a percentage score, divide the total points earned by the number of points possible.)

JOB SKILL 13-7 *(continued)*

Comments:

CHAPTER 14

Banking

OBJECTIVES

After completing the exercises, the student will be able to:

1. Enhance knowledge of medical terminology, interpret abbreviations, and accurately spell medical words.

2. Prepare a bank deposit.

3. Write checks.

4. Endorse a check.

5. Inspect a check.

6. Post payment to a ledger.

7. Post entries to ledger cards and calculate balances.

8. Reconcile a bank statement.

FOCUS ON CERTIFICATION*

CMA Content Summary
- Medical abbreviations
- Banking procedures
- Process accounts receivable
- Preparing bank deposit
- Electronic banking
- Reconciling bank statement
- Maintaining financial records

RMA Content Summary
- Medical terminology and abbreviations
- Collect and post payments
- Patient ledgers and accounts
- Bank deposits
- Checking accounts
- Reconcile bank statements
- Understand check processing procedures
- Process payables and maintain disbursement records
- Perform account calculations

*This *Workbook* and accompanying textbook meet the entry-level administrative and general competencies for the CMA outlined by the AAMA Examination Content Outline and Role Delineation Study and for the RMA and CMAS outlined by the AMT Competencies and Examination Specifications (see Competency Grid in textbook Appendix B).

CMAS Content Summary

- Spell medical terms
- Financial computations
- Accounts payable
- Accounts receivable
- Patient accounts/ledgers
- Banking services and procedures

Abbreviation and Spelling Review

Read the following patient's chart note and write the meanings for the abbreviations listed below the note. To decode any abbreviations you do not understand or that appear unfamiliar to you, refer to the list of abbreviations in Part V of this *Workbook*. Step-by-step directions for this exercise are found in Procedure 1-1 of Chapter 1 in the textbook. Medical terms in the chart note are italicized; study them for spelling. Use your medical dictionary to look up their definitions. Your instructor may give a spelling and definition test that includes these words and abbreviations.

Etta Chan

June 22, 20XX Pt was born with *cystic hydromas* and has had *epileptic seizures* without *vomiting* or *dyspnea*. Pt is on *Dilantin*. Pt is to be started on *phenobarbital* 100 mg t.i.d. i.e., 2 mg/kg per day. Ordered CT scan.

Gerald Practon, MD

Gerald Practon, MD

Pt _____   i.e. _____

mg _____   kg _____

t.i.d. _____   CT _____

Note: i.e. is a Latin abbreviation and may be found in an English dictionary.

Review Questions

Review the objectives, glossary, and chapter information before completing the following review questions.

1. Match the terms in the left column with the definitions in the right column by writing the letters in the blanks.

    _____ debit   a. A check stub

    _____ payee   b. Deposit or addition to a bank account

    _____ voucher   c. The person signing a check to pay out funds from a checking account

    _____ ABA number   d. Withdrawal or subtraction from a bank account

    _____ payer   e. A fee assessed by a bank for processing transactions

    _____credit   f. The person named on a check as the recipient of the amount shown

                             g. Bank or transit number

2. Write the meanings of these abbreviations.

    a. NSF _____

    b. EFTS _____

    c. POS _____

    d. MICR _____

    e. ATM _____

3. Name the most common types of checking accounts.

   a. _____

   b. _____

4. Answer the following questions regarding inspecting a check presented for payment in a physician's office.

   a. What identification should be requested? _____

   _____

   b. What should you do if a patient presents an out-of-state check? _____

   _____

   c. What do you compare the information on the check to when verifying it? _____

   _____

5. What does ABA stand for and what is it used for? _____

   _____

   _____

   _____

6. What is the federal act that grants usage of electronic checks? _____

   _____

7. When calling the bank to use a pay-by-phone system, you would say, "I would like an _____

   _____ ."

8. The following check endorsements are either blank, restrictive, or full. Note next to each statement the type of endorsement.

   a. For deposit only
      Jane Garner _____

   b. Ronald P. Yeager _____

   c. Pay to the order of
      Stationer's Corporation
      Betty T. White
      Harold M. Jeffers _____

9. When accepting a check or making a deposit, how can you tell if the check is from a newly established checking account? _____

   _____

   _____

10. ATMs are open _____ hours a day and _____ days a week; a _____ card is used for transactions.

11. Explain what procedures you should follow if an error is made in writing or typing a check. _____

    _____

    _____

12. Name three options you have when a check is missing the payer's signature.

    a. _____

    b. _____

    c. _____

13. In reconciling the monthly bank statement, indicate whether to *add* or *subtract* the following from (1) the balance appearing on the bank statement, or (2) the balance in the checkbook.

    a. outstanding checks   _____

    b. bank service charges   _____

    c. deposits not shown on the bank statement   _____

14. In adjusting the checkbook balance to obtain a reconciliation with the bank statement, what debits, besides checks, might you list and subtract from the checkbook balance?

    a. _____

    b. _____

    c. _____

15. What number should be used to divide the amount of the difference by to find out if a transposition error has been made on the check stub register? _____

    _____

Critical Thinking Exercises

1. Compare electronic banking and traditional banking methods and summarize the differences between them.

    Features of electronic banking:

    a. _____

    b. _____

    c. _____

    d. _____

    Features of traditional banking:

    a. _____

    b. _____

2. State why you would choose to bank using either electronic banking or traditional banking.

    _____

    _____

    _____

    _____

JOB SKILL 14-1
Prepare a Bank Deposit

Name _____ Date _____ Score _____

Performance Objective

Task: Record checks on a bank deposit slip and calculate total.

Conditions: Use deposit slip (Form 57) and pen or pencil. Refer to textbook Figure 14-3 for a visual example and textbook Procedure 14-1 for step-by-step directions.

Standards: Complete all steps listed in this skill in _____ minutes with a minimum score of _____. (Time element and accuracy criteria may be given by instructor.)

Time: **Start:** _____ **Completed:** _____ **Total:** _____ minutes

Scoring: One point for each step performed satisfactorily unless otherwise listed or weighted by instructor.

Directions with Performance Evaluation Checklist

You open today's mail and find six checks patients have sent to Practon Medical Group, Inc., to pay on their accounts. Record each check on a bank deposit slip, and date and calculate the amount for deposit.

Keith Austin
7637 Concord Circle
Woodland Hills, XY 12345

16-21/1220   6335

Date *March 24, 20xx*

Pay to the order of *Gerald Practon, MD* $ 36.92

Thirty six and 92/100 _____ Dollars

Santa Paula Interstate Bank

Memo *insurance balance*   *Keith Austin*

Hope Wilburn
PO BOX 309
Woodland Hills, XY 12345

55-60/3222   1226

Date *March 26, 20xx*

Pay to the order of *Fran Practon, MD* $ 250.00

Two hundred and fifty dollars and no/100 _____ Dollars

Woodland Hills CITI Bank

Memo *April payment installment*   *Hope Wilburn*

Figure 14-1

JOB SKILL 14-1 (*continued*)

Richard Rickman
444 Platte Place
Woodland Hills, XY 12345

154-20/440   410

Date *March 25, 20xx*

Pay to the
order of   *Practon Medical Group* $ *15.00*

Fifteen and no/100 ———————————————— Dollars

County Bank

Memo *Copay*   *R. Rickman*

Houshang Hutton
8989 Telegraph Rd
Woodland Hills, XY 12345

90-8030/2000   1229

Date *March 26, 20xx*

Pay to the
order of   *Practon Medical Group, Inc.* $ *70.65*

Seventy dollars and 65/100 ———————————— Dollars

Westlake Bank & Trust

Memo *Noncovered services*   *Houshang Hutton*

Carla M. Gafford
613 Redwood Avenue
Woodland Hills, XY 12345

90-4268/1222   4851

Date *March 25, 20xx*

Pay to the
order of   *Gerald Practon, MD* $ *500.00*

Five hundred and no/100 ———————————— Dollars

Intercommercial Bank

Memo *Outpatient surgery deductible*   *Carla Gafford*

Figure 14-1 (*continued*)

JOB SKILL 14-1 (continued)

Dick and Angie Hundley
109 Linden Drive
Woodland Hills, XY 12345

16-24/1220

8203

Date March 26, 20xx

Pay to the order of Dr. Fran Practon

$ 124.00

One hundred and twenty four dollars and no/100 ——————— Dollars

Hillcrest Bank & Mortgage

Memo Medicare deductible

Angie Hundley

Figure 14-1 (continued)

1st Attempt	2nd Attempt	3rd Attempt	
_____	_____	_____	Gather materials (equipment and supplies) listed under "Conditions."
_____	_____	_____	1. Enter the date on the front of the deposit slip; use March 28 (current year).
_____/2	_____/2	_____/2	2. Enter the first check from Keith Austin on the back of the deposit slip, recording the bank number on the left and the amount on the right.
_____/2	_____/2	_____/2	3. Enter the check from Hope Wilburn.
_____/2	_____/2	_____/2	4. Enter the check from Richard Rickman.
_____/2	_____/2	_____/2	5. Enter the check from Houshang Hutton.
_____/2	_____/2	_____/2	6. Enter the check for Carla Gafford.
_____/2	_____/2	_____/2	7. Enter the check for Angie Hundley.
_____	_____	_____	8. Total the amounts from all checks and record.
_____	_____	_____	9. Total the check amounts written on the deposit slip and compare with the total of all checks. If it matches, write the total on the back of the deposit slip.
_____	_____	_____	10. Enter total of all checks from the reverse side on the front of the deposit slip.
_____	_____	_____	11. Enter the subtotal.
_____	_____	_____	12. Enter the total of the deposit, referred to as "net deposit."
_____	_____	_____	Complete within specified time.
_____/20	_____/20	_____/20	**Total points earned** (To obtain a percentage score, divide the total points earned by the number of points possible.)

JOB SKILL 14-1 *(continued)*

Comments:

JOB SKILL 14-2
Write Checks

Name _____ Date _____ Score _____

Performance Objective

Task: Handwrite or type two checks.

Conditions: Use two blank checks and two invoices (Form 58) and pen. Refer to Job Skill 14-2 in the textbook for step-by-step directions and textbook Figures 15-1 and 15-4 for visual illustrations.

Standards: Complete all steps listed in this skill in _____ minutes with a minimum score of _____. (Time element and accuracy criteria may be given by instructor.)

Time: Start: _____ Completed: _____ Total: _____ minutes

Scoring: One point for each step performed satisfactorily unless otherwise listed or weighted by instructor.

Directions with Performance Evaluation Checklist

You have received two invoices for the Practon Medical Group. Handwrite or type two checks for Dr. Practon's signature to pay these bills.

1st Attempt	2nd Attempt	3rd Attempt	
_____	_____	_____	Gather materials (equipment and supplies) listed under "Conditions."
_____	_____	_____	1. Date the first check (No. 485) May 27 of the current year.
____/3	____/3	____/3	2. Make the check payable to Stationer's Corporation; include the company's address.
____/3	____/3	____/3	3. Make the check payable for the amount due indicated on the invoice.
____/3	____/3	____/3	4. Insert the balance forward from the checkbook on the check stub; the amount is $9,825.55.
____/3	____/3	____/3	5. Note the date, what the check is for, and the amount on the check stub.
_____	_____	_____	6. Calculate a new balance and record.
____/3	____/3	____/3	7. Bring the balance forward to the next check, No. 486.
_____	_____	_____	8. Date check No. 486 March 28 of the current year.
____/3	____/3	____/3	9. Make the check payable to Randolph Electrical Supply; include the company's address.
____/3	____/3	____/3	10. Make the check payable for the amount due indicated on the invoice.
____/3	____/3	____/3	11. Note the date, what the check is for, and the amount on the check stub.
_____	_____	_____	12. Calculate a new balance and record.
____/6	____/6	____/6	13. Record the date paid, check number, and amount paid on each invoice.
_____	_____	_____	Complete within specified time.
____/36	____/36	____/36	**Total points earned** (To obtain a percentage score, divide the total points earned by the number of points possible.)

JOB SKILL 14-2 *(continued)*

Comments:

JOB SKILL 14-3
Endorse a Check

Name ______________________________ Date ______________ Score ________

Performance Objective

Task: Enter a restrictive endorsement on a check in the proper location.

Conditions: Use the check from patient Jeffrey Brown shown in *Workbook* Figures 14-2 A and B and pen. Refer to chapter material and Figure 14-2 in the textbook.

Standards: Complete all steps listed in this skill in ________ minutes with a minimum score of ________. (Time element and accuracy criteria may be given by instructor.)

Time: **Start:** ____________ **Completed:** ____________ **Total:** ____________ minutes

Scoring: One point for each step performed satisfactorily unless otherwise listed or weighted by instructor.

Directions with Performance Evaluation Checklist

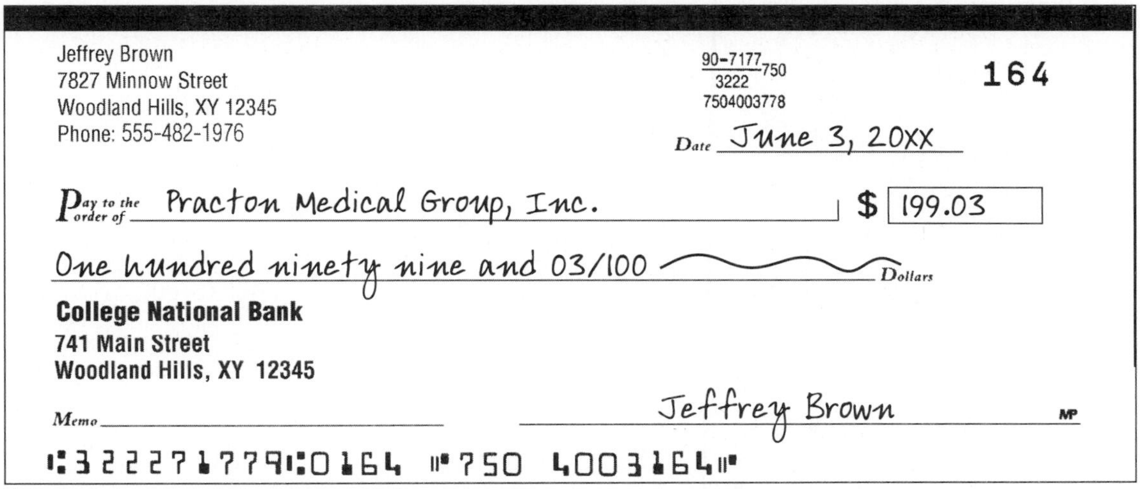
Jeffrey Brown
7827 Minnow Street
Woodland Hills, XY 12345
Phone: 555-482-1976

90-7177/3222 750
7504003778

164

Date June 3, 20XX

Pay to the order of Practon Medical Group, Inc. $ 199.03

One hundred ninety nine and 03/100 Dollars

College National Bank
741 Main Street
Woodland Hills, XY 12345

Memo ______ Jeffrey Brown MP

⑆322271779⑆0164 ⑈750 4003164⑈

Figure 14-2A

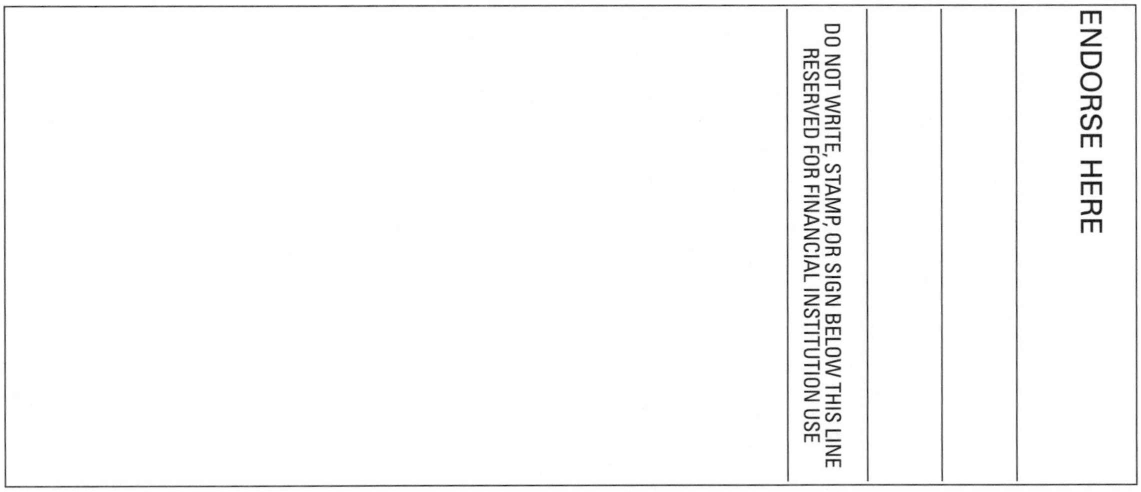
ENDORSE HERE

DO NOT WRITE, STAMP, OR SIGN BELOW THIS LINE
RESERVED FOR FINANCIAL INSTITUTION USE

Figure 14-2B

JOB SKILL 14-3 *(continued)*

1st Attempt	2nd Attempt	3rd Attempt	
_____	_____	_____	Gather materials (equipment and supplies) listed under "Conditions."
___/4	___/4	___/4	1. Enter correct wording for a restrictive endorsement.
_____	_____	_____	2. Place restrictive endorsement in proper location.
_____	_____	_____	Complete within specified time.
___/7	___/7	___/7	**Total points earned** (To obtain a percentage score, divide the total points earned by the number of points possible.)

Comments:

Evaluator's Signature: _____ **Need to Repeat:** _____

JOB SKILL 14-4
Inspect a Check

Name _____ Date _____ Score _____

Performance Objective

Task:　　　　Inspect a check and answer questions.

Conditions:　Use information given for the case, pen or pencil, and illustration of a handwritten check (*Workbook* Figure 14-3).

Standards:　Complete all steps listed in this skill in _____ minutes with a minimum score of _____.
(Time element and accuracy criteria may be given by instructor.)

Time:　　　**Start:** _____ **Completed:** _____ **Total:** _____ minutes

Scoring:　　One point for each step performed satisfactorily unless otherwise listed or weighted by instructor.

Directions with Performance Evaluation Checklist

As you learned after reading Chapter 14 in the textbook, a handwritten check has certain requirements that must be met to be valid. An established patient, Rita Stevens, wrote a check for a Level III office visit totaling $40.20 before leaving the office on May 21, 20XX. Inspect the check and answer the following questions.

RITA STEVENS
126 Sunset Lane
Woodland Hills, XY 12345

$\frac{90-7177}{3222}$750
7504003778

164

Date May 25, 20XX

Pay to the order of Practon Medical Group, Inc.　　　$ 40.00

Forty and 20/100　　　*Dollars*

College National Bank
741 Main Street
Woodland Hills, XY 12345

Memo Level III OV　　　Rita Stevens　　　**MP**

⑈3222717979⑈0164 ⑈⑈750 4003778⑈⑈

Figure 14-3

1st Attempt	2nd Attempt	3rd Attempt	
_____	_____	_____	Gather materials (equipment and supplies) listed under "Conditions."
_____/2	_____/2	_____/2	1. What two personal identification items should be obtained from the patient before accepting a check? _____ _____
_____/2	_____/2	_____/2	2. Does the check list the complete name, address and telephone number of the patient? _____ If not, what is missing? _____ _____
_____/2	_____/2	_____/2	3. Is the check dated correctly? _____ If not, what is the problem? _____
_____	_____	_____	4. Is the check made out to the proper payee? _____
_____	_____	_____	5. Did Mrs. Stevens make the check out for the proper amount? _____

JOB SKILL 14-4 *(continued)*

_____/2   _____/2   _____/2   6. If not, what is the problem? _____

_____

_____   _____   _____   7. How much will Dr. Practon receive? _____

_____   _____   _____   8. Is the check signed? _____

_____   _____   _____   Complete within specified time.

___/14   ___/14   ___/14   **Total points earned** (To obtain a percentage score, divide the total points earned by the number of points possible.)

Comments:

JOB SKILL 14-5
Post a Payment to a Ledger

Name _____ Date _____ Score _____

Performance Objective

Task: Post a payment received by check to a patient's ledger card.

Conditions: Use the check received from patient Jeffrey Brown in *Workbook* Job Skill 14-3 (see *Workbook* Figure 14-1A), ledger card (*Workbook* Figure 14-4), and pen.

Standards: Complete all steps listed in this skill in _____ minutes with a minimum score of _____. (Time element and accuracy criteria may be given by instructor.)

Time: Start: _____ Completed: _____ Total: _____ minutes

Scoring: One point for each step performed satisfactorily unless otherwise listed or weighted by instructor.

Directions with Performance Evaluation Checklist

1st Attempt	2nd Attempt	3rd Attempt	
_____	_____	_____	Gather materials (equipment and supplies) listed under "Conditions."
_____	_____	_____	1. Post the payment using the same date the check was written.
_____	_____	_____	2. Record the check number in the reference column.
_____	_____	_____	3. Use correct abbreviations to describe the payment received on the account.
_____	_____	_____	4. Post the payment in the correct column.
_____	_____	_____	5. Calculate the correct balance and record it in the balance column.
_____	_____	_____	Complete within specified time.
___/7	___/7	___/7	**Total points earned** (To obtain a percentage score, divide the total points earned by the number of points possible.)

Comments:

Evaluator's Signature: _____ **Need to Repeat:** _____

National Curriculum Competency: CAAHEP: III.C.3.a(2)   ABHES: VI.B.1.a.(3)

JOB SKILL 14-5 (*continued*)

STATEMENT

PRACTON MEDICAL GROUP, INC.
4567 Broad Avenue
Woodland Hills, XY 12345-4700
Tel. 555-486-9002
Fax No. 555-488-7815

Mr. Jeffery Brown
230 Main Street
Woodland Hills, XY 12345-0001

DATE	REFERENCE	DESCRIPTION	CHARGES	CREDITS PYMNTS.	ADJ.	BALANCE
1-9-20XX		BALANCE FORWARD ➝				20 00
1-9-20XX	99213	Level III OV	36 80			56 80
1-10-20XX	1-9-20XX	Medicare billed				56 80
3-5-20XX	1-9-20XX	Medicare pmt		24 99		27 36
4-3-20XX	47600	Cholecystectomy	858 35			885 71
4-5-20XX	4-3-20XX	Medicare billed				885 71
6-2-20XX	4-3-20XX	Medicare pmt		686 68		199 03
———	MEDICARE HAS PAID THEIR PORTION OF THIS CLAIM. THE					199 03
———	BALANCE IS YOUR RESPONSIBILITY. PLEASE REMIT.					199 03

RB40BC-2-96

PLEASE PAY LAST AMOUNT IN BALANCE COLUMN ➝

THIS IS A COPY OF YOUR ACCOUNT AS IT APPEARS ON OUR RECORDS

Figure 14-4

JOB SKILL 14-6
Post Entries to Ledger Cards and Calculate Balances

Name _____ Date _____ Score _____

Performance Objective

Task: Post entries to patients' ledger cards and calculate running balances.

Conditions: Use pen or pencil and five ledger cards (*Workbook* Figures 14-5 through 14-9). Refer to the mock Fee Schedule in Part IV of this *Workbook* for procedure codes and charges (find under section titles, i.e., Evaluation and Management for office visits, Pathology and Laboratory for lab tests, and Maternity Care and Delivery for OB care). Refer to Procedure 13-3 in the textbook for step-by-step directions.

Standards: Complete all steps listed in this skill in _____ minutes with a minimum score of _____. (Time element and accuracy criteria may be given by instructor.)

Time: Start: _____ **Completed:** _____ **Total:** _____ minutes

Scoring: One point for each step performed satisfactorily unless otherwise listed or weighted by instructor.

Directions with Performance Evaluation Checklist

Complete the following ledger cards, using the current date to post all transactions.

1. Elizabeth Hooper

DATE	REFERENCE	DESCRIPTION	CHARGES	CREDITS			BALANCE	
				pymnts		Adj		
		BALANCE FORWARD						
6-1-20XX	99203	OV Level III NP	70	92				
6-1-20XX	99000	Handling Pap	5	00				
8-15-20XX	ck# 778	ROA ABC Ins.			69	00		

Figure 14-5

2. Maria Sanchez

DATE	REFERENCE	DESCRIPTION	CHARGES	CREDITS			BALANCE	
				pymnts		Adj		
		BALANCE FORWARD						
7-6-20XX	99244	Consult Level IV	145	05				
7-20-20XX	ck# 432	ROA Pt			25	00		
8-15-20XX	ck# 451	ROA Pt			50	00		
9-18-20XX	ck# 463	ROA Pt			25	00		

Figure 14-6

JOB SKILL 14-6 (*continued*)

3. Brett Walker

DATE	REFERENCE	DESCRIPTION	CHARGES		CREDITS				BALANCE	
					pymnts		Adj			
		BALANCE FORWARD								
7-1-20XX	99203	OV Level III NP	70	92						
7-15-20XX	45308	Proctosigmoidoscopy with removal polyp	135	34						
7-20-20XX	ck 2005	ROA Pt			50	00				
9-1-20XX	Voucher 4006	ROA Blue Cross			165	01				

Figure 14-7

4. Edna Hargrove

DATE	REFERENCE	DESCRIPTION	CHARGES		CREDITS				BALANCE	
					pymnts		Adj			
		BALANCE FORWARD								
8-1-20XX	99213	OV Level III	40	20						
8-1-20XX	58300	IUD insertion	100	00						
8-14-20XX	ck 101	ROA Pt			100	00				

Figure 14-8

5.–9. Beth Jones

DATE	REFERENCE	DESCRIPTION	CHARGES		CREDITS				BALANCE	
					pymnts		Adj			
		BALANCE FORWARD								

Figure 14-9

JOB SKILL 14-6 *(continued)*

1st Attempt	2nd Attempt	3rd Attempt	
_____	_____	_____	Gather materials (equipment and supplies) listed under "Conditions."
____/8	____/8	____/8	1. Elizabeth Hooper has a small uncollected balance due. Dr. Practon said he wishes to write off the balance. Calculate the running balance and post the adjustment entry.
____/4	____/4	____/4	2. Maria Sanchez was in for a consultation and has made several payments on her account. Calculate each posting entry to determine the running balances.
____/9	____/9	____/9	3. Brett Walker paid on his account and his insurance also paid, resulting in an overpayment. The patient is to receive a refund. Calculate the running balances and post the refund (check 2068) to clear the negative balance.
____/14	____/14	____/14	4. Edna Hargrove issued a check for payment toward her last office visit, but it was returned today by ZZZ Bank and marked nonsufficient funds (NSF). Calculate the running balance and post the returned check as well as the $10 bank charge on the ledger card.
____/5	____/5	____/5	5. Beth Jones comes in today for a Level III new patient examination. She is complaining of fatigue, nausea, and dysuria. Post the office visit and calculate the running balance.
____/5	____/5	____/5	6. Dr. Practon feels a laboratory test is needed for Beth (urinalysis, nonautomated without microscopy). Post this service and calculate the running balance.
____/5	____/5	____/5	7. The urinalysis was negative; however, Dr. Practon would like to run a urine pregnancy test. Post this service and calculate a running balance.
____/2	____/2	____/2	8. It is determined that she is pregnant with her first child. The medical assistant discusses maternity care and delivery and advises her of the obstetric fee for a routine vaginal delivery, which includes all antepartum and postpartum visits. The fee is $_____.
____/5	____/5	____/5	9. Her insurance is verified and it is determined that they will pay 85% of Dr. Practon's usual and customary fee for OB care. She pays by check (No. 798) for 15% of the total obstetric fee. Post this payment to her ledger card. Do not post the charge for the OB care; it will be posted at the time of delivery. Her ledger will indicate a negative balance until the obstetric fee is posted.
_____	_____	_____	Complete within specified time.
____/59	____/59	____/59	**Total points earned** (To obtain a percentage score, divide the total points earned by the number of points possible.)

JOB SKILL 14-6 *(continued)*

Comments:

Evaluator's Signature: _____ **Need to Repeat:** _____

| National Curriculum Competency: CAAHEP: III.C.3.a(2)(e), III.C.3.a(2)(f), III.C.3.a(2)(g), III.C.3.a(2)(h) | ABHES: VI.B.1.a.3(p), VI.B.1.a.3(q), VI.B.1.a.3(r), VI.B.1.a.3(s) |

JOB SKILL 14-7
Reconcile a Bank Statement

Name _____ Date _____ Score _____

Performance Objective

Task: Reconcile a bank statement.

Conditions: Use a bank statement (*Workbook* Figure 14-10), pen or pencil, and bank reconciliation worksheet (Form 59). Refer to Procedure 14-3 in the textbook for step-by-step directions.

Standards: Complete all steps listed in this skill in _____ minutes with a minimum score of _____. (Time element and accuracy criteria may be given by instructor.)

Time: **Start:** _____ **Completed:** _____ **Total:** _____ minutes

Scoring: One point for each step performed satisfactorily unless otherwise listed or weighted by instructor.

Directions with Performance Evaluation Checklist

1st Attempt	2nd Attempt	3rd Attempt	
_____	_____	_____	Gather materials (equipment and supplies) listed under "Conditions."
___/10	___/10	___/10	1. You compare and check off each transaction recorded in your checkbook with those listed in this statement and discover the following outstanding checks: No. 318 for $25, No. 337 for $60, No 338 for $78, No. 340 for $15, and No. 341 for $18.20. Record these on the reconciliation form under "Outstanding Checks."
_____	_____	_____	2. Add the total of outstanding checks and record on the reconciliation form.
___/4	___/4	___/4	3. Assume you made deposits of $3,500 on June 30, 20XX, and $1,800 on July 2, 20XX, which do not show on the statement. Record these on the reconciliation form under "Deposits Not Credited."
_____	_____	_____	4. Add the total of deposits not credited and record on the reconciliation form.
_____	_____	_____	5. Enter the ending statement balance on the reconciliation form.
_____	_____	_____	6. Add the total of the deposits not credited to the ending statement balance and record.
_____	_____	_____	7. Subtract the total of the outstanding checks from the figure determined in Step 6 and record.
_____	_____	_____	8. Verify the adjusted total you determined with the checkbook balance, which is $6,807.89
_____	_____	_____	9. Do these figures match and does the checkbook balance? _____ If not, repeat the above steps, recalculating figures.
_____	_____	_____	Complete within specified time.
___/23	___/23	___/23	**Total points earned** (To obtain a percentage score, divide the total points earned by the number of points possible.)

Comments:

Evaluator's Signature: _____ **Need to Repeat:** _____

JOB SKILL 14-7 (*continued*)

COLLEGE NATIONAL BANK
ACCOUNT ACTIVITY

College National Bank
700 West Main Street
Woodland Hills, XY 12345

(800) 540-5060

STATEMENT PERIOD:
FROM: May 17, 20XX
THROUGH June 16, 20XX

PRACTON MEDICAL GROUP, INC   140
4567 BROAD AVENUE
WOODLAND HILLS XY   12345

PAGE	1
ITEM COUNT	30

CHECKING   ACCOUNT 12345-6789

SUMMARY

BEGINNING STATEMENT BALANCE ON 20XX .... $ 633.87

TOTAL OF   4 DEPOSITS/OTHER CREDITS 1414.75

TOTAL OF   15 CHECKS PAID...   271.53
             5 WITHDRAWALS/OTHER CHARGES................................   73.00

ENDING STATEMENT BALANCE ON   20XX 1704.09

CHECKS/ WITHDRAWALS/ OTHER CHARGES

CHECKS:

NUMBER	DATE	AMOUNT	NUMBER	DATE	AMOUNT
0317	06-08	17.40	0328	06-10	29.90
1319	05-25	30.00	0329	05-26	32.05
0320	05-30	7.59	0330	06-02	2.75
0321	05-27	9.00	0331	06-02	30.79
0322	05-24	1.00	0332	06-02	11.47
0323	06-03	6.13			
0324	05-30	1.78			
0325	06-02	67.50			
0326	05-25	21.92			
0327	06-03	2.25			

TOTAL OF 15   CHECKS PAID   271.53

WITHDRAWALS/OTHER CHARGES:

DATE	TRANSACTION DESCRIPTION	AMOUNT
06-10	SURGICAL SUPPLY PAYMENT AT ELECTRONIC BANKING	34.30
06-07	STAR FREE PRESS PAYMENT AT ELECTRONIC BANKING	2.00
06-07	MARINER'S MAIL PAYMENT AT ELECTRONIC BANKING	1.00
06-07	CELLULAR ONE PAYMENT AT ELECTRONIC BANKING	16.00
06-03	CLINT PHARMACY PAYMENT AT ELECTRONIC BANKING	19.70

DEPOSITS/ OTHER CREDITS

DEPOSITS:

DATE	TRANSACTION DESCRIPTION	AMOUNT
06-07	BRANCH DEPOSIT	250.24
06-09	BRANCH DEPOSIT	1000.00
06-15	BRANCH DEPOSIT	156.69
06-16	CHECK DEPOSIT AT BANK BY MAIL	7.82

DAILY BALANCES

DATE	BALANCE	DATE	BALANCE	DATE	BALANCE
05-24	632.87	06-02	418.02	06-09	1605.78
05-25	580.95	06-03	389.94	06-10	1573.88
05-26	548.90	06-07	623.18	06-15	1730.57
05-27	539.90	06-08	605.78	06-16	1704.09
05-30	530.53				

Figure 14-10

CHAPTER 15

Bookkeeping

OBJECTIVES

After completing the exercises, the student will be able to:

1. Enhance knowledge of medical terminology, interpret abbreviations, and accurately spell medical words.

2. Prepare ledger cards, post transactions, and prepare cash receipts.

3. Prepare daily journal (daysheet).

4. Post charges, payments, and adjustments using a daily journal.

5. Prepare bank deposit and balance with monies received.

6. Balance daysheet and carry forward entries.

7. Set up daysheet for new month.

FOCUS ON CERTIFICATION*

CMA Content Summary
- Medical abbreviations
- Calculator
- Bookkeeping systems
- Demographic data
- Daysheets, charge slips, receipts, ledgers
- Financial transactions—charges, payments, and adjustments
- Identify and correct errors
- Petty cash
- Accounts receivable
- Write checks

RMA Content Summary
- Medical terminology and abbreviations
- Bookkeeping terminology
- Accounting procedures
- Balancing procedures
- Accounts receivable and payable
- Post charges, payments, adjustments
- Petty cash
- Bank deposits
- Patient account calculations

*This *Workbook* and accompanying textbook meet the entry-level administrative and general competencies for the CMA outlined by the AAMA Examination Content Outline and Role Delineation Study and for the RMA and CMAS outlined by the AMT Competencies and Examination Specifications (see Competency Grid in textbook Appendix B).

CMAS Content Summary

- Spell medical terms
- Basic accounting principles
- Bookkeeping procedures
- Financial computations
- Accounts receivable/payable

- Monthly trial balance
- Audit controls
- Patient accounts/ledgers
- Petty cash
- Software applications

Abbreviation and Spelling Review

Read the following patient's chart note and write the meanings for the abbreviations listed below the note. To decode any abbreviations you do not understand or that appear unfamiliar to you, refer to the list of abbreviations in Part V of this *Workbook*. Step-by-step directions for this exercise are found in Procedure 1-1 of Chapter 1 in the textbook. Medical terms in the chart note are italicized; study them for spelling. Use your medical dictionary to look up their definitions. Your instructor may give a spelling and definition test that includes these words and abbreviations.

Kevin T. Dusseau

June 30, 20XX Pt has off and on problems with eye. Dx: Acute *bacterial conjunctivitis* L eye. Treat R eye at first sign of *symptoms*. Cold compresses L eye ad lib. for comfort. Retn p.r.n.

Fran Practon, MD

Fran Practon, MD

Pt _____   ad lib. _____

Dx _____   retn _____

L _____   p.r.n. _____

R _____

Review Questions

Review the objectives, glossary, and chapter information before completing the following review questions.

1. Match the terms in the left column with the definitions in the right column and write the letters in the blanks.

   _____ debit

   _____ post

   _____ accounts receivable ledger

   _____ asset

   _____ liability

   _____ daysheet

   _____ credit

   _____ proprietorship

   _____ accounts payable ledger

   a. Bookkeeping entry that decreases the account balance

   b. Record book that lists detailed amounts due to a creditor for supplies, equipment, services rendered, and so on

   c. The owner's net worth

   d. To enter a charge, payment, or adjustment on a ledger or account

   e. Register for recording all daily business accounts payable ledger transactions

   f. That which is owned, tangible or intangible

   g. Legal obligation of one person to another; a debt

   h. Record book that lists all patients' outstanding accounts showing how much each one owes for services rendered

   i. A bookkeeping entry that records increases in assets and expenses and decreases liabilities

2. Name one or more advantages and disadvantages of each of the following bookkeeping systems:

	Advantage	**Disadvantage**
a. single-entry	_____	_____
	_____	_____
b. double-entry	_____	_____
	_____	_____
c. pegboard	_____	_____
	_____	_____
d. computerized	_____	_____
	_____	_____

3. When using a computerized bookkeeping system, you would post charges, payments, and adjustments to a patient _____; in a manual system, you would post to a _____ .

4. Charges are posted on the date _____; payments are posted on the date _____ .

5. Charges are _____ to the account; payments and adjustments are _____ to the account.

6. Write the bookkeeping term that each abbreviation stands for.

   a. B/F _____

   b. pd _____

   c. adj _____

   d. ROA _____

   e. recd_____

7. On the daysheet, the total of what patients have paid by cash and check must equal the total _____ _____ for that day.

8. Explain what calculations need to be made to determine the new accounts receivable figure at the end of the month.

   a. _____

   b. _____

   c. _____

9. An amount evenly divisible by _____ may indicate a transposed figure, and an amount evenly divisible by _____ may indicate posting to the wrong column.

10. If a posting error occurs when writing 900 for 90, this type of error is called _____ _____ .

11. At the end of the day, to reconcile the cash and change drawer, the _____ should equal the cash amount on the _____ , and the remaining amount in the change drawer should be the same as the beginning amount.

12. When is the petty cash fund replenished? _____ or _____ , depending on the demand for funds.

13. When replenishing the petty cash *fund*, add the _____ to the _____ and compare this total to the amount established for the fund; they should equal.

Critical Thinking Exercises

1. Make a list of all forms required when using a pegboard bookkeeping system, and give a brief explanation of the function of each one.

        Form   Function

  a. _____   _____

                                        _____

                                        _____

                                        _____

  b. _____   _____

                                        _____

                                        _____

                                        _____

                                        _____

                                        _____

                                        _____

  c. _____   _____

                                        _____

  d. _____   _____

2. Explain the purposes of a cash or change drawer and a petty cash fund, and tell why a medical practice needs both systems in place.

  a. _____

  b. _____

3. Mrs. Landry's account shows a delinquent balance of $3, and Dr. Practon wants the amount written off the books and the account closed. Explain how you would post this entry on the patient's ledger card.

  _____

  _____

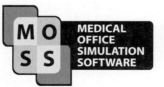

Computer Competency

Go to the Online Companion for this book at www.delmarlearning.com/companions to complete Medical Office Simulation Software activities for this chapter.

Bookkeeping Job Skills 15-1 through 15-12

Job Skills 15-1 through 15-12 take you through step-by-step procedures to gain experience in bookkeeping practices. Although these job skills utilize the pegboard bookkeeping system, the concepts learned apply to computerized bookkeeping and will help you understand posting steps needed in both systems and computations automatically done in computerized systems. Job Skills 15-2 through 15-5 (Project 1), 15-6 through 15-8 (Project 2), and 15-9 through 15-11 (Project 3) may be assigned individually; however, they must be done in order. Instead, the instructor may choose to assign these Job Skills as three projects to be done in class or as homework. Each grouping represents a different day in the medical practice that require various posting, calculating, and balancing of financial records. Job Skill 15-12 involves setting up a daysheet for a new month. With each Job Skill, read it entirely before beginning.

JOB SKILL 15-1
Prepare Ledger Cards

Name _____ Date _____ Score _____

Performance Objective

Task: Insert demographic information and post a balance forward to set up 28 ledger cards and arrange them in alphabetic sequence. These will be used for future Job Skills in this chapter.

Conditions: Use 14 sheets of ledger cards (Forms 60 through 73) for a total of 28 ledgers and typewriter or pen.

Standards: Complete all steps listed in this skill in _____ minutes with a minimum score of _____. (Time element and accuracy criteria may be given by instructor.)

Time: Start: _____ Completed: _____ Total: _____ minutes

Scoring: One point for each step performed satisfactorily unless otherwise listed or weighted by instructor.

Directions with Performance Evaluation Checklist

Set up ledger cards for the following patients by typing or filling in their names, addresses, telephone numbers, dates of birth (DOB), and insurance information; each member of a family has a separate ledger. Indicate the current year in the first "DATE" column and post a balance forward on each ledger card as indicated.

1st Attempt	2nd Attempt	3rd Attempt	
_____	_____	_____	Gather materials (equipment and supplies) listed under "Conditions."
_____/10	_____/10	_____/10	1. Set up ledger card for Mary Lou Chaney 4902 Saviers Road Woodland Hills, XY 12345-0000 Tel: 555-490-8755—home Tel: 555-490-5578—work DOB: 7/30/50 Ins. South West Ins. ID # 459-08-7655 Previous balance: new pt
_____/10	_____/10	_____/10	2. Set up a ledger card for Russell P. Smith 2336 East Manly Street Woodland Hills, XY 12345-0000 Tel: 555-786-0123—home Tel: 555-786-3210—work DOB: 5/6/56 Ins.: Blue Cross/Blue Shield Cert. # 58557AT Group # T84 Previous balance: zero
_____/10	_____/10	_____/10	3. Set up ledger card for Jody F. Swinney 4300 Saunders Road Woodland Hills, XY 12345-0000 Tel: 555-908-6605—home DOB: 1/16/64 Ins: Aetna Casualty Company Policy # 7821-11 Previous balance: $25.00

JOB SKILL 15-1 (*continued*)

_____/10 _____/10 _____/10   4. Set up ledger card for Miss Adrienne Cane
6502 North J Street
Woodland Hills, XY 12345-0000
Tel: 555-498-2110—home
DOB: 7/29/46
Ins: R. L. Kautz & Company
Policy # 7821-1KBM
Previous balance: $85.00

_____/10 _____/10 _____/10   5. Set up ledger card for Mark B. Hanson
2560 South M Street
Woodland Hills, XY 12345-0000
Tel: 555-980-2210—home
Tel: 555-980-0122—work
DOB: 6/22/49
Ins: Prudential Insurance Co.
Policy # 4579
Previous balance: zero

_____/10 _____/10 _____/10   6. Set up ledger card for Robert T. Jenner
1300 Hampshire Road
Woodland Hills, XY 12345-0000
Tel: 555-986-6790—home
Tel: 555-986-0976—work
DOB: 2/28/68
Ins: Guarantee Insurance Company
Policy # 67021
Previous balance: zero

_____/10 _____/10 _____/10   7. Set up ledger card for Harold B. Mason
6107 Harcourt Street
Woodland Hills, XY 12345-0000
Tel: 555-615-0123—home
Tel: 555-615-3201—work
DOB: 8/20/46
Ins: Allstate Insurance Company
Policy # 7632111 BA
Previous balance: zero

_____/10 _____/10 _____/10   8. Set up ledger card for J. B. Haupman
15761 Dickens Street
Woodland Hills, XY 12345-0000
Tel: 555-457-0561—home
DOB: 7/23/28
Ins: Medicare
Medicare ID # 987-XX-0988A
Previous balance: $1,466.56

_____/10 _____/10 _____/10   9. Set up ledger card for Mrs. Betty K. Lawson
6400 Best Way
Woodland Hills, XY 12345-0000
Tel: 555-450-9533—home
DOB: 1/27/69
Ins: TRICARE Extra ID # 5430982XX
Previous balance: zero

JOB SKILL 15-1 (*continued*)

_____/10 _____/10 _____/10 10. Set up ledger card for Miss Carol M. Wolf
2765 Honey Lane Street
Woodland Hills, XY 12345-0000
Tel: 555-892-0651—home
DOB: 8/25/76
Ins: Blue Cross/Blue Shield
Cert. # 76502 AT
Group # T85
Previous balance: zero

_____/10 _____/10 _____/10 11. Set up ledger card for Margaret Jenkins, RN
5692 Rose Avenue
Woodland Hills, XY 12345-0000
Tel: 555-760-3211—home
Tel: 555-760-1123—work
DOB: 6/29/70
Ins: Blue Cross/ Blue Shield
Cert. # 65923AT
Group # T76
Previous balance: new pt

_____/10 _____/10 _____/10 12. Set up ledger card for Roger T. Simpson
792 Baker Street
Woodland Hills, XY 12345-0000
Tel: 555-549-0879—home
Tel: 555-549-9780—work
DOB: 11/2/52
Ins: Farmers Insurance Group
Policy # 56892
Previous balance: $45.00

_____/10 _____/10 _____/10 13. Set up ledger card for Joan Gomez
4391 Wooden Street
Woodland Hills, XY 12345-000
Tel: 555-459-2399—home
Tel: 555-459-9932—work
DOB: 3/15/47
Ins. Fremont Indemnity Company
Policy # 56702111
Previous balance: $60.00

_____/10 _____/10 _____/10 14. Set up ledger card for Maria Bargioni
4892 Simpson Street
Woodland Hills, XY 12345-0000
Tel: 555-549-2344—home
Tel: 555-549-4432—work
DOB: 4/5/76
Ins: Fireman's Fund Insurance Companies
Policy # 568 MB 2111
Previous balance: $25.00

_____/10 _____/10 _____/10 15. Set up ledger card for Jack J. Johnson
5490 Olive Mill Road
Woodland Hills, XY 12345-0000
Tel: 555-857-9920—home
DOB: 5/27/59
Ins: Medicaid
ID # 458962016
Previous balance: zero

JOB SKILL 15-1 *(continued)*

_____/10 _____/10 _____/10 16. Set up ledger card for Lois A. Conrad
                              8920 Canton Street
                              Woodland Hills, XY 12345-000
                              Tel: 555-569-2201—home
                              Tel: 555-569-1022—work
                              DOB: 5/8/55
                              Ins: Gates, McDonald & Company
                              Policy # 4591 XT
                              Previous balance: $31.50

_____/10 _____/10 _____/10 17. Set up ledger card for Miss Marylou Conrad, c/o Lois Conrad
                              8920 Canton Street
                              c/o Lois Conrad
                              Woodland Hills, XY 12345-0000
                              Tel: 555-569-2201—home
                              DOB: 4/22/95
                              Ins: Gates, McDonald & Company
                              Policy # 4591 XT
                              Previous balance: zero

_____/10 _____/10 _____/10 18. Set up ledger card for Hannah F. Riley
                              459 Fifth Avenue
                              Woodland Hills, XY 12345-0000
                              Tel: 555-789-2201—home
                              Tel: 555-789-1022—work
                              DOB: 10/8/62
                              Ins: Hartford Insurance Group
                              Policy # 5601221
                              Previous balance: zero

_____/10 _____/10 _____/10 19. Set up ledger card for Stephen B. Riley Jr.
                              459 Fifth Avenue
                              Woodland Hills, XY 12345-0000
                              Tel: 555-789-2201—home
                              Tel: 555-789-1022—work
                              DOB: 6/29/62
                              Ins: Hartford Insurance Group
                              Policy # 5601221
                              Previous balance: new pt

_____/10 _____/10 _____/10 20. Set up ledger card for Rosa K. Okida
                              7900 Shatto Place
                              Woodland Hills, XY 12345-0000
                              Tel: 555-420-1121—home
                              Tel: 555-420-1211—work
                              DOB: 11/2/58
                              Ins: Home Insurance Company
                              Policy # 789-1191-21K
                              Previous balance: $201.00

_____/10 _____/10 _____/10 21. Set up ledger card for Howard S. Chan
                              3200 Shaw Avenue
                              Woodland Hills, XY 12345-0000
                              Tel: 555-660-3211—home
                              Tel: 555-660-1123—work
                              DOB: 8/3/58
                              Ins: Imperial Insurance Company
                              Policy # 21019KBM
                              Previous balance: zero

JOB SKILL 15-1 (*continued*)

_____/10 _____/10 _____/10 22. Set up ledger card for Rachel T. O'Brien
5598 East 17 Street
Woodland Hills, XY 12345-0000
Tel: 555-566-2199—home
Tel: 555-566-9912—work
DOB: 3/19/68
Ins: North America Health Net POS
Policy # 54901
Previous balance: $50.00

_____/10 _____/10 _____/10 23. Set up ledger card for Martin P. Owens
430 Herndon Place
Woodland Hills, XY 12345-0000
Tel: 555-542-2232—home
Tel: 555-542-2322—work
DOB: 12/3/73
Ins: John Deere Insurance Company
Policy # 67401 J
Previous balance: $25.00

_____/10 _____/10 _____/10 24. Set up ledger card for Joseph C. Smith
P.O. Box 4301
Woodland Hills, XY 12345-0000
Tel: 555-549-1124—home
Tel: 555-549-4211—work
DOB: 6/20/73
Ins: Home Insurance Company
Policy # 589102K
Previous balance: new pt

_____/10 _____/10 _____/10 25. Set up ledger card for Kathryn L. Hope
6680 Bascom Road
Woodland Hills, XY 12345-0000
Tel: 555-210-9980—home
Tel: 555-210-0899—work
DOB: 8/14/60
Ins: Met Life HMO
Policy # 8921
Previous balance: zero

_____/10 _____/10 _____/10 26. Set up ledger card for Russell O. Smith
459 University Avenue
Woodland Hills, XY 12345-0000
Tel: 555-129-1980—home
Tel: 555-129-0891—work
DOB: 2/15/65
Ins: International Insurance Company
Policy # 8901
Previous balance: new pt

_____/10 _____/10 _____/10 27. Set up ledger card for Charlotte J. Brown
769 Sky Park Circle
Woodland Hills, XY 12345-0000
Tel: 555-780-2341—home
Tel: 555-780-1432—work
DOB: 9/5/66
Ins: Kemper Insurance Company
Policy # 5769
Previous balance: $35.00

JOB SKILL 15-1 *(continued)*

_____/3 _____/3 _____/3   28. Set up ledger card with the heading "Miscellaneous Other Income" to be used to record charges and payments for lectures, published articles, and other miscellaneous items; previous balance zero.

_____/28 _____/28 _____/28   29. Cut cards apart and arrange them in alphabetic sequence with the "Miscellaneous Other Income" ledger at the end of the file.

_____ _____ _____   Complete within specified time.

___/303 ___/303 ___/303   **Total points earned** (To obtain a percentage score, divide the total points earned by the number of points possible.)

Comments:

Evaluator's Signature: _____ **Need to Repeat:** _____

National Curriculum Competency: CAAHEP: III.C.3.a(2)   ABHES: VI.B.1.a.8(a)

JOB SKILL 15-2
Bookkeeping Day 1—Post to Patient Ledger Cards and Prepare Cash Receipts

Name _____ Date _____ Score _____

Performance Objective

Task: Post charges and payment to patient ledger cards, calculate running balances and prepare cash receipts.

Conditions: Select ledger cards, which have been alphabetized, from Job Skill 15-1. Use five checks received by Practon Medical Group (Form 74 and 75), cash receipts (Form 76), calculator, and pencil. Refer to textbook Figure 15-3A for posting illustrations and Figure 15-6 for cash receipt example.

Standards: Complete all steps listed in this skill in _____ minutes with a minimum score of _____. (Time element and accuracy criteria may be given by instructor.)

Time: Start: _____ Completed: _____ Total: _____ minutes

Scoring: One point for each step performed satisfactorily unless otherwise listed or weighted by instructor.

Directions with Performance Evaluation Checklist

It is June 28, current year. Pull ledger cards for patients who are on today's schedule (they are highlighted in step-by-step instructions in **bold face**). Post all charges (line by line), referring to the Mock Fee Schedule (Figure A-1; Part IV of this *Workbook*) to obtain fees; calculate running balance for each line of posting. For all commercial (private) insurance programs, Medicaid, and TRICARE, use figures from the "Mock Fees." Cut checks apart and post all payments after charges have been posted; calculate balance due. Complete a receipt for all patients who paid cash.

1st Attempt	2nd Attempt	3rd Attempt	
_____	_____	_____	Gather materials (equipment and supplies) listed under "Conditions."
_____/20	_____/20	_____/20	1. Post charges for patient **Mark B. Hanson.** Est Pt OV Level II Post cash payment (patient paid in full); indicate receipt number in reference column. Complete cash receipt No. 147.
_____/5	_____/5	_____/5	2. Post charges for patient **Russell O. Smith.** NP Office Consult Level III
_____/20	_____/20	_____/20	3. Post charges for patient **Betty K. Lawson.** Est Pt Level I OV Therapeutic injection (IM) Vitamin B12 (medication supply); fee $9 Post payment on account received by check.
_____/10	_____/10	_____/10	4. Post charges for patient **Jody F. Swinney.** Est Pt Level II OV Post copayment received by check.
_____/30	_____/30	_____/30	5. Post charges for patient **Mary Lou Chaney.** NP Level IV OV UA (nonautomated with microscopy) Basic comprehensive audiometry (Medicine Section) Post cash payment (patient paid in full) and indicate receipt number in reference column. Complete cash receipt No. 148.

JOB SKILL 15-2 *(continued)*

_____/15   _____/15   _____/15   6. Post charges for patient **Carol M. Wolf.**
                        Est Pt Level I OV
                        DPT Immunization Injection (product)
                        Immunization administration (DPT); fee $2.50

_____/10   _____/10   _____/10   7. Post charges for patient **Harold B. Mason.**
                        Est Pt Level II OV
                        ECG (Medicine Section)

_____/5   _____/5   _____/5   8. Post charges for patient **Robert T. Jenner.**
                        Initial hospital care (30 minutes—Level I)

INCOMING MAIL: Several checks have been received in the mail today. Some will be posted to the "Miscellaneous Other Income" account. When payments are posted to this account, post the charges the same time the check is received; this is standard office protocol.

_____/6   _____/6   _____/6   9. Post check from *Family Health Magazine* for article written by Dr. Gerald Practon.

_____/6   _____/6   _____/6   10. Post check from **Colony Boys School** for lecture by Dr. Fran Practon.

_____/5   _____/5   _____/5   11. Post personal check from patient **Adrienne Cane;** payment on account.

_____   _____   _____   Complete within specified time.

___/134   ___/134   ___/134   **Total points earned** (To obtain a percentage score, divide the total points earned by the number of points possible.)

Comments:

Evaluator's Signature: _____   **Need to Repeat:** _____

National Curriculum Competency: CAAHEP: III.C.3.a(2)	ABHES: VI.B.1.a.8(a)

JOB SKILL 15-3
Bookkeeping Day 1—Prepare Daily Journal

Name _____ Date _____ Score _____

Performance Objective

Task: Set up daily journal by inserting figures from previous day's totals.

Conditions: Daily Journal—Day 1 (Form 77) and pencil. You may want to use a photocopy machine to enlarge this to legal size to ease handwritten entries. See daily journal posting illustration in textbook Figure 15-5 and step-by-step directions in textbook Procedure 15-1.

Standards: Complete all steps listed in this skill in _____ minutes with a minimum score of _____. (Time element and accuracy criteria may be given by instructor.)

Time: Start: _____ Completed: _____ Total: _____ minutes

Scoring: One point for each step performed satisfactorily unless otherwise listed or weighted by instructor.

Directions with Performance Evaluation Checklist

1st Attempt	2nd Attempt	3rd Attempt	
_____	_____	_____	Gather materials (equipment and supplies) listed under "Conditions."
_____	_____	_____	1. It is June 28, current year. Enter this date on the top of the daysheet and Record of Deposits and use it for all transactions that will occur today.
_____	_____	_____	2. All transactions for June 28, 20XX, will fit on one daysheet; label it page number 1 of 1.
_____	_____	_____	3. Insert the daily journal (daysheet) previous page total ($14,336.60) for Column A from the previous day, June 27, 20XX.
_____	_____	_____	4. Insert the daily journal previous page total ($8,592.41) for Column B-1 from the previous day, June 27, 20XX.
_____	_____	_____	5. Insert the daily journal previous page total ($450.00) for Column B-2 from the previous day, June 27, 20XX.
_____	_____	_____	6. Insert the daily journal previous page total ($1,387.56) for Column C from the previous day, June 27, 20XX.
_____	_____	_____	7. Insert the daily journal previous page total ($980.00) for Column D from the previous day, June 27, 20XX.
_____	_____	_____	8. Enter Accounts Receivable Control, Previous Day's Total: $30,526.32.
_____	_____	_____	9. Enter Accounts Receivable Proof, First of Month figure: $25,232.13.
_____	_____	_____	10. Enter Beginning Cash on Hand figure: $50.00.
_____	_____	_____	11. Insert your name at the bottom of the daysheet in the "Prepared by" area.
_____	_____	_____	Complete within specified time.
___/13	___/13	___/13	**Total points earned** (To obtain a percentage score, divide the total points earned by the number of points possible.)

JOB SKILL 15-3 *(continued)*

Comments:

JOB SKILL 15-4
Bookkeeping Day 1—Post Charges, Payments, and Adjustments Using a Daily Journal

Name _____ Date _____ Score _____

Performance Objective

Task: Post charges, payments, and adjustments on the daily journal; record payments on bank deposit slip and in cash control; endorse checks and prepare bank deposit.

Conditions: Ledgers used in Job Skill 15-2, daysheet prepared in Job Skill 15-3, checks (Form 74 and 75) used in Job Skill 15-3, number 10 envelope, calculator, and pencil. Refer to textbook Procedure 15-1 for step-by-step directions.

Standards: Complete all steps listed in this skill in _____ minutes with a minimum score of _____. (Time element and accuracy criteria may be given by instructor.)

Time: Start: _____ Completed: _____ Total: _____ minutes

Scoring: One point for each step performed satisfactorily unless otherwise listed or weighted by instructor.

Directions with Performance Evaluation Checklist

Daily Journal Instructions

Post all charges, payments, and adjustments for each patient seen on a *single line* of the daysheet. Specific instructions follow:

COLUMNS:

Date: Enter date of posting in first column (e.g., 6/28/20XX).

Reference: This column may be used for various references. For this exercise, all charges and payments for professional services taking place today will be posted on **one line;** use this column to enter the patient's check number when payment is received (e.g., ck 123).

Description: Enter *CPT* codes numbers for all professional services rendered. Enter "Miscellaneous Other Income" to designate the ledger you are posting to for checks received from other sources.

Charges: List **total** charge for **all** professional services rendered by each patient.

Credits—Payments: List payment amount.

Credits—Adjustments: List the amount to be written off the account.

Balance: Add previous balance to charges and subtract credits (payments and adjustments) to obtain the current balance.

Previous Balance: Obtain and enter the amount extended from each patient's ledger card.

Name: Enter last name, first name, and middle initial.

Numbered Lines: Each line is numbered for reference to help with posting accuracy.

Receipt Number: Enter number from cash receipt.

RECORD OF DEPOSITS: Make a photocopy of the "Record of Deposit" section of the daysheet to use as a bank deposit slip. At the top of the *deposit slip,* insert the name of the bank (The First National Bank) and checking account number (12345-6789).

Date: Enter current date on top of Daily Journal form.

   ABA: Enter bank ABA number listed on check.

   Cash: Enter amount of cash payment.

   Checks: Enter amount of check payment.

BUSINESS ANALYSIS SUMMARY: Label and enter copayment amount in Column 1; other columns may be used for various entries depending on the needs of the office.

JOB SKILL 15-4 *(continued)*

For posting information, you can either refer to the ledgers used to post current charges and payments in Job Skill 15-2 or refer once again to specific posting instructions in the step-by-step directions of Job Skill 15-2; you will be posting the same information on the daysheet. In a pegboard bookkeeping system, journal entries will be automatically posted as they are written on ledgers by means of NCR paper. In a computerized system, journal entries will be automatically posted as they are input into the patient's account.

1st Attempt	2nd Attempt	3rd Attempt	
_____	_____	_____	Gather materials (equipment and supplies) listed under "Conditions."
____/7	____/7	____/7	1. Post charge and payment for **Mark B. Hanson.**
____/5	____/5	____/5	2. Post charge for **Russell O. Smith.**
____/10	____/10	____/10	3. Post charges and payment for **Betty K. Lawson.**
____/10	____/10	____/10	4. Post charge and copayment for **Jody F. Swinney.**
____/7	____/7	____/7	5. Post charges and payment for **Mary Lou Chaney.**
____/5	____/5	____/5	6. Post charges for **Carol M. Wolf.**
____/5	____/5	____/5	7. Post charges for **Harold B. Mason.**
____/5	____/5	____/5	8. Post charge for **Robert T. Jenner.**
____/8	____/8	____/8	9. Post check (and charge) from *Family Health Magazine.*
____/8	____/8	____/8	10. Post check (and charge) from **Colony Boys School.**
____/9	____/9	____/9	11. Post personal check from **Adrienne Cane.**
____/3	____/3	____/3	12. Add the proper endorsement for all checks received and put them in an envelope with the bank slip.
_____	_____	_____	Complete within specified time.
____/85	____/85	____/85	**Total points earned** (To obtain a percentage score, divide the total points earned by the number of points possible.)

Comments:

Evaluator's Signature: _____   Need to Repeat: _____

JOB SKILL 15-5
Bookkeeping Day 1—Balance Daysheet

Name _____ Date _____ Score _____

Performance Objective

Task: Total all columns on daysheet, add previous page totals, and enter new figures in month-to-date areas.

Conditions: Daysheet (Day 1) used in Job Skills 15-3 and 15-5, calculator, and pencil. Refer to textbook Procedure 15-1 for step-by-step directions.

Standards: Complete all steps listed in this skill in _____ minutes with a minimum score of _____. (Time element and accuracy criteria may be given by instructor.)

Time: Start: _____ Completed: _____ Total: _____ minutes

Scoring: One point for each step performed satisfactorily unless otherwise listed or weighted by instructor.

Directions with Performance Evaluation Checklist

1st Attempt	2nd Attempt	3rd Attempt	
_____	_____	_____	Gather materials (equipment and supplies) listed under "Conditions."

Daysheet Totals

____/3	____/3	____/3	1. Total Column A, add Previous Page total, and enter Month-to-Date figure.
____/3	____/3	____/3	2. Total Column B-1, add Previous Page total, and enter Month-to-Date figure.
____/3	____/3	____/3	3. Total Column B-2, add Previous Page total, and enter Month-to-Date figure.
____/3	____/3	____/3	4. Total Column C, add Previous Page total, and enter Month-to-Date figure.
____/3	____/3	____/3	5. Total Column D, add Previous Page total, and enter Month-to-Date figure.

Proof of Posting

____/5	____/5	____/5	6. Transfer today's daysheet totals as directed in Proof of Posting section and add or subtract as instructed. If total does not equal Column C, recalculate and look for errors.

Accounts Receivable Control

____/5	____/5	____/5	7. Enter figures from Proof of Posting section as indicated and add or subtract as instructed.

Accounts Receivable Proof

____/5	____/5	____/5	8. Enter Month-to-Date figures and add or subtract as instructed.

Balance Daysheet

___/10	___/10	___/10	9. Compare "Total Accounts Receivable" from accounts receivable control with "Total Accounts Receivable" from accounts receivable proof; they should match. If not, follow instructions on common posting problems to locate the error.

Record Deposit and Balance Cash Control

____/3	____/3	____/3	10. Add all cash received in "Record of Deposits" and enter total cash at bottom.
____/6	____/6	____/6	11. Add all checks received in "Record of Deposits" and enter total checks at bottom.
____/3	____/3	____/3	12. Add total cash received and total checks received to obtain total deposit amount; this amount should equal total of today's payments found in Column B-1.

JOB SKILL 15-5 *(continued)*

_____/5   _____/5   _____/5   13. Balance cash on hand by following the steps listed in "Cash Control."

_____   _____   _____   Complete within specified time.

_____/59   _____/59   _____/59   **Total points earned** (To obtain a percentage score, divide the total points earned by the number of points possible.)

Comments:

Evaluator's Signature: _____ **Need to Repeat:** _____

| National Curriculum Competency: CAAHEP: III.C.3.a(2) | ABHES: VI.B.1.a.3(o), VI.B.1.a.8(a) |

JOB SKILL 15-6
Bookkeeping Day 2—Prepare Daily Journal

Name _____ Date _____ Score _____

Performance Objective

Task: Set up daily journal by inserting figures from previous day's totals.

Conditions: Daily Journal—Day 2 (Form 78) and pencil. You may want to enlarge this on a photocopy machine to legal size to ease handwritten entries. Refer to textbook Procedure 15-1 for step-by-step directions.

Standards: Complete all steps listed in this skill in _____ minutes with a minimum score of _____.
(Time element and accuracy criteria may be given by instructor.)

Time: **Start:** _____ **Completed:** _____ **Total:** _____ minutes

Scoring: One point for each step performed satisfactorily unless otherwise listed or weighted by instructor.

Directions with Performance Evaluation Checklist

1st Attempt	2nd Attempt	3rd Attempt	
_____	_____	_____	Gather materials (equipment and supplies) listed under "Conditions."
_____	_____	_____	1. It is June 29, current year. Enter this date on the top of the daysheet and Record of Deposits and use it for all transactions that will occur today.
_____	_____	_____	2. All transactions for June 29, 20XX, will fit on one daysheet; label it page number 1 of 1.
____/5	____/5	____/5	3. Insert the "Previous Page" (day) totals at the bottom of the daily journal (daysheet) by picking up the figures from June 28, 20XX, "Month-to-Date" totals for Columns A, B-1, B-2, C, and D.
_____	_____	_____	4. Insert the Accounts Receivable Control "Previous Day's Total." This is the "Total Accounts Receivable" figure at the end of the previous day.
_____	_____	_____	5. Carry forward the Accounts Receivable Proof "First of Month" figure as indicated on the previous daysheet.
_____	_____	_____	6. Enter Beginning "Cash on Hand" figure: $50.00.
_____	_____	_____	7. Insert your name at the bottom of the daysheet in the "Prepared by" area.
_____	_____	_____	Complete within specified time.
____/13	____/13	____/13	**Total points earned** (To obtain a percentage score, divide the total points earned by the number of points possible.)

Comments:

Evaluator's Signature: _____ **Need to Repeat:** _____

National Curriculum Competency: CAAHEP: III.C.3.a(2) ABHES: VI.B.1.a.3(a)

JOB SKILL 15-7

Bookkeeping Day 2—Post Charges, Payments, and Adjustments to Patient Ledger Cards and to the Daily Journal; Prepare Cash Receipts and Bank Deposit

Name _____ Date _____ Score _____

Performance Objective

Task: Post charges and payment to patient ledger cards and calculate running balance; prepare cash receipts. Duplicate posting entries on daily journal (daysheet); record payments on bank deposit slip, endorse checks, and prepare bank deposit.

Conditions: Select ledger cards, which have been alphabetized, from Job Skill 15-1 and the daysheet prepared in Job Skill 15-6. Use three checks received by Practon Medical Group (Form 79), cash receipts (Form 76), number 10 envelope, calculator, and pencil. Refer to textbook Figure 15-3A for posting illustrations, Procedure 15-1 for step-by-step directions, and Figure 15-6 for cash receipt example.

Standards: Complete all steps listed in this skill in _____ minutes with a minimum score of _____.
                  (Time element and accuracy criteria may be given by instructor.)

Time: Start: _____ Completed: _____ Total: _____ minutes

Scoring: One point for each step performed satisfactorily unless otherwise listed or weighted by instructor.

Directions with Performance Evaluation Checklist

It is June 29, current year. For this Job Skill, you will be posting to the patient's ledger card and then to the daily journal (daysheet); refer to specific instructions in Job Skill 15-4. Pull ledger cards for patients who are on today's schedule (they are highlighted in step-by-step instructions in bold face) and post entries as done in Job Skills 15-2 and 15-4. Post all charges (line by line) referring to the Mock Fee Schedule (Figure A-1, Part IV of this *Workbook*) to obtain fees; calculate running balance for each line of posting. For all commercial (private) insurance programs, Medicaid, and TRICARE, use figures from the "Mock Fees." Cut checks apart and post all payments after charges have been posted; endorse checks, record on deposit slip, and put into envelope. Complete a receipt for all patients who paid cash; record all payments in the Cash Control section of the daily journal.

1st Attempt	2nd Attempt	3rd Attempt	
_____	_____	_____	Gather materials (equipment and supplies) listed under "Conditions."
_____/11	_____/11	_____/11	1. Post charge on ledger for patient **Margaret Jenkins.** NP Office Consult Level IV Post entry on daysheet.
_____/21	_____/21	_____/21	2. Post charge on ledger for patient **Roger T. Simpson.** Est Pt OV Level IV Post copayment received on ledger; check No. 3000 for $15. Post entries on daysheet. and record payment on bank deposit.
_____/16	_____/16	_____/16	3. Post charges on ledger for patient **Joan Gomez.** ECG in office (Medicine Section) Admit to College Hospital; initial care (50 minutes—Level II) Post entries on daysheet.
_____/11	_____/11	_____/11	4. Post charge on ledger for patient **Harold B. Mason.** Est Pt OV Level II Post entry on daysheet.
_____/11	_____/11	_____/11	5. Post charge on ledger for patient **Maria Bargioni.** Est Pt OV Level III (severe headaches) Post entry on daysheet.

JOB SKILL 15-7 *(continued)*

_____/31 _____/31 _____/31   6. Post charges on ledger for patient **Jack J. Johnson.**
    Est Pt OV Level I
    Tetanus inj (Medicine Section)
    Immunization administration; IM (Medicine Section)
    Post Medicaid copayment (check) on ledger.
    Post entries on daysheet. and record payment on bank deposit.

_____/16 _____/16 _____/16   7. Post charges on ledger for patient **Lois A. Conrad.**
    Est Pt OV Level III
    Pap smear collected and sent to laboratory. Note: the Pap smear is
    bundled into the office visit; however, there is a charge for the handling
    fee (Medicine Section—Special Services and Reports).
    Post entries on daysheet.

_____/21 _____/21 _____/21   8. Post charges on ledger for patient **Marylou Conrad.**
    Est Pt OV Level II
    Poliovirus vaccine; oral immunization (Medicine Section)
    Immunization administration (Medicine Section)
    Post entries on daysheet.

_____/16 _____/16 _____/16   9. Post charges on ledger for patient **Hannah F. Riley.**
    Est Pt OV Level IV
    IUD insertion (Male/Female Genital System)
    Post entries on daysheet.

_____/30 _____/30 _____/30   10. Post charge on ledger for patient **Stephen B. Riley Jr.**
    Office Consult Level IV
    Post cash payment on ledger; $25.
    Complete cash receipt No. 149.
    Post entries on daysheet record payment on bank deposit and cash control.

_____/16 _____/16 _____/16   11. Post charges on ledger for patient **Rosa K. Okida.**
    Est Pt OV Level I
    X-ray R hip (single view)
    Post entries on daysheet.

_____/11 _____/11 _____/11   12. Post charge on ledger for patient **Howard S. Chan.**
    Est Pt OV Level IV
    Post entries on daysheet.

_____/11 _____/11 _____/11   13. Post charge on ledger for patient **Robert T. Jenner.**
    HV (subsequent) Level I
    Post entry on daysheet.

INCOMING MAIL: The morning mail contained a check from Prudential Insurance Company for processing a life insurance examination report.

_____/6 _____/6 _____/6   14. Post check (and charge) on ledger from **Prudential Insurance Company.**
    Post payment on daysheet and record on bank deposit.

_____/3 _____/3 _____/3   15. Add the proper endorsement for all checks received and put them in an
    envelope with the bank slip.

_____ _____ _____   Complete within specified time.

___/233 ___/233 ___/233   **Total points earned** (To obtain a percentage score, divide the total points
    earned by the number of points possible.)

Comments:

Evaluator's Signature: _____   **Need to Repeat:** _____

National Curriculum Competency: CAAHEP: III.C.3.a(2)	ABHES: VI.B.1.a.3(I)

JOB SKILL 15-8
Bookkeeping Day 2—Balance Daysheet

Name _____ Date _____ Score _____

Performance Objective

Task: Total all columns on daysheet, add previous page totals, and enter new figures in month-to-date areas.

Conditions: Daysheet (Day 2) used in Job Skills 15-6 and 15-7, calculator, and pencil. Refer to textbook Procedure 15-1 for step-by-step directions.

Standards: Complete all steps listed in this skill in _____ minutes with a minimum score of _____. (Time element and accuracy criteria may be given by instructor.)

Time: Start: _____ **Completed:** _____ **Total:** _____ minutes

Scoring: One point for each step performed satisfactorily unless otherwise listed or weighted by instructor.

Directions with Performance Evaluation Checklist

1st Attempt	2nd Attempt	3rd Attempt	
_____	_____	_____	Gather materials (equipment and supplies) listed under "Conditions."

Daysheet Totals

1st	2nd	3rd	
____/3	____/3	____/3	1. Total Column A, add Previous Page total, and enter Month-to-Date figure.
____/3	____/3	____/3	2. Total Column B-1, add Previous Page total, and enter Month-to-Date figure.
____/3	____/3	____/3	3. Total Column B-2, add Previous Page total, and enter Month-to-Date figure.
____/3	____/3	____/3	4. Total Column C, add Previous Page total, and enter Month-to-Date figure.
____/3	____/3	____/3	5. Total Column D, add Previous Page total, and enter Month-to-Date figure.

Proof of Posting

____/5	____/5	____/5	6. Transfer today's daysheet totals as directed in Proof of Posting section and add or subtract as instructed. If total does not equal Column C, recalculate and look for errors.

Accounts Receivable Control

____/5	____/5	____/5	7. Enter figures from Proof of Posting section as indicated and add or subtract as instructed.

Accounts Receivable Proof

____/5	____/5	____/5	8. Enter month-to-date figures and add or subtract as instructed.

Balance Daysheet

____/10	____/10	____/10	9. Compare "Total Accounts Receivable" from accounts receivable control with "Total Accounts Receivable" from accounts receivable proof; they should match. If not, follow instructions on common posting problems to locate the error.

Record Deposit and Balance Cash Control

____/3	____/3	____/3	10. Add all cash received in "Record of Deposits" and enter total cash at bottom.
____/6	____/6	____/6	11. Add all checks received in "Record of Deposits" and enter total checks at bottom.
____/3	____/3	____/3	12. Add total cash received and total checks received to obtain total deposit amount; this amount should equal total of today's payments found in Column B-1.

JOB SKILL 15-8 *(continued)*

____/5   ____/5   ____/5   13. Balance cash on hand by following the steps listed in "Cash Control."

_____   _____   _____   Complete within specified time.

____/59   ____/59   ____/59   **Total points earned** (To obtain a percentage score, divide the total points earned by the number of points possible.)

Comments:

Evaluator's Signature: _____ **Need to Repeat:** _____

National Curriculum Competency: CAAHEP: III.C.3.a(2)	ABHES: VI.B.1.a.3(o), VI.B.1.a.8(a)

JOB SKILL 15-9
Bookkeeping Day 3—Prepare Daily Journal

Name _____ Date _____ Score _____

Performance Objective

Task: Set up daily journal by inserting figures from previous day's totals.

Conditions: Daily Journal—Day 3 (Form 80) and pencil. You may want to use a photocopy machine to enlarge this to legal size to ease handwritten entries. Refer to textbook Procedure 15-1 for step-by-step directions.

Standards: Complete all steps listed in this skill in _____ minutes with a minimum score of _____. (Time element and accuracy criteria may be given by instructor.)

Time: **Start:** _____ **Completed:** _____ **Total:** _____ minutes

Scoring: One point for each step performed satisfactorily unless otherwise listed or weighted by instructor.

Directions with Performance Evaluation Checklist

1st Attempt	2nd Attempt	3rd Attempt	
_____	_____	_____	Gather materials (equipment and supplies) listed under "Conditions."
_____	_____	_____	1. It is June 30, current year. Enter this date on the top of the daysheet and Record of Deposits and use it for all transactions that will occur today.
_____	_____	_____	2. All transactions for June 30, 20XX, will fit on one daysheet; label it page number 1 of 1.
_____/5	_____/5	_____/5	3. Insert the "Previous Page" (day) totals at the bottom of the daily journal (daysheet) by picking up the figures from June 29, 20XX, "Month-to-Date" totals for Columns A, B-1, B-2, C, and D.
_____	_____	_____	4. Insert the Accounts Receivable Control "Previous Day's Total." This is the "Total Accounts Receivable" figure at the end of the previous day.
_____	_____	_____	5. Carry forward the Accounts Receivable Proof "First of Month" figure as indicated on the previous daysheet.
_____	_____	_____	6. Enter Beginning "Cash on Hand" figure: $50.00.
_____	_____	_____	7. Insert your name at the bottom of the daysheet in the "Prepared by" area.
_____	_____	_____	Complete within specified time.
_____/13	_____/13	_____/13	**Total points earned** (To obtain a percentage score, divide the total points earned by the number of points possible.)

Comments:

Evaluator's Signature: _____   **Need to Repeat:** _____

JOB SKILL 15-10

Bookkeeping Day 3—Post Charges, Payments, and Adjustments to Patient Ledger Cards and to the Daily Journal; Prepare Cash Receipts and Bank Deposit

Name _____ Date _____ Score _____

Performance Objective

Task: Post charges and payment to patient ledger cards and calculate running balance; prepare cash receipts. Duplicate posting entries on daily journal (daysheet); record payments on bank deposit slip, endorse checks, and prepare bank deposit.

Conditions: Select ledger cards, which have been alphabetized, from Job Skill 15-1 and the daysheet prepared in Job Skill 15-9. Use two checks received by Practon Medical Group (Form 81), cash receipts (Form 76), number 10 envelope, calculator, and pencil. Refer to textbook Figure 15-3A for posting illustrations, Procedure 15-1 for step-by-step directions, and Figure 15-6 for cash receipt example.

Standards: Complete all steps listed in this skill in _____ minutes with a minimum score of _____. (Time element and accuracy criteria may be given by instructor.)

Time: Start: _____ Completed: _____ Total: _____ minutes

Scoring: One point for each step performed satisfactorily unless otherwise listed or weighted by instructor.

Directions with Performance Evaluation Checklist

It is June 30, current year. For this Job Skill, you will be posting to the patient's ledger card and then to the daily journal (daysheet); refer to specific instructions in Job Skill 15-4. Pull ledger cards for patients who are on today's schedule (they are highlighted in step-by-step instructions in **bold face**) and post entries as done in Job Skills 15-2, 15-4, and 15-7. Post all charges (line by line), referring to the Mock Fee Schedule (Figure A-1, Part IV of this *Workbook*) to obtain fees; calculate running balance for each line of posting. Doctors Fran and Gerald Practon are participating physicians in the Medicare program and bill using the "Medicare Participating" provider fee schedule. For all other insurance types, use figures from the "Mock Fees" column. Cut checks apart and post all payments after charges have been posted; endorse checks, record on deposit slip, and put into envelope. Complete a receipt for all patients who paid cash; record all payments in the Cash Control section of the daily journal.

1st Attempt	2nd Attempt	3rd Attempt	
_____	_____	_____	Gather materials (equipment and supplies) listed under "Conditions."
____/11	____/11	____/11	1. Post charge on ledger for patient **J. B. Haupman.** Est Pt OV Level II Post entry on daysheet.
____/21	____/21	____/21	2. Post charge on ledger for patient **Rachel T. O'Brien.** Est Pt OV Level II Post copayment received (check) from managed care plan on ledger. Post entries on daysheet. and record payment on bank deposit.
____/16	____/16	____/16	3. Post charges on ledger for patient **Martin P. Owens.** Est Pt OV Level II Diathermy (Medicine Section—Physical Medicine) Post entries on daysheet.
____/25	____/25	____/25	4. Post charges on ledger for patient **Joseph C. Smith.** NP OV Level III Esophageal intubation (Gastroenterology) Post payment (check) on ledger. Post entries on daysheet.

JOB SKILL 15-10 (*continued*)

_____/20 _____/20 _____/20   5. Post charge on ledger for patient **Kathryn L. Hope.**
Est Pt OV Level II
Post HMO copayment on ledger; $10 cash.
Complete cash receipt No. 150.
Post entries on daysheet.

_____/11 _____/11 _____/11   6. Post charges on ledger for patient **Russell O. Smith.**
Est Pt OV Level II
Post entry on daysheet.

_____/21 _____/21 _____/21   7. Post charge on ledger for patient **Charlotte J. Brown.**
Est Pt OV Level III
Post entry on daysheet.

_____/11 _____/11 _____/11   8. Post charge on ledger for patient **Joan Gomez.**
HV (subsequent) Level I
Post entry on daysheet.

_____/11 _____/11 _____/11   9. Post charge on ledger for patient **Robert T. Jenner.**
Hospital discharge
Post entry on daysheet.

TELEPHONE CALL: Mr. Howard S. Chan telephoned and said he was unable to pay his bill because he lost his job. You spoke with Dr. Practon and he told you to cancel the patient's debt.

_____/12 _____/12 _____/12   10. Post an adjustment on ledger for patient **Howard S. Chan.**
Reference Dr. G. Practon's name on the ledger.
Describe the adjustment as a "hardship."
Post entry on daysheet.

_____ _____ _____   Complete within specified time.

___/161 ___/161 ___/161   **Total points earned** (To obtain a percentage score, divide the total points earned by the number of points possible.)

Comments:

Evaluator's Signature: _____   **Need to Repeat:** _____

National Curriculum Competency: CAAHEP: III.C.3.a(2)   ABHES: VI.B.1.a.3(I)

JOB SKILL 15-11
Bookkeeping Day 3—Balance Daysheet

Name _____ Date _____ Score _____

Performance Objective

Task: Total all columns on daysheet, add previous page totals, and enter new figures in month-to-date areas.

Conditions: Daysheet (Day 3) used in Job Skills 15-9 and 15-10, calculator, and pencil. Refer to textbook Procedure 15-1 for step-by-step directions.

Standards: Complete all steps listed in this skill in _____ minutes with a minimum score of _____. (Time element and accuracy criteria may be given by instructor.)

Time: Start: _____ Completed: _____ Total: _____ minutes

Scoring: One point for each step performed satisfactorily unless otherwise listed or weighted by instructor.

Directions with Performance Evaluation Checklist

1st Attempt	2nd Attempt	3rd Attempt	
_____	_____	_____	Gather materials (equipment and supplies) listed under "Conditions."

Daysheet Totals

1st	2nd	3rd	
____/3	____/3	____/3	1. Total Column A, add Previous Page total, and enter Month-to-Date figure.
____/3	____/3	____/3	2. Total Column B-1, add Previous Page total, and enter Month-to-Date figure.
____/3	____/3	____/3	3. Total Column B-2, add Previous Page total, and enter Month-to-Date figure.
____/3	____/3	____/3	4. Total Column C, add Previous Page total, and enter Month-to-Date figure.
____/3	____/3	____/3	5. Total Column D, add Previous Page total, and enter Month-to-Date figure.

Proof of Posting

____/5	____/5	____/5	6. Transfer today's daysheet totals as directed in Proof of Posting section and add or subtract as instructed. If total does not equal Column C, recalculate and look for errors.

Accounts Receivable Control

____/5	____/5	____/5	7. Enter figures from Proof of Posting section as indicated and add or subtract as instructed.

Accounts Receivable Proof

____/5	____/5	____/5	8. Enter month-to-date figures and add or subtract as instructed.

Balance Daysheet

___/10	___/10	___/10	9. Compare "Total Accounts Receivable" from accounts receivable control with "Total Accounts Receivable" from accounts receivable proof; they should match. If not, follow instructions on common posting problems to locate the error.

Record Deposit and Balance Cash Control

____/3	____/3	____/3	10. Add all cash received in "Record of Deposits" and enter total cash at bottom.
____/6	____/6	____/6	11. Add all checks received in "Record of Deposits" and enter total checks at bottom.
____/3	____/3	____/3	12. Add total cash received and total checks received to obtain total deposit amount; this amount should equal total of today's payments found in Column B-1.

JOB SKILL 15-11 (*continued*)

____/5   ____/5   ____/5   13. Balance cash on hand by following the steps listed in "Cash Control."

_____   _____   _____   Complete within specified time.

____/59   ____/59   ____/59   **Total points earned** (To obtain a percentage score, divide the total points earned by the number of points possible.)

Comments:

Evaluator's Signature: _____ **Need to Repeat:** _____

National Curriculum Competency: CAAHEP: III.C.3.a(2)   ABHES: VI.B.1.a.3(o), VI.B.1.a.8(a)

JOB SKILL 15-12
Bookkeeping Day 4—Set Up Daysheet for New Month

Name _____ Date _____ Score _____

Performance Objective

Task: Set up daily journal for new month by inserting figures from previous day/end-of-month totals.

Conditions: Header and bottom section of daily journal (Form 82), daysheet from previous day/month (Day 3—Job Skill 15-11), and pencil.

Standards: Complete all steps listed in this skill in _____ minutes with a minimum score of _____. (Time element and accuracy criteria may be given by instructor.)

Time: Start: _____ **Completed:** _____ **Total:** _____ minutes

Scoring: One point for each step performed satisfactorily unless otherwise listed or weighted by instructor.

Directions with Performance Evaluation Checklist

1st Attempt	2nd Attempt	3rd Attempt	
_____	_____	_____	Gather materials (equipment and supplies) listed under "Conditions."
_____/3	_____/3	_____/3	1. It is July 1, current year. Enter this date on the top of the daysheet and label it page 1 of 1.
_____/5	_____/5	_____/5	2. Insert zeros (0) in the "Previous Page" (day) totals at the bottom of the daily journal (daysheet) for Columns A, B-1, B-2, C, and D.
_____	_____	_____	3. Insert the Accounts Receivable Control "Previous Day's Total." This is the "Total Accounts Receivable" figure at the end of the previous day.
_____	_____	_____	4. Insert the end-of-month total accounts receivable from June 30, 20XX, in the Accounts Receivable Proof "Accounts Receivable First of Month" area, found in the ending "Total Accounts Receivable." This will be the same total as the previous day's total (i.e., end-of-month total) entered into the Accounts Receivable Control.
_____	_____	_____	5. Insert your name at the bottom of the daysheet in the "Prepared by" area.
_____	_____	_____	Complete within specified time.
_____/13	_____/13	_____/13	**Total points earned** (To obtain a percentage score, divide the total points earned by the number of points possible.)

Comments:

Evaluator's Signature: _____ **Need to Repeat:** _____

National Curriculum Competency: CAAHEP: III.C.3.a(2)	ABHES: VI.B.1.a.3(a)

CHAPTER 16

Health Insurance Systems

OBJECTIVES

After completing the exercises, the student will be able to:

1. Enhance knowledge of medical terminology, interpret abbreviations, and accurately spell medical words.

2. Select proper *CPT* codes using various sections of the codebook for given scenarios and clinical examples.

3. Select proper *ICD-9-CM* codes using various sections of the codebook for given diagnostic statements and scenarios.

4. Complete a managed care authorization form.

5. Abstract information from a patient record and progress notes to code and complete insurance claim forms.

6. Complete a health insurance claim form for a commercial (private) case.

7. Complete a health insurance claim form for a Medicare case.

8. Complete a health insurance claim form for a TRICARE case.

9. Prepare ledger cards, post information, and calculate a running balance.

FOCUS ON CERTIFICATION*

CMA Content Summary

- Medical abbreviations
- Medicare/Medicaid regulations
- HIPAA
- Personal injury
- Workers' compensation
- Coding systems (*CPT, ICD-9-CM* and *HCPCS II*)
- Code linkage
- Capitation

- Medicare, Medicaid, TRICARE, CHAMPVA
- Prepaid health plans (HMO, PPO, POS)
- Manual and electronic claim processing
- Tracing claims, inquiry, and appeals
- Primary/Secondary claims
- Reconciling payments
- Referrals and precertification
- Fee schedules (RVS, RBRVS, DRG)

*This *Workbook* and accompanying textbook meet the entry-level administrative and general competencies for the CMA outlined by the AAMA Examination Content Outline and Role Delineation Study and for the RMA and CMAS outlined by the AMT Competencies and Examination Specifications (see Competency Grid in textbook Appendix B).

RMA Content Summary

- Insurance terminology and abbreviations
- Medical, disability, accident insurance plans
- HMO, PPO, EPO, indemnity plans
- Workers' compensation
- Medicare, Medicaid, TRICARE
- Paper and electronic insurance claims
- HIPAA

- Explanation of benefits
- Claim rejection and follow-up procedures
- Code *ICD-9-CM, CPT, HCPCS II*
- Contractural requirements of insurance plans (time limits)
- Track unpaid claims
- Referral and authorization process

CMAS Content Summary

- Medical and insurance terminology
- Private and managed care plans
- Medicare, Medicaid, Veteran's Administration, TRICARE
- Insurance claims (time limits)
- Workers' compensation and state disability

- Paper and electronic claim submission
- Procedure and diagnostic coding
- Use *CPT, ICD-9-CM,* and *HCPCS II* codebooks
- Process insurance payments
- Track unpaid claims

Abbreviation and Spelling Review

Read the following patient's chart note and write the meanings for the abbreviations listed below the note. To decode any abbreviations you do not understand or that appear unfamiliar to you, refer to the list of abbreviations in Part V of this *Workbook*. Step-by-step directions for this exercise are found in Procedure 1-1 of Chapter 1 in the textbook. Medical terms in the chart note are italicized; study them for spelling. Use your medical dictionary to look up their definitions. Your instructor may give a spelling and definition test that includes these words and abbreviations.

Brad Chieu

May 5, 20XX Pt came into the hosp c̄ a CC of *dyspnea* & pain in the RUQ. He was seen in the ED. Pt has had *diabetes* since childhood/*hypertension* for 3 years. Smoker. Increasing *malaise, nausea, anorexia* for past 5 days. *Polyuria, polydipsia.* The RN took his FH & vitals & recorded his TPR of 96.5°F & BP of 120/70 on the chart. After exam, the Dr. verified that the pt was suffering from COPD & scheduled him for an IPPB TX b.i.d. AP chest x-rays, a TB test and O2 therapy.

Gerald Practon, MD
Gerald Practon, MD

Pt _____

c̄ _____

CC _____

RUQ _____

ED _____

RN _____

FH _____

TPR _____

F _____

BP _____

Dr. _____

COPD _____

IPPB _____

TX _____

b.i.d. _____

AP _____

TB _____

O2 _____

Review Questions

Review the objectives, glossary, and chapter information before completing these review questions.

1. Match the terms in the left column with the definitions in the right column by writing letters in the blanks.

    _____ copayment

    _____ third-party payer

    _____ indemnity

    _____ deductible

    _____ carrier

    _____ adjuster

    _____ fiscal intermediary

    _____ elimination period

    _____ assignment

    _____ partial disability

    a. Employee of an insurance carrier with whom a case is assigned and who follows the case until it is settled

    b. Contractor processes payments to providers on behalf of state or federal agencies or insurance companies

    c. Insurance carrier that intervenes to pay hospital or medical expenses on behalf of beneficiaries or recipients

    d. Benefits paid in a predetermined amount in the event of a covered loss

    e. The transfer of one's right to collect an amount payable under an insurance contract

    f. Organization that offers protection against losses in exchange for a premium

    g. Form of cost sharing in which the insured pays a specific portion toward the amount of the professional services rendered

    h. Period of time after the beginning of a disability for which no benefits are payable

    i. Illness or injury preventing the insured from performing one or more functions of his or her occupation

    j. Amount the insured must pay in a fiscal year before an insurance company will begin the payment of benefits

2. Name and give a brief definition of three types of commercial (private) health insurance plans.

    a. _____

    _____

    b. _____

    _____

    c. _____

    _____

3. The insured is also known as a/an _____ or
    _____ .

4. An elimination period written in an insurance policy may also be known as a/an _____ or
    _____ .

5. An attachment to a policy excluding certain illnesses or disabilities is called a/an _____
    _____ .

6. Managed care plans pay the physician by _____ .

7. Dr. Practon wants to know if Mrs. Snow's managed care plan covers a particular surgical procedure. This is a process known as _____ .

8. Dr. Practon completes a form for preauthorization of a diagnostic test to be ordered for Lee Cho. This process may also be called _____ or _____.

9. Before scheduling elective surgery on Phyllis Horton, Dr. Practon wants to know the maximum amount the insurance plan will pay. This is a process known as _____ .

10. Name five popular types of managed care health plans and list their abbreviations.

   a. _____

   b. _____

   c. _____

   d. _____

   e. _____

11. Nonparticipating and participating physicians accept _____ percent of the allowable fee paid by Medicare.

12. A [participating or nonparticipating] physician may not bill more than the Medicare limiting charge.

13. What is the time limit for submission of a Medicare claim? _____

_____

14. A document from the insurance company that arrives with a check for payment of an insurance claim is called a/an _____ . In the Medicare program, this document is called a/an _____ , and the one sent to patients is called a/an

_____ .

15. Medicare Part D is [voluntary or involuntary] prescription drug coverage offered by [government or private] insurance carriers.

16. When submitting a Medicare/Medicaid claim, the physician [should, should not, must always] accept assignment or payment will go to the patient.

17. A claim processed by Medicare and automatically processed by Medicaid is referred to as a/an _____ claim.

18. The TRICARE fiscal year is from _____ to _____ .

19. Define the following terms in relation to disability insurance.

   a. Temporary disability: _____

   _____

   b. Partial disability: _____

   _____

   c. Total disability: _____

   _____

20. After an initial workers' compensation report, insurance carriers want progress reports submitted on the injured worker each time the patient is seen, or on a/an _____ basis.

21. The insurance claim form that is accepted by most commercial (private) insurance companies, Medicare, Medicaid, and TRICARE is called _____ .

22. If a patient signs an assignment of benefits statement, where is the insurance check sent? _____

_____

23. The new standard unique health identifier that all health care providers use when submitting claims is called the _____ .

24. A service that receives insurance claims, edits and sorts them, and then electronically transmits them to insurance companies is called a/an _____ .

25. When completing health insurance claims electronically, list the types of codes required on the claim according to the Standard Code Set.

    a. _____

    b. _____

    c. _____

26. For coding purposes, the definition of *new patient* is _____

    _____

    _____ .

27. Procedure codes consist of _____-digit number(s) with _____-digit modifiers.

28. Explain the difference between a consult and referral of a patient.

    a. Consult: _____

    _____

    b. Referral: _____

    _____

29. Write the definition of these three symbols that appear in the *Current Procedural Terminology** codebook.

    a. + _____

    b. • _____

    c. Δ _____

30. Repairs of lacerations are coded according to:

    a. _____

    b. _____

    c. _____

31. The documentation required in a patient's medical record when an injection is given includes:

    a. _____

    b. _____

    c. _____

32. Diagnostic codes using *ICD-9-CM* can vary from _____ to _____ digits.

33. Mrs. Gary Waxman has brought in a Prudential insurance form that has an employer section for completion. You wish to use the health insurance claim form, CMS-1500. Describe the procedure for submission of the claim. _____

    _____

    _____

    _____

**Current Procedural Terminology* codes, descriptions, and two-digit numeric modifiers only are from *CPT 2007*. ©2006, American Medical Association. All rights reserved.

34. Indicate whether the following statements are true (T) or false (F).

   a. _____ Only an original CMS-1500 claim form may be optically scanned.

   b. _____ It is permissible to type data in lowercase for claims being optically scanned.

   c. _____ When entering data on a claim that is to be optically scanned, dates are keyed using six digits.

   d. _____ Staples and paper clips may be used for attachments when sending insurance claims.

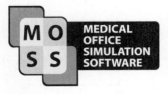

Computer Competency

Go to the Online Companion for this book at www.delmarlearning.com/companions to complete Medical Office Simulation Software activities for this chapter.

JOB SKILL 16-1
Review *Current Procedural Terminology* Codebook Sections

Name _____ Date _____ Score _____

Performance Objective

Task: Locate procedure codes in various sections of the *Current Procedural Terminology (CPT)**
                 codebook.

Conditions: *Current Procedural Terminology* codebook and pen or pencil.

Standards: Complete all steps listed in this skill in _____ minutes with a minimum score of _____.
                (Time element and accuracy criteria may be given by instructor.)

Time: **Start:** _____ **Completed:** _____ **Total:** _____ minutes

Scoring: One point for each step performed satisfactorily unless otherwise listed or weighted by instructor.

Directions with Performance Evaluation Checklist

Insert the section of *CPT* where each of the following codes are located.

1st Attempt	2nd Attempt	3rd Attempt	
_____	_____	_____	Gather materials (equipment and supplies) listed under "Conditions."
_____	_____	_____	1. 99202 _____
_____	_____	_____	2. 27500 _____
_____	_____	_____	3. 73500 _____
_____	_____	_____	4. 00500 _____
_____	_____	_____	5. 80055 _____
_____	_____	_____	6. 90713 _____
_____	_____	_____	7. 75970 _____
_____	_____	_____	8. 41872 _____
_____	_____	_____	9. 86805 _____
_____	_____	_____	10. 95004 _____
_____	_____	_____	11. 99281 _____
_____	_____	_____	12. 01810 _____
_____	_____	_____	Complete within specified time.
___/14	___/14	___/14	**Total points earned** (To obtain a percentage score, divide the total points earned by the number of points possible.)

JOB SKILL 16-1 *(continued)*

Comments:

Evaluator's Signature: _____ **Need to Repeat:** _____

National Curriculum Competency: CAAHEP: III.C.3.a(3)(c)   ABHES: VI.B.1.a.8(b)

JOB SKILL 16-2
Code Evaluation and Management Services

Name _____ Date _____ Score _____

Performance Objective

Task: Locate evaluation and management codes in various subsections of the E/M section of *CPT*.

Conditions: *Current Procedural Terminology** codebook, "Evaluation and Management Services Guidelines" found at the beginning of the E/M section, and *CPT* notes that appear prior to the subsections and within categories of the E/M section. Refer to the section "Coding for Professional Services" in the textbook and Procedure 16-1 for step-by-step directions.

Standards: Complete all steps listed in this skill in _____ minutes with a minimum score of _____. (Time element and accuracy criteria may be given by instructor.)

Time: Start: _____ **Completed:** _____ **Total:** _____ minutes

Scoring: One point for each step performed satisfactorily unless otherwise listed or weighted by instructor.

Directions with Performance Evaluation Checklist

The following divisions in this Job Skill are designed to acquaint you with various subsections in the Evaluation and Management (E/M) section of *CPT*. The problems become more difficult as you progress.

E/M codes are used by physicians to report a significant portion of their services. Some physicians rank E/M codes on a scale of 1 to 5, with 5 as the highest, most complex level, and 1 as the lowest, least-complex level. This terminology appears on multipurpose billing forms. The levels are determined by the last digit and are broken down as follows:

	OFFICE VISITS		CONSULTATIONS	
	New	Established	Office	Hospital
Level 1	99201	99211	99241	99251
Level 2	99202	99212	99242	99252
Level 3	99203	99213	99243	99253
Level 4	99204	99214	99244	99254
Level 5	99205	99215	99245	99255

Remember, it is the physician's responsibility to assign E/M codes, and this Job Skill is for familiarization purposes. The problems will acquaint you with terminology for this section of the *CPT* codebook.

1st Attempt	2nd Attempt	3rd Attempt	
_____	_____	_____	Gather materials (equipment and supplies) listed under "Conditions."

New Patient Office Visit Codes: Select by level of service and key components.

_____	_____	_____	1. This is a level 2 case: Expanded problem-focused history Expanded problem-focused examination Straightforward medical decision making	_____
_____	_____	_____	2. This is a level 4 case: Comprehensive examination Comprehensive history Moderate complexity medical decision making	_____
_____	_____	_____	3. This is a level 1 case: Problem-focused history Problem-focused examination Straightforward decision making	_____

**Current Procedural Terminology* codes, descriptions, and two-digit numeric modifiers only are from *CPT 2007*. ©2006, American Medical Association. All rights reserved.

JOB SKILL 16-2 *(continued)*

Established Patient Office Visit Codes: Select by level of service and key components, taking into consideration the rule that states you need "two out of three" key components to assign a code for an established patient.

_____   _____   _____   4. This is a level 2 case:
                               Problem-focused history   _____
                               Problem-focused examination
                               Straightforward medical decision making

_____   _____   _____   5. This is a level 4 case:
                               Detailed history   _____
                               Detailed examination
                               Moderate complexity medical decision making

_____   _____   _____   6. This is a level 5 case:
                               Comprehensive history   _____
                               Comprehensive examination
                               High-complexity decision making

Code Range 99201 to 99238—Services provided in physician's office, hospital inpatient/outpatient, or other ambulatory facility. Select codes according to key components.

____/3 ____/3 ____/3   7. Office visit for a four-year-old male, established patient,   _____
                               with an expanded problem-focused history and physical
                               examination for earache and dyshidrosis of feet and low-
                               complexity medical decision making.

____/3 ____/3 ____/3   8. Office visit for a 35-year-old male, established patient, with   _____
                               a detailed history and examination for a new onset RLQ
                               pain. Medical decision making was of moderate complexity.

____/3 ____/3 ____/3   9. Initial hospital visit for a 15-year-old male with a detailed   _____
                               history and examination for infectious mononucleosis and
                               dehydration. Medical decision making was of low
                               complexity.

____/3 ____/3 ____/3   10. Subsequent hospital visit for a nine-year-old female   _____
                               admitted for lobar pneumonia with vomiting and
                               dehydration. A problem-focused interval history was made
                               because she is becoming afebrile but tolerates oral fluids.
                               An expanded problem-focused examination was done,
                               with straightforward decision making.

____/3 ____/3 ____/3   11. Office visit for a nine-year-old male, established patient, who _____
                               has been taking swimming lessons and now presents with a
                               two-day history of left ear pain with purulent drainage. This
                               visit required a problem-focused history and examination,
                               with straightforward decision making.

Code Range 99241 to 99275—Consultation services provided in the physician's office, hospital inpatient/outpatient, or other ambulatory facility. Select codes according to key components.

____/3 ____/3 ____/3   12. Office consultation for a 67-year-old male with chronic low   _____
                               back pain radiating to the left leg requiring a detailed history
                               and examination and low-complexity decision making.

____/3 ____/3 ____/3   13. Initial office consultation for a 21-year-old female with acute _____
                               upper respiratory tract symptoms that required an expanded
                               problem-focused history and examination with straightforward
                               decision making.

____/3 ____/3 ____/3   14. Office consult for 30-year-old female with chronic pelvic   _____
                               inflammatory disease who now has left lower quadrant
                               pain with a palpable pelvic mass. This visit required a
                               comprehensive history and examination and moderate-
                               complexity decision making.

JOB SKILL 16-2 *(continued)*

_____/3 _____/3 _____/3 15. Initial office consultation for a 60-year-old carpenter with _____
olecranon bursitis requiring a problem-focused history and
examination. Medical decision making was straightforward.

_____/3 _____/3 _____/3 16. Hospital consultation for a highly functional 70-year-old _____
male to review laboratory studies. A problem-focused
history and examination was performed. Medical decision
making was straightforward.

Code Range 99281 to 99499—Services provided in a hospital emergency or critical care department, nursing facility, rest home or custodial care facility, and patient's home as well as prolonged physician standby, case management, care plan, and preventive medicine services. Select codes according to key components or time.

_____/3 _____/3 _____/3 17. First hour of critical care of a 16-year-old male with acute _____
respiratory failure from asthma.

_____/3 _____/3 _____/3 18. A child is seen in the emergency department with rash on _____
both legs after exposure to poison ivy. This visit required
an expanded problem-focused history and examination but
low-complexity medical decision making.

_____/3 _____/3 _____/3 19. Initial nursing facility visit to evaluate a 70-year-old male _____
found confused and wandering, admitted by Adult
Protective Services without a qualifying stay or inpatient
diagnostic work-up. Patient lives alone and has no relatives
in the area. A comprehensive history and examination was
performed. Medical decision making was of moderate
complexity.

_____/3 _____/3 _____/3 20. Subsequent visit in a skilled nursing facility to a female with _____
controlled dementia, hypertension, and diabetes. During
the visit, she seemed to exhibit flu symptoms. An expanded
problem-focused interval history and examination was
performed. Medical decision making was straightforward.

_____/3 _____/3 _____/3 21. Emergency department visit for a female who received _____
an abrasion and needs a tetanus toxoid immunization. A
problem-focused history and examination was performed,
and medical decision making was straightforward.

_____ _____ _____ Complete within specified time.

_____/53 _____/53 _____/53 **Total points earned** (To obtain a percentage score, divide the total points earned
by the number of points possible.)

Comments:

Evaluator's Signature: _____ **Need to Repeat:** _____

National Curriculum Competency: CAAHEP: III.C.3.a(3)(c)	ABHES: VI.B.1.a.8(b)

JOB SKILL 16-3
Code Surgical Procedures and Services

Name _____ Date _____ Score _____

Performance Objective

Task: Locate the correct procedure code within the Surgery section of *CPT* for each description listed.

Conditions: *Current Procedural Terminology** codebook, "Surgery Guidelines" found at the beginning of the Surgery section, *CPT* notes that appear prior to and within the subsections and categories of the Surgery section, and pen or pencil. Refer to the section "Coding for Professional Services" in the textbook and Procedure 16-1 for step-by-step directions.

Standards: Complete all steps listed in this skill in _____ minutes with a minimum score of _____. (Time element and accuracy criteria may be given by instructor.)

Time: **Start:** _____ **Completed:** _____ **Total:** _____ minutes

Scoring: One point for each step performed satisfactorily unless otherwise listed or weighted by instructor.

Directions with Performance Evaluation Checklist

Surgery codes 10021 to 69990 are divided according to body systems, then anatomic parts of the body. Use the *CPT* codebook to obtain the correct code number for each descriptor given. Critical thinking enters this Job Skill as you use your judgment to determine the correct code, since some cases do not contain full details. Read each case and code description carefully.

1st Attempt	2nd Attempt	3rd Attempt	
_____	_____	_____	Gather materials (equipment and supplies) listed under "Conditions."

INTEGUMENTARY SYSTEM 10021–19499

_____/5	_____/5	_____/5	1. Excision, benign lesion, face, 0.5 cm	_____
_____/5	_____/5	_____/5	2. Repair layered closure of lt leg 2.7 cm laceration	_____

MUSCULOSKELETAL SYSTEM 20000–29999

_____/5	_____/5	_____/5	3. Closed reduction of rt humeral shaft fracture, no manipulation	_____
_____/5	_____/5	_____/5	4. Subsequent application of long leg cast (walker)	_____

RESPIRATORY SYSTEM 30000–32999

_____/5	_____/5	_____/5	5. Remove fried potato from left nostril of child	_____
_____/5	_____/5	_____/5	6. Simple excision of small nasal polyp	_____

CARDIOVASCULAR SYSTEM 33010–37799

_____/5	_____/5	_____/5	7. Introduction of catheter into superior vena cava	_____
_____/5	_____/5	_____/5	8. Coronary artery bypass using single arterial graft	_____

HEMIC/LYMPHATIC MEDIASTINUM/DIAPHRAGM 38100–39599

_____/5	_____/5	_____/5	9. Biopsy of cervical lymph nodes; open, deep	_____
_____/5	_____/5	_____/5	10. Open excision for removal of total spleen	_____

JOB SKILL 16-3 *(continued)*

DIGESTIVE SYSTEM 40490–49999

_____/5 _____/5 _____/5   11. Liver biopsy; needle; percutaneous   _____

_____/5 _____/5 _____/5   12. Open excision to remove gallbladder (cholecystectomy)   _____

URINARY SYSTEM 50010–53899

_____/5 _____/5 _____/5   13. Drainage of deep periurethral abscess   _____

_____/5 _____/5 _____/5   14. Aspiration of bladder by needle   _____

MALE GENITAL/INTERSEX/FEMALE GENITAL/MATERNITY CARE AND DELIVERY 54000–59899

_____/5 _____/5 _____/5   15. Removal of IUD   _____

_____/5 _____/5 _____/5   16. Cesarean delivery including obstetric/antepartum/   _____
                                          postpartum care

ENDOCRINE/NERVOUS SYSTEMS 60000–64999

_____/5 _____/5 _____/5   17. Complete thyroidectomy   _____

_____/5 _____/5 _____/5   18. Cervical laminoplasty with decompression of spinal   _____
                                          cord; two segments

EYE AND OCULAR ADNEXA/AUDITORY/OPERATING MICROSCOPE 65091–69990

_____/5 _____/5 _____/5   19. Subconjunctival injection   _____

_____/5 _____/5 _____/5   20. Removal of temporal bone tumor   _____

_____ _____ _____   Complete within specified time.

___/102 ___/102 ___/102   **Total points earned** (To obtain a percentage score, divide the total points
                                          earned by the number of points possible.)

Comments:

Evaluator's Signature: _____ **Need to Repeat:** _____

National Curriculum Competency: CAAHEP: III.C.3.c(3)(c)	ABHES: VI.B.1.a.8.(b)

JOB SKILL 16-4
Code Radiology and Laboratory Procedures and Services

Name _____ Date _____ Score _____

Performance Objective

Task: Locate the correct procedure code in the Radiology and Pathology/Laboratory section of *CPT* for each description.

Conditions: *Current Procedural Terminology** codebook, "Radiology" and "Pathology/Laboratory" Guidelines found at the beginning of each section of *CPT*, *CPT* notes that appear prior to and within the subsections and categories of each section, and pen or pencil. Refer to the section "Coding for Professional Services" in the textbook and Procedure 16-1 for step-by-step directions.

Standards: Complete all steps listed in this skill in _____ minutes with a minimum score of _____.
(Time element and accuracy criteria may be given by instructor.)

Time: Start: _____ **Completed:** _____ **Total:** _____ minutes

Scoring: One point for each step performed satisfactorily unless otherwise listed or weighted by instructor.

Directions with Performance Evaluation Checklist

1st Attempt	2nd Attempt	3rd Attempt	
_____	_____	_____	Gather materials (equipment and supplies) listed under "Conditions."

RADIOLOGY 70010–79999 AND PATHOLOGY/LABORATORY 80048–89356

____/5	____/5	____/5	1. X-rays of hand, four views	_____
____/5	____/5	____/5	2. Bilateral renal angiography	_____
____/5	____/5	____/5	3. Lipid panel	_____
____/5	____/5	____/5	4. Bacterial culture quantitative, urine	_____
_____	_____	_____	Complete within specified time.	
___/22	___/22	___/22	**Total points earned** (To obtain a percentage score, divide the total points earned by the number of points possible.)	

Comments:

Evaluator's Signature: _____ **Need to Repeat:** _____

National Curriculum Competency: CAAHEP: III.C.3.a(3)(c) ABHES: VI.B.1.a.8(b)

JOB SKILL16-5
Code Procedures and Services in the Medicine Section

Name _____ Date _____ Score _____

Performance Objective

Task: Locate the correct procedure code from the Medicine section of *CPT* for each scenario.

Conditions: *Current Procedural Terminology** codebook, "Medicine Guidelines" found at the beginning of the Medicine section, *CPT* notes that appear prior to and within the subsections and categories of the Medicine section, and pen or pencil. Refer to the section "Coding for Professional Services" in the textbook and Procedure 16-1 for step-by-step directions.

Standards: Complete all steps listed in this skill in _____ minutes with a minimum score of _____. (Time element and accuracy criteria may be given by instructor.)

Time: Start: _____ Completed: _____ Total: _____ minutes

Scoring: One point for each step performed satisfactorily unless otherwise listed or weighted by instructor.

Directions with Performance Evaluation Checklist

1st Attempt	2nd Attempt	3rd Attempt		
_____	_____	_____	Gather materials (equipment and supplies) listed under "Conditions."	
____/10	____/10	____/10	1. Immune globulin injection, botulism, intravenous	
			Product:	_____
			Administration:	_____
____/10	____/10	____/10	2. Influenza virus vaccine (split virus) intramuscular injection (IM), to a 62-year-old patient	
			Product:	_____
			Administration:	_____
____/5	____/5	____/5	3. Replacement of contact lens	_____
____/5	____/5	____/5	4. Cardiovascular stress test (treadmill) with continuous electrocardiographic monitoring with physician supervision, interpretation, and report	_____
____/5	____/5	____/5	5. Handling of specimen for transfer from the physician's office to a laboratory	_____
_____	_____	_____	Complete within specified time.	
____/37	____/37	____/37	**Total points earned** (To obtain a percentage score, divide the total points earned by the number of points possible.)	

Comments:

Evaluator's Signature: _____ **Need to Repeat:** _____

National Curriculum Competency: CAAHEP: III.C.3.a(3)(c)	ABHES: VI.B.1.a.8(b)

JOB SKILL 16-6
Code Clinical Examples

Name _____ Date _____ Score _____

Performance Objective

Task: Read each scenario, select the correct *CPT* or *HCPCS Level II* procedure code.

Conditions: Use *Current Procedure Terminology** codebook or Tables 16-5 and 16-6 in the textbook, Mock Fee Schedule and *HCPCS Level II* codes found in Part IV of the *Workbook,* and pen or pencil.

Standards: Complete all steps listed in this skill in _____ minutes with a minimum score of _____.
         (Time element and accuracy criteria may be given by instructor.)

Time: **Start:** _____ **Completed:** _____ **Total:** _____ minutes

Scoring: One point for each step performed satisfactorily unless otherwise listed or weighted by instructor.

Directions with Performance Evaluation Checklist

This Job Skill will familiarize you with the parts of the CMS-1500 claim form, coding from SOAP chart notes, and *HCPCS Level II* codes. All sections of *CPT* will be used. Answer the questions and insert data in Field 24 of the CMS-1500 claim form.

1st Attempt	2nd Attempt	3rd Attempt	
_____	_____	_____	Gather materials (equipment and supplies) listed under "Conditions."

CMS-1500 Claim Form—Scenario A: On February 3, current year, a private insurance patient is taken to an ambulatory surgery center with effusion of fluid (hydrathrosis) of the right knee. The physician does an arthrocentesis and aspirates. Applied dressing and patient is to return to office in one week.

_____/7 _____/7 _____/7   1. What is the correct procedure code?
                 Insert this in the unshaded area of Field 24D (*CPT/HCPCS*).

_____/7 _____/7 _____/7   2. What is the mock fee for this service?
                 Insert this in the unshaded area of Field 24F.

_____/7 _____/7 _____/7   3. How many times was this procedure performed?
                 Indicate this in the unshaded area of Field 24G (DAYS OR UNITS).

_____/7 _____/7 _____/7   4. What is the date of the service or procedure?
                 Indicate the eight-digit date in the unshaded area of Field 24A (left portion only).

24. A. DATE(S) OF SERVICE						B. PLACE OF SERVICE	C. EMG	D. PROCEDURES, SERVICES, OR SUPPLIES (Explain Unusual Circumstances)		E. DIAGNOSIS POINTER	F. $ CHARGES	G. DAYS OR UNITS	H. EPSDT Family Plan	I. ID. QUAL.	J. RENDERING PROVIDER ID. #
From			To					CPT/HCPCS	MODIFIER						
MM	DD	YY	MM	DD	YY										
														NPI	

CMS-1500 Claim Form—Scenario B: On May 6, a new patient is seen in the office of an otologist after referral by a family physician to evaluate and treat diminished hearing in right ear. The physician performed an expanded problem-focused history and examination. A comprehensive audiometry threshold evaluation and speech recognition was performed, revealing a conductive right ear low-frequency loss of hearing. Patient was referred to an audiologist for hearing aid examination and selection. Decision making was straightforward. Patient asked to return in one month.

_____/7 _____/7 _____/7   5. What are the correct procedure codes?
                 Insert these in the unshaded area of Field 24D (*CPT/HCPCS*).

*Current Procedural Terminology codes, descriptions, and two-digit numeric modifiers only are from *CPT 2007.* ©2006, American Medical Association. All rights reserved.

JOB SKILL 16-6 *(continued)*

_____/7   _____/7   _____/7   6. What are the mock fees for these services?
Insert these in the unshaded area of Field 24F.

_____/7   _____/7   _____/7   7. How many times were theses procedures performed?
Indicate this in the unshaded area of Field 24G (DAYS OR UNITS).

_____/7   _____/7   _____/7   8. What is the date of the service for each procedure?
Indicate the eight-digit date in the unshaded area of Field 24A (left portion only).

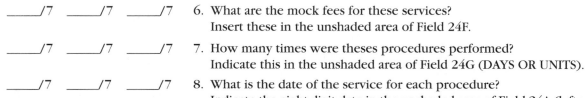

SOAP Chart Note A:

4/15/XX Maria Gomez

S: A 35-year-old female established patient is seen for a new complaint of left lower quadrant pain; 1 wk. duration. Symptoms: mild fever, decreased appetite, and mild constipation for 1 wk. Pt denies abdominal injury, change in urination, or abnormal menstruation. LMP: 3/12/XX.

O: Temp: 100.2°F; BP 130/80, HR 80; RR 18.
Lungs: Clear.
Abdomen: Both sides mildly hyperactive, flat, mild guarding LLQ, rebound neg; fullness LLQ; no discrete masses; no HSM.
Rectal: Normal tone; no masses; guaiac positive.
Pelvic: Cervix closed, uterus and ovaries normal, fullness lt lat adnexa c̄ tenderness.
CBC, elevated. WBC c̄ mild lt shift; UA, normal; HCG, pregnancy test negative.

A: Probable diverticulitis of sigmoid colon based on clinical picture.

P: Obtain barium enema to R/O diverticulitis. Begin antibiotics and dietary restriction during acute phase and follow up in three days.

_____/5   _____/5   _____/5   9. Read the SOAP note and select the correct E/M code.   _____

Chart Note B:

A physician does a history and examination on an established patient for 5 minutes, performs acne surgery (code 10040), and counsels the patient on skin care and diet for 10 minutes.

_____/5   _____/5   _____/5   10. Read the chart note and select the correct E/M code.   _____

HCPCS Level II Codes

_____/3   _____/3   _____/3   11. Select the correct *HCPCS* Level II code for one sterile eye pad.   _____

_____/3   _____/3   _____/3   12. Select the correct *HCPCS* Level II code for underarm crutches.   _____

_____/3   _____/3   _____/3   13. Select the correct *HCPCS* Level II code for 2cc gamma globulin inj IM.   _____

_____/3   _____/3   _____/3   14. Select the correct *HCPCS* Level II code for the physician interpretation of a screening Pap smear.   _____

_____   _____   _____   Complete within specified time.

_____/80   _____/80   _____/80   **Total points earned** (To obtain a percentage score, divide the total points earned by the number of points possible.)

JOB SKILL 16-6 *(continued)*

Comments:

JOB SKILL 16-7
Code Diagnosis from Chapters 1, 2, 3, 4, and 5 in *ICD-9-CM*

Name _____ Date _____ Score _____

Performance Objective

Task: Code diagnoses from the first five chapters of *ICD-9-CM*, Volumes I and II.

Conditions: Use *International Classification of Diseases—9th Revision—Clinical Modification,* Volumes I and II; and pen or pencil. Refer to Procedure 16-2 in the textbook for step-by-step directions.

Standards: Complete all steps listed in this skill in _____ minutes with a minimum score of _____. (Time element and accuracy criteria may be given by instructor.)

Time: **Start:** _____ **Completed:** _____ **Total:** _____ minutes

Scoring: One point for each step performed satisfactorily unless otherwise listed or weighted by instructor.

Directions with Performance Evaluation Checklist

Read the following statements, look up main terms in Volume II of the diagnostic codebook, and then confirm the code selection in Volume I.

1st Attempt	2nd Attempt	3rd Attempt		
_____	_____	_____	Gather materials (equipment and supplies) listed under "Conditions."	
____/5	____/5	____/5	1. Code human immunodeficiency virus.	_____
____/5	____/5	____/5	2. Code blackwater fever malaria.	_____
____/5	____/5	____/5	3. Code melanoma of the arm.	_____
____/5	____/5	____/5	4. Code benign neoplasm of the testes.	_____
____/5	____/5	____/5	5. Code type II diabetes mellitus without complications.	_____
____/5	____/5	____/5	6. Code rickets.	_____
____/5	____/5	____/5	7. Code hereditary hemolytic anemia.	_____
____/5	____/5	____/5	8. Code primary thrombocytopenia.	_____
____/5	____/5	____/5	9. Code anxiety.	_____
____/5	____/5	____/5	10. Code mild mental retardation.	_____
_____	_____	_____	Complete within specified time.	
____/52	____/52	____/52	**Total points earned** (To obtain a percentage score, divide the total points earned by the number of points possible.)	

Comments:

Evaluator's Signature: _____ **Need to Repeat:** _____

National Curriculum Competency: CAAHEP: III.C.3.a(3)(d) ABHES: VI.B.1.a.3(w), VI.B.1.a.8(b)

JOB SKILL 16-8
Code Diagnoses from Chapters 6, 7, 8, 9, and 10 in *ICD-9-CM*

Name _____ Date _____ Score _____

Performance Objective

Task: Code diagnoses from Chapters 6 through 10 of *ICD-9-CM*, Volumes I and II.

Conditions: Use *International Classification of Diseases—9th Revision—Clinical Modification,* Volumes I and II; and pen or pencil. Refer to Procedure 16-2 in the textbook for step-by-step directions.

Standards: Complete all steps listed in this skill in _____ minutes with a minimum score of _____.
                 (Time element and accuracy criteria may be given by instructor.)

Time: Start: _____ **Completed:** _____ **Total:** _____ minutes

Scoring: One point for each step performed satisfactorily unless otherwise listed or weighted by instructor.

Directions with Performance Evaluation Checklist

Read the following statements, look up main terms in Volume II of the diagnostic codebook, and then confirm the code selection in Volume I.

1st Attempt	2nd Attempt	3rd Attempt		
_____	_____	_____	Gather materials (equipment and supplies) listed under "Conditions."	
____/5	____/5	____/5	1. Code epileptic seizure.	_____
____/5	____/5	____/5	2. Code intraocular elevated tension.	_____
____/5	____/5	____/5	3. Code malignant hypertension.	_____
____/5	____/5	____/5	4. Code cerebral hemorrhage.	_____
____/5	____/5	____/5	5. Code viral pneumonia.	_____
____/5	____/5	____/5	6. Code chronic bronchitis.	_____
____/5	____/5	____/5	7. Code ulcerative stomatitis.	_____
____/5	____/5	____/5	8. Code peptic ulcer.	_____
____/5	____/5	____/5	9. Code stage II chronic renal disease.	_____
____/5	____/5	____/5	10. Code fibroadenosis of the breast.	_____
_____	_____	_____	Complete within specified time.	
____/52	____/52	____/52	**Total points earned** (To obtain a percentage score, divide the total points earned by the number of points possible.)	

Comments:

Evaluator's Signature: _____ **Need to Repeat:** _____

National Curriculum Competency: CAAHEP: III.C.3.a(3)(d)   ABHES: VI.B.1.a.3(w), VI.B.1.a.8(b)

JOB SKILL 16-9
Code Diagnoses from Chapters 11, 12, 13, 14, and 15 in *ICD-9-CM*

Name _____ Date _____ Score _____

Performance Objective

Task: Code diagnoses from Chapters 11 through 15 of *ICD-9-CM*, Volumes I and II.

Conditions: Use *International Classification of Diseases—9th Revision—Clinical Modification,* Volumes I and II; and pen or pencil. Refer to Procedure 16-2 in the textbook for step-by-step directions.

Standards: Complete all steps listed in this skill in _____ minutes with a minimum score of _____. (Time element and accuracy criteria may be given by instructor.)

Time: Start: _____ Completed: _____ Total: _____ minutes

Scoring: One point for each step performed satisfactorily unless otherwise listed or weighted by instructor.

Directions with Performance Evaluation Checklist

Read the following statements, look up main terms in Volume II of the diagnostic codebook, and then confirm the code selection in Volume I.

1st Attempt	2nd Attempt	3rd Attempt		
_____	_____	_____	Gather materials (equipment and supplies) listed under "Conditions."	
____/5	____/5	____/5	1. Code excessive vomiting in early pregnancy causing dehydration.	_____
____/5	____/5	____/5	2. Code postpartum condition of retained placenta without hemorrhage.	_____
____/5	____/5	____/5	3. Code impetigo.	_____
____/5	____/5	____/5	4. Code dermatitis due to cold weather.	_____
____/5	____/5	____/5	5. Code Kaschin-Beck disease affecting multiple sites.	_____
____/5	____/5	____/5	6. Code spondylosis of the lumbar spine.	_____
____/5	____/5	____/5	7. Code complete bilateral cleft palate.	_____
____/5	____/5	____/5	8. Code accessory toe on the right foot.	_____
____/5	____/5	____/5	9. Code incompetent cervix (that caused fetal mortality).	_____
____/5	____/5	____/5	10. Code neonatal diabetes mellitus.	_____
_____	_____	_____	Complete within specified time.	
____/52	____/52	____/52	**Total points earned** (To obtain a percentage score, divide the total points earned by the number of points possible.)	

Comments:

Evaluator's Signature: _____ **Need to Repeat:** _____

National Curriculum Competency: CAAHEP: III.C.3.a(3)(d)   ABHES: VI.B.1.a.3(w), VI.B.1.a.8(b)

JOB SKILL 16-10
Code Diagnoses from Chapters 16 and 17 Plus V and E Codes in *ICD-9-CM*

Name _____ Date _____ Score _____

Performance Objective

Task: Code diagnoses from Chapters 16 and 17 of *ICD-9-CM,* Volumes I and II, code factors that influence health care status using V codes, and code external causes of injury and poisoning using E codes.

Conditions: Use *International Classification of Diseases—9th Revision—Clinical Modification,* Volumes I and II; and pen or pencil. Refer to Procedure 16-2 in the textbook for step-by-step directions.

Standards: Complete all steps listed in this skill in _____ minutes with a minimum score of _____. (Time element and accuracy criteria may be given by instructor.)

Time: Start: _____ Completed: _____ Total: _____ minutes

Scoring: One point for each step performed satisfactorily unless otherwise listed or weighted by instructor.

Directions with Performance Evaluation Checklist

Read the following statements, look up main terms in Volume II of the diagnostic codebook, and then confirm the code selection in Volume I. Use the Index to External Causes of Injury when selecting E codes, found at the end of Volume II.

1st Attempt	2nd Attempt	3rd Attempt		
_____	_____	_____	Gather materials (equipment and supplies) listed under "Conditions."	
____/5	____/5	____/5	1. Code frequency of urination.	_____
____/5	____/5	____/5	2. Code microcalcification found on mammogram.	_____
____/5	____/5	____/5	3. Code fracture of two ribs.	_____
____/5	____/5	____/5	4. Code left ankle sprain.	_____
____/5	____/5	____/5	5. Code supervision of first normal pregnancy.	_____
____/5	____/5	____/5	6. Code personal history of blood disease.	_____
____/5	____/5	____/5	7. Code influenza vaccination.	_____
____/5	____/5	____/5	8. Code positive HIV test result with no symptoms.	_____
____/5	____/5	____/5	9. Code rattlesnake bite.	_____
____/5	____/5	____/5	10. Code an accidental poisoning using tranquilizers.	_____
_____	_____	_____	Complete within specified time.	
____/52	____/52	____/52	**Total points earned** (To obtain a percentage score, divide the total points earned by the number of points possible.)	

Comments:

Evaluator's Signature: _____ **Need to Repeat:** _____

National Curriculum Competency: CAAHEP: III.C.3.a(3)(d)	ABHES: VI.B.1.a.3(w), VI.B.1.a.8(b)

JOB SKILL 16-11
Complete a Managed Care Authorization Form

Name _____ Date _____ Score _____

Performance Objective

Task: Complete a managed care authorization form coding diagnosis and procedure.

Conditions: Use Managed Care Plan Treatment Authorization Request (Form 83), computer or typewriter, *ICD-9-CM* codebook, and *CPT* codebook.* Refer to textbook Figure 16-1 for a visual example.

Standards: Complete all steps listed in this skill in _____ minutes with a minimum score of _____.
                  (Time element and accuracy criteria may be given by instructor.)

Time: Start: _____ **Completed:** _____ **Total:** _____ minutes

Scoring: One point for each step performed satisfactorily unless otherwise listed or weighted by instructor.

Directions with Performance Evaluation Checklist

Read the following scenario and complete the Managed Care Authorization Form: On August 3, (current year), Antoyan Gagonian comes into Dr. Gerald Practon's office complaining of low back pain of two weeks' duration. He has difficulty walking, moving to a sitting position, and standing from a sitting position. Mr. Gagonian, born on October 10, 1963, lives at 2345 West Bath Street, Woodland Hills, XY 12345-0324; telephone number (555) 765-0720.

After taking a history and complete physical examination, Dr. Practon orders x-rays of the lower back and determines a working diagnosis of lumbago due to displacement of lumbar intervertebral disc. However, Mr. Gagonian's symptoms exceed typical criteria for this diagnosis. The patient is given a prescription for pain medication and muscle relaxant for muscle spasm. Dr. Practon recommends a magnetic resonance imaging (MRI) scan of the lumbar spine (without contrast) to investigate the problem further. The scan is to be done at College Hospital outpatient radiology.

Dr. Practon is the primary care physician for the managed care program, Health Net, of which Mr. Gagonian is a member. Dr. Practon's state license number is his member identification number with the insurance company. An authorization must be obtained for this study; the patient's insurance eligibility is verified today.

1st Attempt	2nd Attempt	3rd Attempt	
_____	_____	_____	Gather materials (equipment and supplies) listed under "Conditions."
_____/6	_____/6	_____/6	1. Complete the patient's demographic information on the authorization form.
_____/5	_____/5	_____/5	2. Complete the information for the primary care physician, referring physician, and managed care plan.
_____/8	_____/8	_____/8	3. Code the diagnosis and list the description.
_____/5	_____/5	_____/5	4. Indicate the treatment plan.
_____/7	_____/7	_____/7	5. Code the requested procedure or test and list the description.
_____/3	_____/3	_____/3	6. Indicate the facility information.
_____	_____	_____	7. Obtain the physician's signature.
_____/4	_____/4	_____/4	8. Have Dr. Practon complete the primary care physician portion of the form.
_____	_____	_____	Complete within specified time.
_____/41	_____/41	_____/41	**Total points earned** (To obtain a percentage score, divide the total points earned by the number of points possible.)

Current Procedural Terminology codes, descriptions, and two-digit numeric modifiers only are from *CPT 2007*. ©2006, American Medical Association. All rights reserved.

JOB SKILL 16-11 *(continued)*

Comments:

JOB SKILL 16-12
Complete a Health Insurance Claim Form for a Commercial Case

Name _____ Date _____ Score _____

Performance Objective

Task: Abstract information from a patient record and progress note to code diagnoses and procedures and complete a health insurance claim form for a commercial case. Determine fees and post the information to the patient's ledger card.

Conditions: 1. Complete one health insurance claim form (Form 84).
2. Refer to Cathy B. Maywood's patient record and progress notes (*Workbook* Figure 16-1).
3. Use *CPT* codebook* to code procedures and services (or Tables 16-5 and 16-6 in the textbook for E/M services).
4. Use *ICD-9-CM* codebook to code diagnoses.
5. Locate physician information and charges in the fee schedule in Part IV of the *Workbook*.
6. Refer to CMS-1500 field instructions for commercial insurance in Appendix A of the textbook.
7. View insurance template for a visual example of a completed commercial (private) insurance claim form (Figure A-1 in Appendix A of the textbook).
8. Complete a ledger card (Figure 16-2 in the *Workbook*).
9. Use typewriter, pen, or pencil.

Standards: Complete all steps listed in this skill in _____ minutes with a minimum score of _____.
(Time element and accuracy criteria may be given by instructor.)

Time: Start: _____ Completed: _____ Total: _____ minutes

Scoring: One point for each step performed satisfactorily unless otherwise listed or weighted by instructor.

Directions with Performance Evaluation Checklist

1st Attempt	2nd Attempt	3rd Attempt	
_____	_____	_____	Gather materials (equipment and supplies) listed under "Conditions."

CMS-1500 Claim Form

____/3	____/3	____/3	1. Address the claim form to the insurance carrier.
____/19	____/19	____/19	2. Obtain patient and insured information from the patient record, and complete the top portion of the claim form.
____/3	____/3	____/3	3. On the initial date of service, obtain the patient's signature on the claim form indicating authorization to release medical information to the insurance carrier and assignment of benefits to the physician.
_____	_____	_____	5. Answer the question in Field 20 and mark the correct box.
____/7	____/7	____/7	6. Code the office consult and complete the first line of service for June 2, 20XX.
____/7	____/7	____/7	7. Code for the handling of two specimens and complete the second line of service. Note: Multiply the charge by the number of units (2) and list the total in Field 24F. Indicate 2 units in Field 24G.
____/7	____/7	____/7	8. Complete the third line of service for the procedure on June 9, 20XX.
____/7	____/7	____/7	9. Complete the fourth line of service for the procedure on June 12, 20XX.
____/18	____/18	____/18	10. Total the claim and complete Fields 25 through 33 on the claim form; date the claim June 30, current year.

Current Procedural Terminology codes, descriptions, and two-digit numeric modifiers only are from *CPT 2007.* ©2006, American Medical Association. All rights reserved.

JOB SKILL 16-12 *(continued)*

Ledger Card

____/4	____/4	____/4	11. List procedure codes in the Reference column on ledger card.
____/4	____/4	____/4	12. List charges in the Charge column on ledger card.
____/4	____/4	____/4	13. Calculate and record running balance for each charge posted.
____/5	____/5	____/5	14. Indicate when the insurance company has been billed.
_____	_____	_____	Complete within specified time.
____/93	____/93	____/93	**Total points earned** (To obtain a percentage score, divide the total points earned by the number of points possible.)

Comments:

Evaluator's Signature: _____   **Need to Repeat:** _____

National Curriculum Competency: CAAHEP: III.C.3.a(3)(b), III.C.3.a(3)(e)   ABHES: VI.B.1.a.3(x), VI.B.1.a.8(c)

JOB SKILL 16-12 *(continued)*

No. 1612

PATIENT RECORD

Maywood	Cathy	B.	11-24-62	F	(555) 592-1841
LAST NAME	**FIRST NAME**	**MIDDLE NAME**	**BIRTH DATE**	**SEX**	**HOME PHONE**
384 Gary Street		Woodland Hills	XY		12345
ADDRESS		**CITY**	**STATE**		**ZIP CODE**
(555) 206-7788			Cmaywood@EM.com		
CELL PHONE	**PAGER NO.**	**FAX NO.**	**E-MAIL ADDRESS**		
458-XX-2601			CP22498X		
PATIENT'S SOC. SEC. NO.			**DRIVER'S LICENSE**		
public relations secretary		St. Joseph's Hospital			
PATIENT'S OCCUPATION		**NAME OF COMPANY**			
4501 Main Street Woodland Hills, XY 1234				(555) 581-2600	
ADDRESS OF EMPLOYER				**PHONE**	
Robert M. Maywood		supervisor			
SPOUSE OR PARENT		**OCCUPATION**			
United Parcel		261 Jeffers Street, Woodland Hills, XY 12345		(555) 521-8011	
EMPLOYER		**ADDRESS**		**PHONE**	
Colonial Health Ins. Co. 11 Royal St. Woodland Hills, 12345			self		
NAME OF INSURANCE		**INSURED OR SUBSCRIBER**			
265012B		687SJ			
POLICY/CERTIFICATE NO.		**GROUP NO.**			

REFERRED BY: Bert B. Evans, MD, NPI 00065411XX

DATE	PROGRESS
6/2/20XX	New patient was referred for consultation (comprehensive history and examination with moderate medical decision making) with complaints of irregular vaginal bleeding after intercourse. Pelvic exam showed cervicitis and cervical erosion. Pap smear and cervical mucosa smear taken and sent to outside laboratory. Patient to return in one week for possible cauterization of cervix. llf *Fvan Pvactom, MD*
6/9/20XX	Lab results indicate Class 1IB PAP. Patient has cryocauterization of cervix performed. Recommend endometrial biopsy. Pt. scheduled for outpatient surgery at College Hospital on June 12, 20XX. llf *Fvan Pvactom, MD*
6/12/20XX	Pt reports to outpatient surgery at College Hospital at 5:30 a.m. Endometrial biopsy performed. Diagnosis: Postcoital bleeding. llf *Fvan Pvactom, MD*

Figure 16-1

JOB SKILL 16-12 *(continued)*

STATEMENT
PRACTON MEDICAL GROUP, INC.
4567 Broad Avenue
Woodland Hills, XY 12345-4700
Tel. 555-486-9002
Fax No. 555-488-7815

Cathy B. Maywood
384 Gary Street
Woodland Hills, XY 12345

Phone No.(H) 555-592-1841 (W) 555-581-2600   Birthdate 11-24-62
Insurance Co. Colonial Health Ins. Co.   Policy No. 265012B / 687SJ

DATE	REFERENCE	DESCRIPTION	CHARGES	Pymnts	Adj	BALANCE	
		BALANCE FORWARD					
6-2-XX		Consult NP					
6-2-XX		Handling of Specimens					
6-9-XX		Cauterization of Cervix					
6-12-XX		Endometrial Bx					

CREDITS

Pay last amount in balance column ↑

Figure 16-2

JOB SKILL 16-12 *(continued)*

CMS-1500 Comment Sheet for Job Skills 16-12, 16-13, and 16-14

INSTRUCTOR: This comment sheet may be used to grade insurance claim forms instead of, or in addition to the Performance Evaluation Checklist that appears within these job skills; make copies as needed.

TOTAL POINTS EARNED:_____   TOTAL POINTS POSSIBLE: 100

Evaluator's Signature:_____

BLOCK	INCORRECT	MISSING	NOT NEEDED	REMARKS	BLOCK	INCORRECT	MISSING	NOT NEEDED	REMARKS
Top					18				
1					19				
1a									
2					20				
3					21				
4									
5					22				
6					23				
7					24a				
8					24b				
					24c				
9					24d				
9a									
9b									
9c					24e				
9d									
					24f				
10a					24g				
10b					24h,				
10c					24i				
10d					24j				
11					25, 26				
11a					27				
11b					28				
11c					29				
11d									
12					30				
13									
14					31				
15									
16					32				
17									
17a					33				
					Refererence Initials				

JOB SKILL 16-13
Complete a Health Insurance Claim Form for a Medicare Case

Name _____ Date _____ Score _____

Performance Objective

Task: Abstract information from a patient record and progress note to code diagnoses and procedures and complete a health insurance claim form for a Medicare case. Determine fees and post the information to the patient's ledger card.

Conditions: 1. Complete one health insurance claim form (Form 85).
2. Refer to Michael T. Donlevy's patient record and progress notes (*Workbook* Figure 16-3).
3. Use *CPT* codebook* to code procedures and services (or Tables 16-5 and 16-6 in the textbook for E/M services).
4. Use *ICD-9-CM* codebook to code diagnoses.
5. Locate physician information and charges in the fee schedule in Part IV of the *Workbook*.
6. Refer to CMS-1500 field instructions for the Medicare program in Appendix A of the textbook.
7. View insurance template for a visual example of a completed Medicare claim form in Figure 16-3 of the textbook.
8. Complete a ledger card (Figure 16-4 in the *Workbook*).
9. Use typewriter, pen, or pencil.

Standards: Complete all steps listed in this skill in _____ minutes with a minimum score of _____.
(Time element and accuracy criteria may be given by instructor.)

Time: Start: _____ Completed: _____ Total: _____ minutes

Scoring: One point for each step performed satisfactorily unless otherwise listed or weighted by instructor.

Directions with Performance Evaluation Checklist

Dr. Gerald Practon is a participating physician with the Medicare program, so he accepts assignment; bill using the participating physician fees. After completing the claim form and ledger card, refer to the Mock Fee Schedule in the *Workbook* and answer the fee-related questions.

1st Attempt	2nd Attempt	3rd Attempt	
_____	_____	_____	Gather materials (equipment and supplies) listed under "Conditions."

CMS-150 Claim Form

____/3	____/3	____/3	1.	Address the claim form to the Medicare Fiscal Intermediary.
____/16	____/16	____/16	2.	Obtain patient and insured information from the patient record and complete the top portion of the claim form.
____/3	____/3	____/3	3.	On the initial date of service, obtain the patient's signature on the claim form indicating authorization to release medical information to the insurance carrier and assignment of benefits to the physician.
____/2	____/2	____/2	4.	Fill in Field 14 and answer the question in Field 20; mark the correct box.
____/7	____/7	____/7	5.	Code the emergency room visit and complete the first line of service for June 3, 20XX.
____/7	____/7	____/7	6.	Code the procedure and complete the second line of service for June 3, 20XX.
_____	_____	_____	7.	Determine whether or not you would bill for the follow-up office visit, and state the logic for your answer.
____/17	____/17	____/17	8.	Total the claim and complete Fields 25 through 33 on the claim form.
_____	_____	_____	9.	Date the claim June 30, current year.

Current Procedural Terminology codes, descriptions, and two-digit numeric modifiers only are from *CPT 2007*. ©2006, American Medical Association. All rights reserved.

JOB SKILL 16-13 *(continued)*

Ledger Card

_____/2 _____/2 _____/2   10. List procedure codes in Reference column on ledger card.

_____/2 _____/2 _____/2   11. List charges in Charge column on ledger card.

_____/2 _____/2 _____/2   12. Calculate and record running balance for each charge posted.

_____/4 _____/4 _____/4   13. Indicate when the insurance company has been billed.

Fee Schedule

_____/2 _____/2 _____/2   14. If Dr. Practon is *participating* in the Medicare program, how much will he receive for the emergency room visit?

From Medicare: $ _____

From the patient: $ _____

_____ _____ _____   15. If Dr. Practon is *not participating* in the Medicare program, how much will he receive for the emergency room visit from Medicare? $ _____

_____/2 _____/2 _____/2   16. If Dr. Practon is *not participating* in the Medicare program and charges the maximum *limiting charge,* how much will he receive for the emergency room visit?

From Medicare: $ _____

From the patient: $ _____

_____ _____ _____   Complete within specified time.

____/74 ____/74 ____/74   **Total points earned** (To obtain a percentage score, divide the total points earned by the number of points possible.)

Comments:

JOB SKILL 16-13 *(continued)*

No. 1613

PATIENT RECORD

Donlevy	Michael	T.		3/10/17	M	(555) 421-0015
LAST NAME	**FIRST NAME**	**MIDDLE NAME**		**BIRTH DATE**	**SEX**	**HOME PHONE**

2821 Georgia Street	Woodland Hills	XY	12345
ADDRESS	**CITY**	**STATE**	**ZIP CODE**

CELL PHONE	**PAGER NO.**	**FAX NO.**	**E-MAIL ADDRESS**
451-XX-9003			D033123X
PATIENT'S SOC. SEC. NO.			**DRIVER'S LICENSE**

Retired truck driver

PATIENT'S OCCUPATION	**NAME OF COMPANY**

ADDRESS OF EMPLOYER		**PHONE**

Patricia M. Donlevy	retired	
SPOUSE OR PARENT	**OCCUPATION**	

EMPLOYER	**ADDRESS**	**PHONE**

Medicare Fiscal Intermediary PO Box 123, Anytown, XY 12345	self
NAME OF INSURANCE	**INSURED OR SUBSCRIBER**

451-XX-9003A	
POLICY/CERTIFICATE NO.	**GROUP NO.**

REFERRED BY: Harry Donlevy (brother)

DATE	**PROGRESS**
6/3/20XX	Called to ER at the request of patient who fell at home and cut his head (EPF HX & PX, LC MDM). Sutured a 3.5 cm scalp wound (intermediate repair laceration). RTO in 4 days for dressing change. llf *Gerald Practon, MD*
6/7/20XX	Dressing changed. Wound healing well, no signs of infection. Pt RTO next week for suture removal. llf *M. Athims, CMA*

Figure 16-3

JOB SKILL 16-13 *(continued)*

STATEMENT
PRACTON MEDICAL GROUP, INC.
4567 Broad Avenue
Woodland Hills, XY 12345-4700
Tel. 555 -486-9002
Fax No. 555 -488-7815

Michael T. Donlevy
2821 Georgia Street
Woodland Hills, XY 12345

Phone No.(H) 555-421-0015 (W)_____ Birthdate 3/10/17_____
Insurance Co. Medicare_____ Policy No. 451-xx-9003A____

DATE	REFERENCE	DESCRIPTION	CHARGES	CREDITS		BALANCE
				Pymnts	Adj	
		BALANCE FORWARD				
6-3-xx		ER Visit				
6-3-xx		Laceration repair				

Pay last amount in balance column   ↑

Figure 16-4

JOB SKILL 16-14
Complete a Health Insurance Claim Form for a TRICARE Case

Name _____ Date _____ Score _____

Performance Objective

Task: Abstract information from a patient record and progress note to code diagnoses and procedures and complete a health insurance claim form for a TRICARE case. Determine fees and post the information to the patient's ledger card.

Conditions: 1. Complete one health insurance claim form (Form 86).
2. Refer to Frances O. Davidson's patient record and progress notes (*Workbook* Figure 16-5).
3. Use *CPT* codebook* to code procedures and services (or Tables 16-5 and 16-6 in the textbook for E/M services).
4. Use *ICD-9-CM* codebook to code diagnoses.
5. Locate physician information and charges in the fee schedule in Part IV of the *Workbook*.
6. Refer to CMS-1500 field instructions for the TRICARE program in Appendix A of the textbook.
7. View insurance template for a visual example of a completed TRICARE claim form in Figure 16-9 of the textbook.
8. Complete a ledger card (Figure 16-6 in the *Workbook*).
9. Use typewriter, pen, or pencil.

Standards: Complete all steps listed in this skill in _____ minutes with a minimum score of _____.
(Time element and accuracy criteria may be given by instructor.)

Time: Start: _____ Completed: _____ Total: _____ minutes

Scoring: One point for each step performed satisfactorily unless otherwise listed or weighted by instructor.

Directions with Performance Evaluation Checklist

Dr. Gerald Practon is a participating physician with the TRICARE program, so he accepts assignment; bill using the mock fees.

1st Attempt	2nd Attempt	3rd Attempt	
_____	_____	_____	Gather materials (equipment and supplies) listed under "Conditions."

CMS-1500 Claim Form

_____/3	_____/3	_____/3	1. Address the claim form to TRICARE.
_____/26	_____/26	_____/26	2. Obtain patient and insured information from the patient record, and complete the top portion of the claim form.
_____/3	_____/3	_____/3	3. On the initial date of service, obtain the patient's signature on the claim form indicating authorization to release medical information to the insurance carrier and assignment of benefits to the physician.
_____	_____	_____	4. Answer the question in Field 20 and mark the correct box.
_____/7	_____/7	_____/7	5. Code the office visit and complete the first line of service for June 4, 20XX.
_____/7	_____/7	_____/7	6. Code the electrocardiogram and complete the second line of service for June 4, 20XX.
_____/7	_____/7	_____/7	7. Code the spirometry and complete the third line of service for June 4, 20XX.
_____/7	_____/7	_____/7	8. Code the blood draw and complete the fourth line of service for June 4, 20XX.
_____/7	_____/7	_____/7	9. Code the handling fee and complete the fifth line of service for June 4, 20XX.
_____/7	_____/7	_____/7	10. Code the urinalysis and complete the sixth line of service for June 4, 20XX.
_____/18	_____/18	_____/18	11. Total the claim and complete Fields 25 through 33 on the claim form; date the claim June 30, current year .

Current Procedural Terminology codes, descriptions, and two-digit numeric modifiers only are from *CPT 2007*. ©2006, American Medical Association. All rights reserved.

JOB SKILL 16-14 *(continued)*

Ledger Card

_____/6 _____/6 _____/6   12. List procedure codes in Reference column on ledger card.

_____/6 _____/6 _____/6   13. List charges in Charge column on ledger card.

_____/6 _____/6 _____/6   14. Calculate and record running balance for each charge posted.

_____/4 _____/4 _____/4   15. Indicate when the insurance company has been billed.

_____ _____ _____   Complete within specified time.

___/117 ___/117 ___/117   **Total points earned** (To obtain a percentage score, divide the total points earned by the number of points possible.)

Comments:

Evaluator's Signature: _____ **Need to Repeat:** _____

National Curriculum Competency: CAAHEP: III.C.3.a(3)(b), III.C.3.a(3)(e)   ABHES: VI.B.1.a.3(v), VI.B.1.a.3(y), VI.B.1.a.8(c)

JOB SKILL 16-14 (*continued*)

No. 1614

PATIENT RECORD

Davidson	Frances	O.	4/10/50	F	(555) 217-8105
LAST NAME	**FIRST NAME**	**MIDDLE NAME**	**BIRTH DATE**	**SEX**	**HOME PHONE**
128 Watson Street		Woodland Hills	XY		12345
ADDRESS		**CITY**	**STATE**		**ZIP CODE**
(555) 324-0088		(555) 217-8105	Fdavidson@EM.com		
CELL PHONE	**PAGER NO.**	**FAX NO.**	**E-MAIL ADDRESS**		
283-XX-1651			D034963X		
PATIENT'S SOC. SEC. NO.			**DRIVER'S LICENSE**		
tailor		Sampson Department Store			
PATIENT'S OCCUPATION		**NAME OF COMPANY**			
7841 Broadway St. Woodland Hills, XY 12345				(555) 289-7811	
ADDRESS OF EMPLOYER				**PHONE**	
Lieutenant William C. Davidson		U.S. Navy Lieutenant/Active Status NY		DOB 11/4/51	
SPOUSE OR PARENT		**OCCUPATION**			
USN		PO Box 1878, APO New York, NY 09194			
EMPLOYER		**ADDRESS**		**PHONE**	
TRICARE Standard, PO Box 444, Anytown, XY 12345			husband/sponsor		
NAME OF INSURANCE			**INSURED OR SUBSCRIBER**		
Social Security no. 821-XX-2601					
POLICY/CERTIFICATE NO.		**GROUP NO.**			

REFERRED BY: Martha B. Emory (friend)

DATE	PROGRESS
6/4/20XX	New patient comes in with CC of chest pain (moderate to severe), difficulty breathing, weakness, fatigue, & dizziness (Level 4 E/M). Performed ECG; normal sinus rhythm. Performed spirometry total and timed capacity; reduced lung capacity. Took blood specimen and sent to outside lab for CBC and basic metabolic panel. UA (non-automated with microscopy) neg. Edema throughout lower extremities. Dx: congestive heart failure. Start patient on diuretic; may need hospitalization. RTO tomorrow. llf <div style="text-align:right">Gerald Practon, MD</div>

Figure 16-5

JOB SKILL 16-14 *(continued)*

STATEMENT
PRACTON MEDICAL GROUP, INC.
4567 Broad Avenue
Woodland Hills, XY 12345-4700
Tel. 555-486-9002
Fax No. 555-488-7815

Frances O. Davidson
128 Watson Street
Woodland Hills, XY 12345

Phone No.(H) _555-217-8105_ (W) _555-289-7811_   Birthdate _4/10/50_
Insurance Co. _TRICARE Standard_   Policy No. _821-xx-2601_

DATE	REFERENCE	DESCRIPTION	CHARGES	CREDITS		BALANCE	
				Pymnts	Adj		
		BALANCE FORWARD					
6-4-XX		OV NP					
6-4-XX		ECG					
6-4-XX		Spirometry					
6-4-XX		Venipuncture					
6-4-XX		Handling Spec					
6-4-XX		UA					

Pay last amount in balance column   ↑

Figure 16-6

Office Managerial Responsibilities

After completing the exercises, the student will be able to:

1. Enhance knowledge of medical terminology, interpret abbreviations, and accurately spell medical words.

2. Write an agenda for an office meeting.

3. Prepare material for an office procedures manual.

4. Abstract data from a catalog and key an order form.

5. Complete an order form for office supplies.

6. Perform mathematic calculations required for office management.

7. Prepare a travel expense report.

FOCUS ON CERTIFICATION*

CMA Content Summary

- Medical abbreviations
- Professional organizations
- Group dynamics
- Office policies
- Professional communication and behavior
- Interviewing techniques
- Legal restrictions
- Personnel standards, hiring, and termination
- OSHA compliance
- Americans with Disabilities Act
- HIPAA

- Employment laws
- Maintenance agreements and repairs of equipment
- Management report generation
- Managing physician's professional schedule and travel
- Maintain physical plant
- Office environment
- Recruit, interview, hire, evaluate, discipline, and terminate employees
- Inventory control; purchasing and storage

*This *Workbook* and accompanying textbook meet the entry-level administrative and general competencies for the CMA outlined by the AAMA Examination Content Outline and Role Delineation Study and for the RMA and CMAS outlined by the AMT Competencies and Examination Specifications (see Competency Grid in textbook Appendix B).

- Liability coverage
- Time management
- Office policies and procedures manual
- Patient brochure
- Personnel manual

- Ordering goods, monitoring invoices, tracking merchandise, paying accounts
- Maintain employee immunization records
- Preplanned emergency actions

RMA Content Summary

- HIPAA
- Laws, regulations, and acts pertaining to the practice of medicine
- Professional development; continuing education
- Interpersonal relations
- Patient brochures
- Office policies and procedures
- Family medical leave act
- Maintain practice accounts

- Supplies and equipment management
- OSHA regulations
- Computer hardware and software
- Office sanitation, safety, and comfort
- Emergency protocols and procedures
- Training employees
- Biohazardous waste controls
- Procedures to prevent infectious pathogens by employees

CMAS Content Summary

- Medical and insurance terminology
- Basic laws pertaining to the medical practice
- Continuing education
- Prevention of disease transmission
- Medical office emergencies
- Patient information materials
- Business functions
- Vendors and supplies
- Manage and supervise staff
- Performance reviews and disciplinary action
- Office procedural manual

- Recruit, orient, and train new staff members
- Manage employee benefits
- Office safety and emergency instructions
- Biohazardous waste
- OSHA
- Supply, ordering, and inventory
- Office equipment, maintenance, and repair
- Medical office environment
- Oversee facility
- Staff meetings and in-service

Abbreviation and Spelling Review

Read the following patient's chart note and write the meanings for the abbreviations listed below the note. To decode any abbreviations you do not understand or that appear unfamiliar to you, refer to the list of abbreviations in Part V of this *Workbook*. Step-by-step directions for this exercise are found in Procedure 1-1 of Chapter 1 in the text. Medical terms in the chart note are italicized; study them for spelling. Use your medical dictionary to look up their definitions. Your instructor may give a spelling and definition test that includes these words and abbreviations.

DATE	PROGRESS
12-14-20XX	Helen P Craig CC: Back pain originating in the *flank* + radiating across the *abdomen* Pt complains of *abdominal distention* & difficulty *urinating*. Exam reveals increased *sensitivity* in *lumbar* & *groin* areas. Considerable discomfort c̄ marked *urethral stenosis* U/A: 5-10 RBC occ wbc s gr 1.012 X: KUB & IVP revealed small *calculus* in R UPJ dilat to 24F c̄ Brer Inc fluid intake, low *calcium* diet Rx *Aluminum hydroxide* gel 60 ml q.i.d. RTC 1 wk. for FU + decision on whether to operate. G Practon, MD

CC _____   UPJ _____

Pt _____   dilat _____

c̄ _____   F _____

U/A _____   Brev _____

RBC _____   inc _____

occ _____   RX _____

wbc _____   ml _____

sp gr _____   q.i.d. _____

X _____   RTC _____

KUB _____   wk. _____

IVP _____   FU _____

R _____

Review Questions

Review the objectives, glossary, and chapter information before completing the following review questions.

1. Why is it important for the office manager to be a mentor and coach? _____
_____

2. What two mechanisms can be put into place in a medical office to help patient relations, promote patient satisfaction, and learn what policies and procedures need improvement? _____
_____

3. To boost job performance, what three things should be emphasized during a staff meeting?

   a. _____

   b. _____

   c. _____

4. As a new employee, where would you look to find your job description? _____
_____

5. List one federal agency that administers statutes and regulations that employers must adhere to, and name a resource it publishes that can be used to determine which statutes apply to your office. _____
_____
_____

6. What is the name of the act that covers most benefit plans in the private sector? _____
_____

7. Define *disaster response plan*. _____
_____

8. What laws prohibit job discrimination based on race, color, religion, sex, or national origin? _____
_____

9. How would you know if the Family and Medical Leave Act applies to your job in a medical office? _____
_____

10. Write the "general duty" clause from the OSH Acts, which is the basis of compliance mandated by the Occupational Safety and Health Administration. _____

    _____

    _____

    _____

    _____

    _____

11. As an office manager, what two questions will you be expected to answer if a case of sexual harassment goes to court? _____

    _____

    _____

12. What is the purpose of an office policies and procedures manual? _____

    _____

    _____

13. When hiring a new employee, what are four responsibilities of an office manager? What would you do first, second, third, and fourth? _____

    _____

14. After an employee has been hired and before he or she is expected to perform all tasks, what are two responsibilities of the office manager? _____

15. What observations should be included when an office manager evaluates a new employee? _____

    _____

    _____

16. Before selecting a housecleaning service, what must be done? _____

    _____

17. When selecting a new piece of equipment for the medical office, what are some things to consider?

    a. _____

    b. _____

    c. _____

    d. _____

    e. _____

    f. _____

    g. _____

18. What are three important points to consider when selecting a vendor to order office or medical supplies from?

    a. _____

    b. _____

    c. _____

19. State four reasons why it may be unsatisfactory to order supplies in bulk.

    a. _____

    b. _____

    c. _____

    d. _____

20. When an order for merchandise arrives, what steps should be taken after the package is opened? _____

    _____

    _____

21. Name three items that must appear on a running inventory card.

    a. _____

    b. _____

    c. _____

22. If the physician is planning to attend a medical convention, at what point should the office manager start

    making the arrangements? _____

    _____

Critical Thinking Exercises

1. As an office manager, what strategy would you use to correct an employee who is a gossip and spreads a

   harmful rumor about another employee? _____

   _____

   _____

   _____

   _____

   _____

2. List some methods that an office manager might implement to promote open and honest communication.

   _____

   _____

   _____

   _____

   _____

   _____

3. As an office manager, describe how you would make a new employee feel more relaxed during his or her first

   week at work. _____

   _____

   _____

   _____

   _____

JOB SKILL 17-1
Write an Agenda for an Office Meeting

Name _____ Date _____ Score _____

Performance Objective

Task: Assemble information and key or type an outline for an office meeting agenda.

Conditions: One sheet of white paper, computer or typewriter, example of an agenda outlining items covered in the previous staff meeting (textbook Figure 17-4), agenda suggestions posted on a bulletin board seen in *Workbook* Figure 17-1, and step-by-step directions found in Procedure 17-2 in the textbook.

Standards: Complete all steps listed in this skill in _____ minutes with a minimum score of _____. (Time element and accuracy criteria may be given by instructor.)

Time: **Start:** _____ **Completed:** _____ **Total:** _____ minutes

Scoring: One point for each step performed satisfactorily unless otherwise listed or weighted by instructor.

Directions with Performance Evaluation Checklist

Refer to textbook Figure 17-4 to learn what occurred at the previous meeting and to determine unfinished business. Study the notes in *Workbook* Figure 17-1, gathered from members of the staff, indicating actions they wish to introduce at the meeting and when the meeting is scheduled. List all subject matter for the agenda in rough draft outline form.

Mon.
I want to discuss possibility of moving transcription station to Rm. A, which is away from reception room interruptions.
Amy Fluor

from the desk of Gerald Practon...
I will present summer vacation schedule for sign-ups.
G.P.

Staff meeting scheduled for 2/25/XX in conference room at 12 noon. Lunch will be provided. Please make plans to attend.
Jane Paulsen-OM

I PLAN TO INTRODUCE GARY KLEIN, FROM MEDICAL ARTS PRESS, WHO WILL PRESENT THE ADVANTAGES OF ALPH/COLOR FILING SYSTEM. (I THINK HIS REPORT SHOULD BE SCHEDULED LAST ON THE AGENDA.)
CARLA HASKINS

F.P. and G.P.
At our last meeting I was asked to investigate cleaning services. I'm going to recommend we hire Todd's Cleaning to begin on March 15, and I'll make a motion to this effect.
Also, someone needs to notify Martha's Maids soon that we are terminating their services. Would you like me to do this?
Jane Paulsen-OM

I am going to suggest hiring an accting firm to audit the books yearly on Jan. 1.
Mike O'Shea
bookkeeper

From the desk of Fran Practon...
I will suggest that since flex-time is to be initiated in May, a committee should be named to spell out scheduling, compensation, and benefits for the staff and incorporate it into the office procedures manual; also there should be a discussion of circumstances under which an alternative work schedule will be used.

Figure 17-1

JOB SKILL 17-1 (*continued*)

1st Attempt	2nd Attempt	3rd Attempt	
_____	_____	_____	Gather materials (equipment and supplies) listed under "Conditions."
_____	_____	_____	1. Key a heading for the staff meeting agenda.
____/3	____/3	____/3	2. Indicate when the meeting will take place.
_____	_____	_____	3. Indicate that the office manager, Jane Paulsen, will act as the chairperson and will call the meeting to order.
_____	_____	_____	4. Indicate that the minutes from the previous meeting are read.
_____	_____	_____	5. Indicate who is present (all staff members are present).
____/3	____/3	____/3	6. Under Committee Reports, indicate that staff members Amy Fluor (transcription) and Mike O'Shea (bookkeeping) will be reporting as committee chairpersons.
____/3	____/3	____/3	7. Indicate that Jane Paulsen and Dr. Fran Practon will be reposting unfinished business.
____/3	____/3	____/3	8. Indicate that Dr. Gerald Practon and Carla Haskins will be reporting new business.
_____	_____	_____	9. Note that the next meeting is scheduled at 8:30 a.m. on March 20, 20XX.
_____	_____	_____	10. Indicate that the meeting is adjourned.
_____	_____	_____	Complete within specified time.
____/20	____/20	____/20	**Total points earned** (To obtain a percentage score, divide the total points earned by the number of points possible.)

Comments:

Evaluator's Signature: _____ **Need to Repeat:** _____

National Curriculum Competency: CAAHEP: III.C.3.c(1)(a)	ABHES: VI.B.1.a.6(f)

JOB SKILL 17-2
Prepare Material for an Office Procedures Manual

Name _____ Date _____ Score _____

Performance Objective

Task: Assemble information on office appointments for Practon Medical Group, Inc., and key or type a sample reference sheet for an office procedures manual.

Conditions: One or two sheets of white paper; computer or typewriter. Refer to Procedure 17-4 in the text-book for step-by-step directions. Refer to the Appointment section of "Office Policies" listed in Part IV of the *Workbook* to obtain specific appointment information. Refer to Chapter 6 for general appointment guidelines and textbook Figure 17-7 to help you plan a well-organized reference sheet.

Standards: Complete all steps listed in this skill in _____ minutes with a minimum score of _____. (Time element and accuracy criteria may be given by instructor.)

Time: **Start:** _____ **Completed:** _____ **Total:** _____ minutes

Scoring: One point for each step performed satisfactorily unless otherwise listed or weighted by instructor.

Directions with Performance Evaluation Checklist

Doctors Gerald and Fran Practon have asked you to prepare a reference sheet for the office procedures manual detailing appointment procedures. Create a page listing information regarding appointments that is easy for all employees to follow.

1st Attempt	2nd Attempt	3rd Attempt	
_____	_____	_____	Gather materials (equipment and supplies) listed under "Conditions."
_____	_____	_____	1. Key a heading for the reference sheet.
_____	_____	_____	2. Key a heading for "Appointment Office Hours."
____/3	____/3	____/3	3. List appointment days and times as well as office policy for routine appointments.
____/3	____/3	____/3	4. List appointment days and times as well as office policy for emergency appointments, work-ins, call-backs, and dictation.
____/3	____/3	____/3	5. List hospital surgery days and times for doctors Gerald and Fran Practon.
____/2	____/2	____/2	6. List the appropriate times for house calls.
_____	_____	_____	7. Create a heading for time allotment for office visits and procedures.
_____	_____	_____	8. List the time allotment for initial office visits.
_____	_____	_____	9. List the time allotment for consultations.
_____	_____	_____	10. List the time allotment for follow-up office visits.
____/6	____/6	____/6	11. List the time allotment for brief office visits for such things as suture removal; name various procedures that fit into this category.
_____	_____	_____	12. List the time allotment for office surgeries.
_____	_____	_____	13. List the office policy for house calls.
_____	_____	_____	14. Create a heading for questions to be asked when an appointment is made over the telephone.

JOB SKILL 17-2 *(continued)*

____/5 ____/5 ____/5   15. List five basic questions to ask when an appointment is made over the telephone.

      a. _____

      b. _____

      c. _____

      d. _____

      e. _____

_____ _____ _____   Complete within specified time.

____/33 ____/33 ____/33   **Total points earned** (To obtain a percentage score, divide the total points earned by the number of points possible.)

Comments:

Evaluator's Signature: _____ **Need to Repeat:** _____

National Curriculum Competency: CAAHEP: III.C.3.c(1)(a)   ABHES: VI.B.1.a.2(o)

JOB SKILL 17-3
Abstract Data from a Catalog and Key an Order Form

Name _____ Date _____ Score _____

Performance Objective

Task: Abstract information from catalog data sheets, determine charges, accurately key or type an order form, calculate discounts and sales tax, and compute a total.

Conditions: Order form (Form 87), catalog sheets (*Workbook* Figures 17-2 and 17-3), calculator, and pen or pencil. Refer in the textbook to Procedure 17-7 for step-by-step directions and Example 17-2 for an example of calculating sales tax.

Standards: Complete all steps listed in this skill in _____ minutes with a minimum score of _____. (Time element and accuracy criteria may be given by instructor.)

Time: **Start:** _____ **Completed:** _____ **Total:** _____ minutes

Scoring: One point for each step performed satisfactorily unless otherwise listed or weighted by instructor.

Directions with Performance Evaluation Checklist

Doctors Fran and Gerald Practon want to order some printed letterhead, second sheets, and envelopes from Medical Arts Press. Study and abstract the correct information from the catalog sheets, noting the discount offered for second sheets. Then, complete the order form using the name, address, and so forth of Practon Medical Group, Inc. Determine the cost for each item, calculate discounts, and insert this information on the order form.

1st Attempt	2nd Attempt	3rd Attempt	
_____	_____	_____	Gather materials (equipment and supplies) listed under "Conditions."
____/6	____/6	____/6	1. Complete the "Bill to" information on the order form.
_____	_____	_____	2. Fill in the e-mail address for Practon Medical Group, Inc., (PMGI@aol.com) on both forms.
_____	_____	_____	3. Indicate "SAME" in the "Ship to" location on the order form.
____/2	____/2	____/2	4. Fill in the customer order number (0001002345) and the source code (BTGF) from the catalog.
____/2	____/2	____/2	5. List your name as the person to call for questions and the office telephone number; you are at extension 12.
_____	_____	_____	6. List the practice specialty and number of doctors.
_____	_____	_____	7. Indicate the method of shipping as UPS 2nd Day.
____/7	____/7	____/7	8. List the first item ordered: 2,000 raised-printed 25% rag content bond paper (8½″ by 11″); black ink, type style NR, product color ivory.
____/5	____/5	____/5	9. List the second item ordered: 1,000 Hammermill bond raised printed second sheets (8½″ by 11″), color ivory; apply the discount and indicate "Unprinted."
____/7	____/7	____/7	10. List the third item ordered: 1,000 raised-printed 25% rag content bond envelopes (number 10); black ink, type style NR, color ivory.
_____	_____	_____	11. Total the merchandise order and insert figure.
_____	_____	_____	12. Calculate 7% sales tax and insert figure.
_____	_____	_____	13. Add the sales tax to the total of the order and insert figure.
_____	_____	_____	Complete within specified time.
____/38	____/38	____/38	**Total points earned** (To obtain a percentage score, divide the total points earned by the number of points possible.)

JOB SKILL 17-3 *(continued)*

Comments:

Evaluator's Signature: _____ **Need to Repeat:** _____

National Curriculum Competency: CAAHEP: III.C.3.a(1), III.C.3.a(1)(a)   ABHES: VI.B.1.a.6(d)

JOB SKILL 17-3 *(continued)*

letterheads

Distinctive. Dignified. Four popular sizes in your choice of paper stocks with flat or raised printing. Select either Hammermill Bond, an extremely popular paper noted for its bright white, smooth surface or 25% Rag Content Bond with Its cockle surface and crisp finish. We take an Intense pride In these papers and the craftsmanship of the printing. All copy in black ink.

SECOND SHEETS
Unprinted. Available at 60% of the Hammermill Bond price. Choice of onlonskin or Hammermill.

555 896 1114

RAYMOND S. STRONG, M.D.
SUITE 315 PROFESSIONAL BUILDING
1616 SHERIDAN WAY   LAKESIDE CITY XY 12345-0000

Raymond S. Strong, M.D.
1616 Sheridan Way
Suite 315, Professional Building
Lakeside City, XY 12345-0000
(555) 896-1114

Raymond S Strong MD
1616 Sheridan Way
Suite 315 Professional Building
Lakeside City XY 12345-0000
555-896-1114

555/896-1114   Suite 315 Professional Bldg
Raymond S. Strong
1616 Sheridan Way
Lakeside City XY 12345-0000

5½ 8½ inches   6¼ 9¼ inches   7¼ 10½ inches   8½ 11 inches

	HAMMERMILL BOND STOCK					25% RAG CONTENT BOND			
	Quantity	5½×8½ HB-407	6¼×9¼ HB-690	7¼×10½ HB-403	8½×11 HB-401	Quantity	5½×8½ NB-675	6¼×9¼ NB-69	7¼×10½ NB-70	8½×11 NB-81
FLAT-PRINTED	500	$9.85	$12.25	$13.55	$15.95	500	$11.35	$13.55	$16.40	$18.65
	1000	13.95	18.35	20.70	23.10	1000	16.25	22.00	24.55	26.80
	2000	24.95	30.65	34.95	39.60	2000	27.25	37.55	42.10	48.60
	5000	58.15	70.60	80.10	83.65	5000	59.55	82.15	93.25	113.50
	Quantity	5½×8½ PE-144	6¼×9¼ PE-695	7¼×10½ PE-146	8½×11 PE-140	Quantity	5½×8½ PNB-560	6¼×9¼ PNB-695	7¼×10½ PNB-540	8½×11 PNB-530
RAISED-PRINTED	500	$11.70	$14.50	$16.00	$17.65	500	$13.15	$16.00	$17.60	$21.50
	1000	16.45	20.45	22.75	25.25	1000	18.70	22.15	26.15	29.65
	2000	28.35	35.40	40.65	45.15	2000	32.80	40.75	45.50	51.15
	5000	56.30	75.15	86.90	99.65	5000	71.90	92.50	104.65	114.40

Figure 17-2

JOB SKILL 17-3 *(continued)*

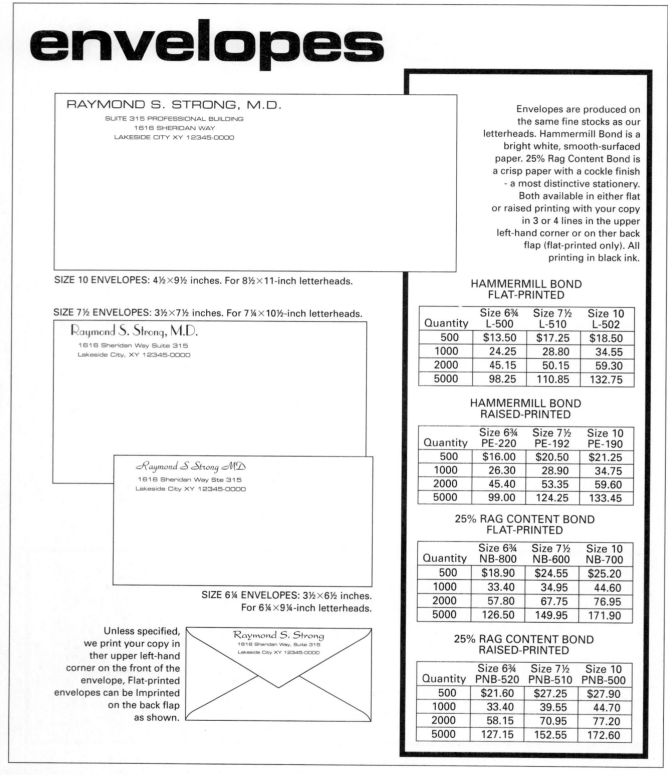

envelopes

RAYMOND S. STRONG, M.D.
SUITE 315 PROFESSIONAL BUILDING
1616 SHERIDAN WAY
LAKESIDE CITY XY 12345-0000

SIZE 10 ENVELOPES: 4½×9½ inches. For 8½×11-inch letterheads.

SIZE 7½ ENVELOPES: 3½×7½ inches. For 7¼×10½-inch letterheads.

Raymond S. Strong, M.D.
1616 Sheridan Way Suite 315
Lakeside City, XY 12345-0000

Raymond S Strong MD
1616 Sheridan Way Ste 315
Lakeside City XY 12345-0000

SIZE 6¼ ENVELOPES: 3½×6½ inches.
For 6¼×9¼-inch letterheads.

Unless specified, we print your copy in ther upper left-hand corner on the front of the envelope, Flat-printed envelopes can be Imprinted on the back flap as shown.

Raymond S. Strong
1616 Sheridan Way, Suite 315
Lakeside City XY 12345-0000

Envelopes are produced on the same fine stocks as our letterheads. Hammermill Bond is a bright white, smooth-surfaced paper. 25% Rag Content Bond is a crisp paper with a cockle finish - a most distinctive stationery. Both available in either flat or raised printing with your copy in 3 or 4 lines in the upper left-hand corner or on ther back flap (flat-printed only). All printing in black ink.

HAMMERMILL BOND FLAT-PRINTED

Quantity	Size 6¾ L-500	Size 7½ L-510	Size 10 L-502
500	$13.50	$17.25	$18.50
1000	24.25	28.80	34.55
2000	45.15	50.15	59.30
5000	98.25	110.85	132.75

HAMMERMILL BOND RAISED-PRINTED

Quantity	Size 6¾ PE-220	Size 7½ PE-192	Size 10 PE-190
500	$16.00	$20.50	$21.25
1000	26.30	28.90	34.75
2000	45.40	53.35	59.60
5000	99.00	124.25	133.45

25% RAG CONTENT BOND FLAT-PRINTED

Quantity	Size 6¾ NB-800	Size 7½ NB-600	Size 10 NB-700
500	$18.90	$24.55	$25.20
1000	33.40	34.95	44.60
2000	57.80	67.75	76.95
5000	126.50	149.95	171.90

25% RAG CONTENT BOND RAISED-PRINTED

Quantity	Size 6¾ PNB-520	Size 7½ PNB-510	Size 10 PNB-500
500	$21.60	$27.25	$27.90
1000	33.40	39.55	44.70
2000	58.15	70.95	77.20
5000	127.15	152.55	172.60

Figure 17-3

JOB SKILL 17-4
Complete an Order Form for Office Supplies

Name _____ Date _____ Score _____

Performance Objective

Task: Complete an order form for office supplies, filling in designated spaces and computing total amount ordered.

Conditions: Order form (Form 88) and pen or pencil. Refer to Procedure 17-7 in the textbook for step-step directions and Figure 17-9 in the textbook for a visual example.

Standards: Complete all steps listed in this skill in _____ minutes with a minimum score of _____. (Time element and accuracy criteria may be given by instructor.)

Time: Start: _____ Completed: _____ Total: _____ minutes

Scoring: One point for each step performed satisfactorily unless otherwise listed or weighted by instructor.

Directions with Performance Evaluation Checklist

Doctors Fran and Gerald Practon have asked you to order some office supplies. Neatly and accurately complete the order form.

1st Attempt	2nd Attempt	3rd Attempt	
_____	_____	_____	Gather materials (equipment and supplies) listed under "Conditions."
_____	_____	_____	1. Fill in the customer number (0001002345).
____/5	____/5	____/5	2. Complete the customer contact information.
____/7	____/7	____/7	3. Order four 1,000 single-sheet cartons of CMS-1500 laser-printed insurance claim forms (8½″ by 11″), $29.95/carton, Cat. No. RED-25104, page 53.
____/7	____/7	____/7	4. Order four boxes of end-tab file folders with two fasteners (blue, letter size), ¾″ expansions, $40.90/box, Cat No. GLW-FF113, page 32.
____/7	____/7	____/7	5. Order six daily group practice wirebound appointment books with 15- minute appointments, four columns per page, appointments from 8 a.m. to 7:45 p.m. (11″ by 7 ⅞″), $29.15 each (price break: for each five ordered, one is free), Cat. No. GLW-AB402, page 65.
____/7	____/7	____/7	6. Order five packages of large envelopes (9″ by 12″) with clasp, 28 lb heavyweight Kraft, 25/pkg., $3.75 pkg., Cat No. 42SH-11, page 61.
____/7	____/7	____/7	7. Order two packages of double-prong clasp envelopes (9″ by 12″), reinforced eyelet, gummed flaps, $4.25/pkg., Cat. No. 387-ACJ, page 62.
____/7	____/7	____/7	8. Order two dozen packages of Post-it flags, Style No. 680-1 (1″ by 1.7″), one dozen red, one dozen yellow, $1.49 pkg., Cat. No. 49WEX-52, page 50.
_____	_____	_____	9. Total order and insert figure.
_____	_____	_____	10. Calculate and insert sales tax at 6%.
_____	_____	_____	11. Determine the two-day shipping and handling fee, which is 5% of the total order. This is waived for orders over $400; and a flat fee of $15.00 is charged.
_____	_____	_____	12. Add the sales tax and shipping and handling fee to determine the total amount for the order; insert this figure on the order form.
____/4	____/4	____/4	13. You will be paying for the order with the company credit card, which is a Visa card, number 2222-3333-4444-XXXX, expiration date August, 2014. You have signature authority on the card; complete this section.
_____	_____	_____	Complete within specified time.
____/58	____/58	____/58	**Total points earned** (To obtain a percentage score, divide the total points earned by the number of points possible.)

JOB SKILL 17-4 *(continued)*

Comments:

National Curriculum Competency: CAAHEP: III.C.3.a(1), III.C.3.c(1)(a)   ABHES: VI.B.1.a.6(d)

JOB SKILL 17-5
Perform Mathematic Calculations of an Office Manager

Name _____ Date _____ Score _____

Performance Objective

Task:　　　　Perform basic mathematic calculations when ordering supplies to determine the cost, taking advantage of special discounts, and applying sales tax.

Conditions:　Calculator, paper, and pencil.

Standards:　Complete all steps listed in this skill in _____ minutes with a minimum score of _____.
　　　　　　(Time element and accuracy criteria may be given by instructor.)

Time:　　　　Start: _____ Completed: _____ Total: _____ minutes

Scoring:　　One point for each step performed satisfactorily unless otherwise listed or weighted by instructor.

Directions with Performance Evaluation Checklist

The office manager may be responsible for ordering supplies, and he or she should be able to perform basic mathematics to calculate discounts and sales tax amounts. Wise purchasing and correct math procedures can save the office added expense. Solve the following problems, assuming that you pay all bills within the discount period stated. Discounts are subtracted before sales tax is added.

1st Attempt	2nd Attempt	3rd Attempt	
_____	_____	_____	Gather materials (equipment and supplies) listed under "Conditions."
_____/2	_____/2	_____/2	1. The laundry bill is $33.80. If paid within 10 days, the company allows a 2.5% discount. Calculate the amount of the bill. $ _____
_____/5	_____/5	_____/5	2. Mr. Carl McFadden had five office visits at $25 each, three injections at $8.50 each, an x-ray at $26.60, and a home visit at $40.00. He has a $4.60 credit on his account. What will be the amount of his next bill? $ _____
_____/2	_____/2	_____/2	3. Mr. Bill Nelson is scheduled to have corrective surgery, which will be $385. He is asked to make a down payment of $50 before the operation, and then his payments will be divided into six equal installments. What will be the amount of each installment? $ _____
____/10	____/10	____/10	4. The following items are on an invoice that arrived today. You are required to check to see that the bill is correct and that the supplies received are the ones ordered. The physician will receive a 3% discount, and sales tax is 6%. The total shown on the invoice is $26.14. Calculate and verify that the amount is correct.

                    4 bottles rubbing alcohol @ $2.25 each

                    3 thermometers @ $1.95 each

                    6 boxes cotton @ $.29 each

                    6 bottles mouthwash @ $.89 each

                    11 cartons cotton swabs @ $.39 each

                    3 hypodermic needles @ $.39 each

      The correct amount for which the check would be written is $ _____.

1st Attempt	2nd Attempt	3rd Attempt	
_____/5	_____/5	_____/5	5. Paper towels are sold at the rate of $6.50 per dozen rolls. Figure the cost of 10 dozen rolls of towels with a 3.5% discount and a 6% sales tax. $ _____

JOB SKILL 17-5 (*continued*)

____/6   ____/6   ____/6   6. Dr. Fran Practon needs 500 needles priced at $2.60 per hundred. If she pays within 10 days, she receives a 2% discount; sales tax is 5.5%. What amount would you pay with the discount? $ _____

____/6   ____/6   ____/6   7. An advertisement states that eight thermometers cost $12.42 minus a 3% discount. Dr. Practon wants to order a dozen to take advantage of the savings; sales tax is 5%. What would the cost be? $ _____

____/3   ____/3   ____/3   8. Robert Mason's account of $98.50 has been delinquent for three months. According to the office procedures manual, after 90 days a 2% service charge, compounded monthly, is added to future bills. What will be the amount owed after nine months? $ _____

____/2   ____/2   ____/2   9. Steri-strips cost $4.95 per box; there are 100 in a box.

    a. How much would 300 Steri-strips cost? $ _____

    b. How much would 700 Steri-strips cost? $ _____

____/12   ____/12   ____/12   10. If the Steri-strips are purchased in large lots of 1,000 or more, the manufacturer allows a discount of 15%.

    a. How much would 3,000 Steri-strips cost? $ _____

    b. How much would 14,000 Steri-strips cost? $ _____

    c. If an orthopedic surgical group uses 200 Steri-strips a month, how much would be saved in a year by making a single purchase for a year's supply rather than 12 monthly purchases? $ _____

_____   _____   _____   Complete within specified time.

____/55   ____/55   ____/55   **Total points earned** (To obtain a percentage score, divide the total points earned by the number of points possible.)

Comments:

Evaluator's Signature: _____   **Need to Repeat:** _____

National Curriculum Competency: CAAHEP: III.C.3.c(4)(d)   ABHES: VI.B.1.a.6(d)

JOB SKILL 17-6
Prepare Two Order Forms

Name _____ Date _____ Score _____

Performance Objective

Task: Key or type two order forms for medical supplies using the given information and determine the total amount owed after taking advantage of all discounts.

Conditions: Order forms (Form 89 and 90) and computer or typewriter. Refer to Procedure 17-7 in the textbook for step-by-step directions and Figure 17-9 in the textbook for a visual example.

Standards: Complete all steps listed in this skill in _____ minutes with a minimum score of _____. (Time element and accuracy criteria may be given by instructor.)

Time: Start: _____ Completed: _____ Total: _____ minutes

Scoring: One point for each step performed satisfactorily unless otherwise listed or weighted by instructor.

Directions with Performance Evaluation Checklist

Use the following information to order office and medical supplies. Determine the total for all merchandise, subtract the physician's discount, and then add the sales tax. The supplies are to be shipped to Practon Medical Group, Inc. Note: Photocopies would be made before sending off the order; all prices are fictitious.

1st Attempt	2nd Attempt	3rd Attempt	
_____	_____	_____	Gather materials (equipment and supplies) listed under "Conditions."
____/10	____/10	____/10	1. Complete the "Bill to" information on both order forms.
____/2	____/2	____/2	2. Fill in the e-mail address for Practon Medical Group, Inc., (PMGI@aol.com) on both forms.
____/2	____/2	____/2	3. Indicate "SAME" in the "Ship to" location on both order forms.
____/4	____/4	____/4	4. Fill in the customer order number (0001002345) and the source code (BTGF) from the catalog.
____/4	____/4	____/4	5. List your name as the person to call for questions and the office telephone number; you are at extension 12.
____/2	____/2	____/2	6. List the practice specialty and number of doctors.
____/2	____/2	____/2	7. Indicate the method of shipping as UPS 2nd Day.

Order No. 1

1st	2nd	3rd	
____/6	____/6	____/6	8. Order four reams of white 8½″ by 11″ bond paper, 20# weight, catalog number P20, unit price $12.95.
____/5	____/5	____/5	9. Order five boxes security-lined envelopes, 500/box, no. 6¾, catalog number E60, unit price 19.99.
____/5	____/5	____/5	10. Order 1,500 large no. 10 envelopes, catalog number E10, unit price $5.50M.*
____/5	____/5	____/5	11. Order six boxes red fine-line ballpoint pens, catalog number B23, unit price $3.95.
_____	_____	_____	12. Subtotal the merchandise order and insert figure.
_____	_____	_____	13. Calculate 2% discount and insert figure.
_____	_____	_____	14. Subtract discount from subtotal.
_____	_____	_____	15. Insert total on order form.
_____	_____	_____	16. Calculate 5.5% sales tax and insert figure.
_____	_____	_____	17. Add the sales tax and insert total for order.

*M is the Roman numeral that means one thousand.

JOB SKILL 17-6 *(continued)*

Order No. 2

_____/4 _____/4 _____/4 18. Order three surgeon's blade handles (Model No. B872C), catalog number BH3, unit price $2.95.

_____/4 _____/4 _____/4 19. Order two dozen scalpel blades (No. F112), 12 to a box, catalog number SB2, unit price $1.39.

_____/4 _____/4 _____/4 20. Order four Oval Duplex thermometers, rectal, catalog number T66, unit price $2.95.

_____/4 _____/4 _____/4 21. Order 3M* tongue blades, catalog number RB2, unit price $2.50M.

_____/8 _____/8 _____/8 22. Order 5,000 laser (8.5″ by 11″), OCR-scannable red ink insurance claim forms (single sheets) for Dr. Fran Practon with her state license number printed on the form. Catalog number CMS29, unit prices: $43.99/1,000; $77.99/2,000; $144.99/5,000; $239.99/10,000; $389.99/20,000.

_____ _____ _____ 23. Subtotal the merchandise order and insert figure.

_____ _____ _____ 24. Calculate a 3% discount and subtract it from the subtotal.

_____ _____ _____ 25. List the merchandise total.

_____ _____ _____ 26. Calculate 4% sales tax and insert figure.

_____ _____ _____ 26. Add the sales tax to the total of the order and insert figure.

_____ _____ _____ Complete within specified time.

_____/84 _____/84 _____/84 **Total points earned** (To obtain a percentage score, divide the total points earned by the number of points possible.)

Comments:

Evaluator's Signature: _____ **Need to Repeat:** _____

National Curriculum Competency: CAAHEP: III.C.3.a(1), III.C.3.c(1)(a)	ABHES: VI.B.1.a.6(d)

*M is the Roman numeral that means one thousand.

JOB SKILL 17-7
Prepare a Travel Expense Report

Name _____ Date _____ Score _____

Performance Objective

Task: Complete a Travel Expense Report for the accountant.

Conditions: Travel Expense Report (Form 91) and pen or pencil. Refer to textbook Procedure 17-10 for step-by-step directions and textbook Figure 17-15 for a visual example.

Standards: Complete all steps listed in this skill in _____ minutes with a minimum score of _____.
(Time element and accuracy criteria may be given by instructor.)

Time: Start: _____ Completed: _____ Total: _____ minutes

Scoring: One point for each step performed satisfactorily unless otherwise listed or weighted by instructor.

Directions with Performance Evaluation Checklist

Dr. Gerald Practon presented a research paper at a medical convention in Boston, Massachusetts. He kept a detailed record of all expenses for the week of May 9 (Sat.) through May 16 (Sat.). Set up a Travel Expense Report, transferring the following figures and placing them in the proper columns. Calculate totals.

1st Attempt	2nd Attempt	3rd Attempt	
_____	_____	_____	Gather materials (equipment and supplies) listed under "Conditions."
_____/2	_____/2	_____/2	1. Enter beginning and ending dates of trip.
_____/8	_____/8	_____/8	2. Record dates for column headings that will be used on the travel report.
_____	_____	_____	3. Record parking fees for Monday: $5.20.
_____	_____	_____	4. Record parkway toll fees for Monday: $4.00.
_____/5	_____/5	_____/5	5. Record tips for the week: $2 on Saturday, $3 on Sunday, $6 on Wednesday, $5.50 on Friday, and $6.25 on Saturday.
_____/7	_____/7	_____/7	6. Record the discounted Hertz car rental, which was $25 per day for seven days.
_____/2	_____/2	_____/2	7. Record gasoline expenses, which were $30.90 on Monday and $44.20 on Saturday.
_____/7	_____/7	_____/7	8. Record the hotel expenses: Conroy Hotel was $150 per night for the first four nights, Commonwealth Hotel was $135 per night for the next two nights, and Shoreham Hotel was $165 per night for the last night.
_____	_____	_____	9. Record one telephone call ($1.91) on Sunday, May 10, which was made to confirm the time for the speaking engagement.
_____/16	_____/16	_____/16	10. Record all meal expenses.

Day	Breakfast	Lunch	Dinner
Sunday	$8.90	$15.40	$36.20
Monday	5.10	—	26.14
Tuesday	3.40	10.90	31.50
Wednesday	—	13.98	48.14
Thursday	9.15	10.00	20.02
Friday	10.82	22.08	36.33

1st Attempt	2nd Attempt	3rd Attempt	
_____/7	_____/7	_____/7	11. Calculate and record total for Lodging.
_____/5	_____/5	_____/5	12. Calculate and record total for Breakfasts.
_____/5	_____/5	_____/5	13. Calculate and record total for Lunches.
_____/6	_____/6	_____/6	14. Calculate and record total for Dinners.

JOB SKILL 17-7 *(continued)*

_____	_____	_____	15. Calculate and record total for Local Fares.
_____/7	_____/7	_____/7	16. Calculate and record total for Auto Expenses.
_____	_____	_____	17. Calculate and record total for Parking Fees.
_____	_____	_____	18. Calculate and record total for Phone and E-mail.
_____	_____	_____	19. Calculate and record total for Entertainment.
_____/5	_____/5	_____/5	20. Calculate and record total for Tips.
_____	_____	_____	21. Calculate and record total for Toll Charges.
_____/2	_____/2	_____/2	22. Calculate and record total for Other/Miscellaneous.
_____/3	_____/3	_____/3	23. Calculate and record total for May 9.
_____/7	_____/7	_____/7	24. Calculate and record total for May 10.
_____/7	_____/7	_____/7	25. Calculate and record total for May 11.
_____/5	_____/5	_____/5	26. Calculate and record total for May 12.
_____/5	_____/5	_____/5	27. Calculate and record total for May 13.
_____/5	_____/5	_____/5	28. Calculate and record total for May 14.
_____/6	_____/6	_____/6	29. Calculate and record total for May 15.
_____/2	_____/2	_____/2	30. Calculate and record total for May 16.
_____/10	_____/10	_____/10	31. Add and record all totals in the right column.
_____/8	_____/8	_____/8	32. Add and record all totals listed for each day and verify against the figure obtained in step 31; they should be the same. If not, recalculate and compare again.
_____/2	_____/2	_____/2	33. Write a brief description for the purpose of the trip and enter on report.
_____	_____	_____	Complete within specified time.
___/154	___/154	___/154	**Total points earned** (To obtain a percentage score, divide the total points earned by the number of points possible.)

Comments:

CHAPTER 18

Financial Management of the Medical Practice

OBJECTIVES

After completing the exercises, the student will be able to:

1. Enhance knowledge of medical terminology, interpret abbreviations, and accurately spell medical words.

2. Write checks for disbursements.

3. Record expenditures, pay bills, and replenish and balance petty cash fund.

4. Reconcile a bank statement.

5. Prepare payroll.

6. Complete a payroll register.

7. Complete an employee earning record.

8. Complete an employee's withholding allowance certificate.

9. Complete an employee benefit form.

FOCUS ON CERTIFICATION*

CMA Content Summary

- Medical abbreviations
- Professionalism
- Working as a team member
- Internal Revenue Service forms
- Employment laws
- Personnel records
- Aging accounts receivable
- Write checks
- Employee payroll records
- Calculate wages and taxes
- Prepare payroll checks and earnings statements
- Deposit taxes, file, and mail tax reports

*This *Workbook* and accompanying textbook meet the entry-level administrative and general competencies for the CMA outlined by the AAMA Examination Content Outline and Role Delineation Study and for the RMA and CMAS outlined by the AMT Competencies and Examination Specifications (see Competency Grid in textbook Appendix B).

RMA Content Summary
- Medical terminology and abbreviations
- Accounting procedures
- Accounts payable
- Disbursement accounts

- Employee payroll procedures
- Payroll withholding and deductions
- Payroll tax forms and deposits
- Payroll calculations

CMAS Content Summary
- Medical and insurance terminology
- Accounting principles
- Financial computations
- Accounts payable

- Check writing
- Employee payroll and reports
- Payroll tax deductions and records

Abbreviation and Spelling Review

Read the following patient's chart notes and write the meanings for the abbreviations listed below the note. To decode any abbreviations you do not understand or that appear unfamiliar to you, refer to the list of abbreviations in Part V of this *Workbook*. Step-by-step directions for this exercise are found in Procedure 1-1 of Chapter 1 in the textbook. Medical terms in the chart note are italicized; study them for spelling. Use your medical dictionary to look up their definitions. Your instructor may give a spelling and definition test that includes these words and abbreviations.

Bernice Saxon

April 10, 20XX Pt had closed reduction of *telescoping* nasal *ethmoidal fracture* with sutures and application of an *external nasal* splint. When pt ret'nd from surg, she was given 100 mg of *Demerol* q. 3h. IM. Her vital signs were taken q.i.d. for the first 2 days & then b.i.d. p̄ that. Sleeping medication was given h.s. She will be seen in the office in 4 days for follow-up.

Gerald Practon, MD

Gerald Practon, MD

Pt _____	IM _____
ret'nd _____	q.i.d. _____
surg _____	b.i.d. _____
mg _____	p̄ _____
q. 3h. _____	h.s. _____

Lucy Corsentino

July 7, 20XX Pt, a 3-year-old, has had temp 100.1° for 2 days. Exam reveals strep throat. DX: Acute *streptococcal pharyngitis*. Plan: *Penicillin V potassium* 250 mg/tsp to be taken in a dose of 1 tsp q.i.d. x 10 days, *Tylenol* up to 1 gm q. 4h. for pain & fever. Mother advised not to give ASA.

Fran Practon, MD

Fran Practon, MD

Pt _____	1 gm _____
DX _____	q. 4h. _____
mg/tsp _____	ASA _____
q.i.d. x 10 days _____	

Review Questions

Review the objectives, glossary, and chapter information before completing the following review questions.

1. List several ways a computerized financial management system benefits a medical practice.

   a. _____

   b. _____

   c. _____

   d. _____

   e. _____

2. What important report is used to begin a financial analysis of a medical practice? _____

   _____

3. What projection does the office manager look at to determine how much actual cash should be available each month? _____

   _____

4. An office manager calculates the accounts receivable ratio in order to determine how well which person is performing his or her job? _____

   _____

   _____

5. Income received and expenses paid are presented in a report called a _____

   _____ .

6. What are some of the things that are looked at and learned when an office manager analyzes a medical practice's productivity?

   a. _____

   b. _____

   c. _____

   d. _____

7. To track the accounts payable, expenditures are recorded in a _____ .

8. What law covers minimum wage and overtime standards? _____

9. The office manager must post notices in the medical office according to the _____ .

10. Name some responsibilities of the office manager or medical assistant when he or she is in complete charge of the payroll.

    a. _____

    b. _____

    c. _____

    d. _____

    e. _____

    f. _____

11. Explain how to obtain a tax identification number for a physician-employer. _____

    _____

12. Explain how an employee obtains a tax identification number. _____

    _____

13. Why do you have an employee complete an Employee's Withholding Allowance Certificate, Form W-4?

_____

14. Under FICA, both the _____ and _____ contribute at a rate specified by law.

15. Name three programs financed under Social Security (FICA) from one payroll tax, and list what they provide.

    a. Program 1: _____

       Provides: _____

    b. Program 2: _____

       Provides: _____

    c. Program 3: _____

       Provides: _____

16. List three names used for state disability insurance deductions.

    a. _____

    b. _____

    c. _____

17. List several optional payroll deductions; also called _____.

    a. _____

    b. _____

    c. _____

    d. _____

    e. _____

    f. _____

    g. _____

18. a. How often are federal unemployment tax deposits made and reported on Form 508? _____

    b. How often must employers report payments by using Form 940? _____

19. In what publication does the Department of the Treasury, Internal Revenue Service, publish submission guidelines and requirements for quarterly reports, federal tax deposits, and unemployment tax payments?

_____

20. The employer's quarterly federal tax return must be filed by an employer on or before _____,

_____, _____, and _____ on Form _____.

21. Spell out the following payroll abbreviations.

    FICA_____

    FUTA_____

    UCD_____

Critical Thinking Exercises

1. Explain an insurance aging report and list ways it can be broken down for analysis. _____

_____

_____

_____

_____

_____

2. Agnes Baker terminated her employment with Dr. Jeffries on August 31. What document must be given to her by the employer and what is the time limit?_____

_____

3. Name the documents related to payroll that are required in each employee's personnel file and state their purposes.

a. _____

_____

b. _____

_____

4. Why is it a federal requirement that the Wage and Tax Statement (W-2) Tax Form be sent by the employer to both the IRS and to each employee? _____

_____

5. You may have difficulty remembering whether *biweekly* means "twice a week" or "every two weeks"; it can mean both. However, *semiweekly* is usually used for "twice a week," and in accounting *biweekly* is used for "every two weeks." In the following list, check the correct definitions.

biyearly _____ a. twice a year   semiannually _____ a. every six months

_____ b. once a year   _____ b. every two years

_____ c. every two years   _____ c. once a year

biweekly _____ a. twice a week   semimonthly _____ a. every half month

_____ b. every two weeks   _____ b. twice a month

_____ c. semiweekly   _____ c. twice monthly

quarterly _____ a. twice a year   weekly _____ a. every day

_____ b. every four weeks   _____ b. once a week

_____ c. four times a year   _____ c. every week

6. State the deductions from a payroll check required in your state.

a. _____

b. _____

c. _____

d. _____

e. _____

7. Looking ahead to when you are employed as an administrative medical assistant, list what kind of fringe benefits you would prefer and why. _____

_____

JOB SKILL 18-1
Write Checks for Disbursement

Name _____ Date _____ Score _____

Performance Objective

Task: Write checks for disbursement, enter transactions on the check register, and post deposits.

Conditions: Check register (Forms 92, 93, and 94), twelve checks (four sheets: Forms 95 through 98), calculator, and pencil. Refer to Procedure 18-1 in the textbook for step-by-step directions. Note: Job Skills 18-1, 18-2, and 18-3 will use the same information and check register.

Standards: Complete all steps listed in this skill in _____ minutes with a minimum score of _____. (Time element and accuracy criteria may be given by instructor.)

Time: Start: _____ Completed: _____ Total: _____ minutes

Scoring: One point for each step performed satisfactorily unless otherwise listed or weighted by instructor.

Directions with Performance Evaluation Checklist

Read the entire Job Skill before beginning. You may want to enlarge Forms 92, 93, and 94 onto legal size paper to make it easier to handwrite entries.

Check Stub: List date and record deposit(s), and then add to the balance forward; list the check amount and a brief description subtracting the amount to determine the checkbook balance; always carry the balance forward to the next check.

Check Entries: Write out the amount of the check and enter the numerical figure in the "Check Amount." Record the company name and address to which the check is written; use the date indicated.

Check Register: Study the column headings to familiarize yourself with the various categories. Write the amount of the check in the "Gross" column and in the "Amount of Check" column (Page 1); indicate the check number. Then, post each check amount on the appropriate line in the correct disbursement column on Page 2 or 3 of the check register.

1st Attempt	2nd Attempt	3rd Attempt	
_____	_____	_____	Gather materials (equipment and supplies) listed under "Conditions."
_____/5	_____/5	_____/5	1. Prepare pages 1, 2, and 3 of the check register (Forms 92, 93, and 94) for checks drawn on "The First National Bank" for the month of June 20XX.
_____/2	_____/2	_____/2	2. Record the beginning checkbook balance of $9,745.45 on the first check stub (No. 479) and on Page 2 of the check register bank deposit slip.
_____/2	_____/2	_____/2	3. Record a deposit of $130 on June 1, 20XX, on the first check stub (no. 479) and on the bank deposit slip.
_____/8	_____/8	_____/8	4. Make out check no. 479 on June 1, 20XX, for rent to Security Pacific Company, 2091 Mission Street, Woodland Hills, XY 12345, in the amount of $1,900.00, and make the appropriate calculations on the check stub.
_____/6	_____/6	_____/6	5. Record check no. 479 on the check register.
_____/2	_____/2	_____/2	6. Record a deposit of $95 on June 3, 20XX, on check stub no. 480 and on the bank deposit slip.
_____/8	_____/8	_____/8	7. Make out check no. 480 on June 3, 20XX, for medical supplies to Central Laboratories, 351 Robin Avenue, Woodland Hills, XY 12345, in the amount of $74.50, and make the appropriate calculations on the check stub.
_____/6	_____/6	_____/6	8. Record check no. 480 on the check register.
_____/8	_____/8	_____/8	9. Make out check no. 481 on June 3, 20XX, for parking fees to Broadway Garage, 4560 Broad Avenue, Woodland Hills, XY 12345, in the amount of $300.00, and make the appropriate calculations on the check stub.
_____/6	_____/6	_____/6	10. Record check no. 481 on the check register.

JOB SKILL 18-1 (*continued*)

_____/2   _____/2   _____/2   11. Record a deposit of $195 on June 4, 20XX, on check stub no. 482 and on the bank deposit slip.

_____/8   _____/8   _____/8   12. Make out check no. 482 on June 4, 20XX, for diesel fuel to Union Oil Company, PO Box 232, Woodland Hills, XY 12345, in the amount of $87.75, and make the appropriate calculations on the check stub.

_____/6   _____/6   _____/6   13. Record check no. 482 on the check register.

_____/2   _____/2   _____/2   14. Record a deposit of $80 on June 15, 20XX, on check stub no. 483 and on the bank deposit slip.

_____/8   _____/8   _____/8   15. Make out check no. 483 on June 15, 20XX, for quarterly city tax to Woodland Hills Tax Commission, 2200 James Street, Woodland Hills, XY 12345, in the amount of $162.00, and make the appropriate calculations on the check stub.

_____/6   _____/6   _____/6   16. Record check no. 483 on the check register.

_____/8   _____/8   _____/8   17. Make out check no. 484 on June 15, 20XX, for medications to Eli Lilly and Company, Lilly Corporate Center, Indianapolis, IN 46285, in the amount of $226.00, and make the appropriate calculations on the check stub.

_____/6   _____/6   _____/6   18. Record check no. 484 on the check register.

_____/2   _____/2   _____/2   19. Record a deposit of $160 on June 20, 20XX, on check stub no. 485 and on the bank deposit slip.

_____/8   _____/8   _____/8   20. Make out check no. 485 on June 20, 20XX, for utilities to Woodland Hills Gas Company, 50 South M Street, Woodland Hills, XY 12345, in the amount of $87.80, and make the appropriate calculations on the check stub.

_____/6   _____/6   _____/6   21. Record check no. 485 on the check register.

_____/8   _____/8   _____/8   22. Make out check no. 486 on June 20, 20XX, for drugs and medical supplies to Sargents Pharmacy, 711 Wheeler Road, Woodland Hills, XY 12345, in the amount of $38.75, and make the appropriate calculations on the check stub.

_____/6   _____/6   _____/6   23. Record check no. 486 on the check register.

_____/8   _____/8   _____/8   24. Make out check no. 487 on June 20, 20XX, for a donation to United Fund, PO Box 400, New York, NY 10015, in the amount of $200.00, and make the appropriate calculations on the check stub.

_____/6   _____/6   _____/6   25. Record check no. 487 on the check register.

_____/2   _____/2   _____/2   26. Record a deposit of $105 on June 25, 20XX, on check stub no. 488 and on the bank deposit slip.

_____/8   _____/8   _____/8   27. Make out check no. 488 on June 25, 20XX, for utilities to Woodland Hills Telephone Company, 505 Peppermint Street, Woodland Hills, XY 12345, in the amount of $79.60, and make the appropriate calculations on the check stub.

_____/6   _____/6   _____/6   28. Record check no. 488 on the check register.

_____/8   _____/8   _____/8   29. Make out check no. 489 on June 25, 20XX, for utilities to Woodland Hills Electric Company, 320 Banyon Avenue, Woodland Hills, XY 12345, in the amount of $85.78, and make the appropriate calculations on the check stub.

_____/6   _____/6   _____/6   30. Record check no. 489 on the check register.

_____/8   _____/8   _____/8   31. Make out check no. 490 on June 25, 20XX, for office linens to Rite-Way Laundry, 2500 Torrance Way, Woodland Hills, XY 12345, in the amount of $45.00, and make the appropriate calculations on the check stub.

_____/6   _____/6   _____/6   32. Record check no. 490 on the check register.

_____   _____   _____   Complete within specified time.

___/189   ___/189   ___/189   **Total points earned** (To obtain a percentage score, divide the total points earned by the number of points possible.)

JOB SKILL 18-1 *(continued)*

Comments:

Evaluator's Signature: _____ **Need to Repeat:** _____

JOB SKILL 18-2
Record Expenditures, Pay Bills, Replenish and Balance Petty Cash Fund

Name _____ Date _____ Score _____

Performance Objective

Task: Write checks for invoices received, complete the check register, enter deposit, and replenish petty cash.

Conditions: Four invoices (*Workbook* Figure 18-1), check register used in Job Skill 18-1 (Forms 92, 93, and 94), five checks (Forms 99 and 100), petty cash receipt envelope (Form 101), calculator, and pencil. Refer to Procedure 18-1 in the textbook for step-by-step directions.

Standards: Complete all steps listed in this skill in _____ minutes with a minimum score of _____. (Time element and accuracy criteria may be given by instructor.)

Time: Start: _____ Completed: _____ Total: _____ minutes

Scoring: One point for each step performed satisfactorily unless otherwise listed or weighted by instructor.

Directions with Performance Evaluation Checklist

Read the entire Job Skill before beginning. Use the date June 30, 20XX.

1st Attempt	2nd Attempt	3rd Attempt	
_____	_____	_____	Gather materials (equipment and supplies) listed under "Conditions."

Check Register

1st	2nd	3rd	
_____	_____	_____	1. Carry checkbook balance forward from the previous Job Skill to check no. 491.
____/6	____/6	____/6	2. You have deposited money on the following dates for the amounts listed: 6/28 $410.99, 6/29 $70, 6/30 $95. Include these deposits on the first check stub that you will be using (No. 491) and on Page 2 of the check register bank deposit slip.
____/2	____/2	____/2	3. If possible, copy the invoices in Figure 18-1 (page 349) and cut them apart.
____/56	____/56	____/56	4. Write checks for the invoices shown in Figure 18-1 and record the information on the check register as in Job Skill 18-1.
____/12	____/12	____/12	5. Indicate the following on each invoice: date paid, check number, and check amount.

Petty Cash

1st	2nd	3rd	
____/2	____/2	____/2	6. Indicate on the petty cash receipt envelope (Form 101) the beginning petty cash amount of $100 for June 1, 20XX.
____/30	____/30	____/30	7. Enter the following expenses that occurred during the month of June on the petty cash receipt envelope listing the date paid, voucher number, to whom it was paid, a brief description of the item, under which account heading it would be listed (i.e., office supplies, postage, medical supplies, miscellaneous), and the amount.

Date	Voucher	Vendor	Item	Amount
6/3/XX	103	Crown Stationers	stationery supplies	$5.70
6/7/XX	104	U.S. Postal Service	postage due	.95
6/15/XX	105	Thrifty Drug Store	medical supplies	10.32
6/20/XX	106	TG & Y Store	miscellaneous (office plant)	3.40
6/22/XX	107	U.S. Postal Service	postage	39.00
6/27/XX	108	Thrifty Drug Store	medical supplies	2.62

JOB SKILL 18-2 *(continued)*

____/6	____/6	____/6	8. Total the amount of all items and record on the last line.
____/4	____/4	____/4	9. List the following headings in the "Distribution of Petty Cash": Office Supplies, Postage, Medical Supplies, Miscellaneous.
____/6	____/6	____/6	10. Itemize each of the expenditures under the correct heading.
____/4	____/4	____/4	11. Total each column under "Distribution of Petty Cash" and list the total on the last line.
____/4	____/4	____/4	12. Add all totals listed and record on the last line under "Totals." This number should be the same as the total in step 8.
_____	_____	_____	13. List the amount of all vouchers paid under "Receipts Paid."
_____	_____	_____	14. Count the cash in the cash drawer and list under "Cash on Hand."
____/2	____/2	____/2	15. Add the receipts paid and the cash on hand; it should equal the beginning amount in the office fund account.
_____	_____	_____	16. List this amount in "Total Receipts and Cash."
____/2	____/2	____/2	17. Subtract the "Total Receipts and Cash" from the "Office Fund Amount" and list the amount of money that is over or short.
____/6	____/6	____/6	18. Write check no. 495, made out to "Petty Cash," for the amount necessary to replenish the petty cash.
____/11	____/11	____/11	19. List petty cash amounts on the check register. Note: Add together items in the same category; office supplies and postage will be combined and listed under "Office Supplies."
_____	_____	_____	20. Indicate this transaction on the "Petty Cash Receipt Envelope."

Balance Check Register

____/17	____/17	____/17	21. Total both columns on page 1 of the check register and record at bottom of form; they should equal.
____/8	____/8	____/8	22. Total the bank deposit and all columns on page 2 of the check register and record at bottom of form.
____/6	____/6	____/6	23. Total all columns on page 3 of the check register and record at bottom of form.
____/14	____/14	____/14	24. Balance check register by adding all disbursement column totals on pages 2 and 3; they should equal Total C listed on page 1.
_____	_____	_____	Complete within specified time.
____/205	____/205	____/205	**Total points earned** (To obtain a percentage score, divide the total points earned by the number of points possible.)

Comments:

Evaluator's Signature: _____   **Need to Repeat:** _____

National Curriculum Competency: CAAHEP: III.C.3.a.2(a), III.C.3.a.2(b)   ABHES: VI.B.1.a.3(j), VI.B.1.a.3(n), VI.B.1.a.3(o) , VI.B.1.a.8(e)

JOB SKILL 18-2 *(continued)*

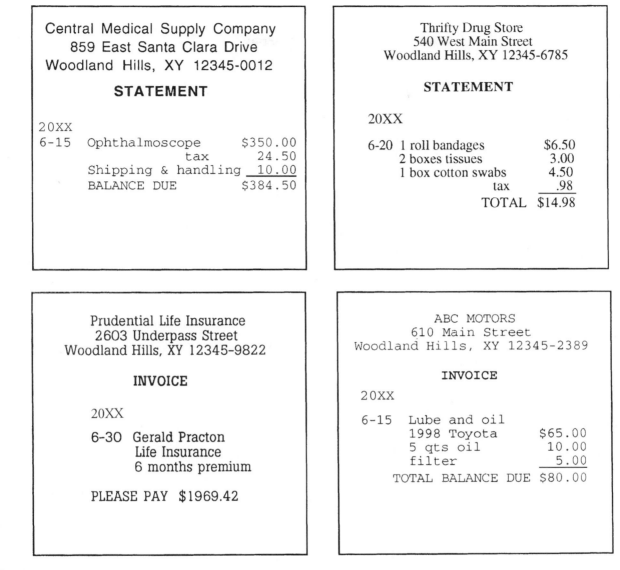

Central Medical Supply Company
859 East Santa Clara Drive
Woodland Hills, XY 12345-0012

STATEMENT

20XX
6-15   Ophthalmoscope $350.00
                    tax   24.50
        Shipping & handling   10.00
        BALANCE DUE $384.50

Thrifty Drug Store
540 West Main Street
Woodland Hills, XY 12345-6785

STATEMENT

20XX

6-20 1 roll bandages $6.50
      2 boxes tissues   3.00
      1 box cotton swabs   4.50
                    tax   .98
            TOTAL $14.98

Prudential Life Insurance
2603 Underpass Street
Woodland Hills, XY 12345-9822

INVOICE

20XX

6-30 Gerald Practon
      Life Insurance
      6 months premium

PLEASE PAY $1969.42

ABC MOTORS
610 Main Street
Woodland Hills, XY 12345-2389

INVOICE

20XX

6-15   Lube and oil
        1998 Toyota $65.00
        5 qts oil   10.00
        filter   5.00
    TOTAL BALANCE DUE $80.00

Figure 18-1

JOB SKILL 18-3
Reconcile a Bank Statement

Name _____ Date _____ Score _____

Performance Objective

Task: Reconcile a bank statement.

Conditions: One bank account reconciliation form (Form 102), checkbook stubs completed in Job Skill 18-1 and 18-2, bank statement (*Workbook* Figure 18-2), calculator, and pen or pencil. Refer to Job Skill 14-7 to review the steps for reconciling a bank statement.

Standards: Complete all steps listed in this skill in _____ minutes with a minimum score of _____. (Time element and accuracy criteria may be given by instructor.)

Time: Start: _____ Completed: _____ Total: _____ minutes

Scoring: One point for each step performed satisfactorily unless otherwise listed or weighted by instructor.

Directions with Performance Evaluation Checklist

You have received the bank statement from The First National Bank for June 20XX. Use the checks written for the month of June 20XX (no. 479 through 495), and the bank statement shown in *Workbook* Figure 18-2 to reconcile the bank statement.

1st Attempt	2nd Attempt	3rd Attempt	
_____	_____	_____	Gather materials (equipment and supplies) listed under "Conditions."
____/9	____/9	____/9	1. Mark off all checks made out during the month of June that have been returned by the bank and appear on the bank statement.
____/16	____/16	____/16	2. List all checks that have not been returned on the reconciliation form under "Outstanding Checks or Other Withdrawals."
____/8	____/8	____/8	3. Add all outstanding checks and record the total on the reconciliation form.
____/6	____/6	____/6	4. Check off all deposits that have been made during the month of June that appear on the bank statement.
____/6	____/6	____/6	5. List all deposits that do not appear on the statement on the reconciliation form under "Deposits Not Credited."
____/3	____/3	____/3	6. Add all deposits not credited to the account and record the total on the reconciliation form.
____/4	____/4	____/4	7. Balance the checking account using the steps indicated on the reconciliation form under "Balance Your Account."
____/2	____/2	____/2	8. Compare this figure with the ending figure in the checkbook (see check no. 495); they should match.
_____	_____	_____	Complete within specified time.
____/56	____/56	____/56	**Total points earned** (To obtain a percentage score, divide the total points earned by the number of points possible.)

Comments:

Evaluator's Signature: _____ **Need to Repeat:** _____

National Curriculum Competency: CAAHEP: III.C.3.a(2)	ABHES: VI.B.1.a.3(k)

JOB SKILL 18-3 (*continued*)

Account Statement ⬡ THE FIRST NATIONAL BANK

CHECKING ACCOUNT #00012345   WOODLAND HILLS 140

0020
100

PRACTON MEDICAL GROUP, INC   140
4567 BROAD AVENUE
WOODLAND HILLS XY   12345

CHECKING ACCOUNT SUMMARY AS OF 06-27-20XX   3

BEGINNING BALANCE	TOTAL DEPOSITS	TOTAL WITHDRAWALS	SERVICE CHARGES	ENDING BALANCE
9,754 45	765 00	3076 80	00	7,442 65

- - - - - - - - - - - - - -CHECKING ACCOUNT TRANSACTIONS- - - - - - - - - - - - - -

DEPOSITS   DATE   AMOUNT

	DATE	AMOUNT
BRANCH DEPOSIT	06-01	130.00
BRANCH DEPOSIT	06-03	95.00
BRANCH DEPOSIT	06-04	195.00
BRANCH DEPOSIT	06-15	80.00
BRANCH DEPOSIT	06-20	160.00
BRANCH DEPOSIT	06-25	105.00

- - - -CHECKS- - - -			- - - -CHECKS- - - -			- - - -BALANCES- - - -	
ITEM	DATE	AMOUNT	ITEM	DATE	AMOUNT	DATE	BALANCES
479	06-01	1,900.00	484	06-15	226.00	06-01	7,984.45
480	06-03	74.50	485	06-20	87.80	06-03	7,704.95
481	06-03	300.00	486	06-20	38.75	06-04	7,812.20
482	06-04	87.75	487	06-20	200.00	06-15	7,504.20
483	06-15	162.00				06-20	7,337.65
						06-25	7,442.65

Figure 18-2

JOB SKILL 18-4
Prepare Payroll

Name _____ Date _____ Score _____

Performance Objective

Task: Prepare payroll for seven employees; calculate gross pay and all deductions to determine net pay.

Conditions: Income tax tables (*Workbook* Figures 18-3 through 18-11), calculator, and pen or pencil. Refer to Procedure 18-2 in the textbook for step-by-step directions and textbook Figures 18-18 and 18-19 for examples of a completed employee earning record and monthly payroll register.

Standards: Complete all steps listed in this skill in _____ minutes with a minimum score of _____. (Time element and accuracy criteria may be given by instructor.)

Time: Start: _____ Completed: _____ Total: _____ minutes

Scoring: One point for each step performed satisfactorily unless otherwise listed or weighted by instructor.

Directions with Performance Evaluation Checklist

It is May 28, 20XX, and you will be preparing the payroll for seven employees. Following are payroll guidelines:

1. Hourly employees are paid once each month, on the first.

2. Salaried employees are paid semimonthly.

3. A few employees have elected to pay 2% of their gross pay into the Practon Medical Group, Inc., insurance plan.

4. If you reside in California, Hawaii, New Jersey, New York, Puerto Rico, or Rhode Island, assume state disability insurance (SDI) is 1% of gross pay; in all other states, disregard this deduction.

5. Determine the employee's status and refer to the tax tables that follow this exercise to determine federal and state deductions. If the amount of income is shown on two lines (e.g., at least $540 but less than $560 and at least $560 but less than $580), use the higher deduction.

6. Calculate FICA deductions at 6.2% of gross earnings.

7. Calculate Medicare deductions at 1.45% of gross earnings.

8. Divorced persons are considered "single" on federal tax tables and "head of household" on state tax tables that appear in this exercise.

9. Single persons with a dependent parent are considered "unmarried head of household" with the state.

10. Read the following scenarios and use the worksheet provided to indicate whether the person is single (S), married (M), or divorced (D); the number of exemptions claimed; whether the employee is on salary or hourly and number of hours worked, if hourly, and frequency of pay (e.g., semimonthly, monthly). Then calculate and record the gross pay, all necessary deductions, and net pay.

1st Attempt	2nd Attempt	3rd Attempt	
			Gather materials (equipment and supplies) listed under "Conditions."
___/13	___/13	___/13	1. Prepare payroll for Hillary Sheehan who is the physician's bookkeeper. She is married and claims herself as an exemption. She earns $13 an hour and worked 168 hours this month with no overtime.

JOB SKILL 18-4 (*continued*)

Status	Exemptions	Salary/hrs Worked	Frequency of Pay
S M D	0 1 2 3	_____	Monthly/Semimonthly

Gross Pay	FICA	Fed. Inc. Tax	State Inc. Tax	SDI	Medicare	Other	Total Deduc.	Net Pay

____/13   ____/13   ____/13

2. Prepare payroll for Roger Young, who works part-time as a custodian on weekends. He is single and claims himself and a dependent mother. He is paid $6.50 per hour. He worked 18 hours this month.

Status	Exemptions	Salary/hrs Worked	Frequency of Pay
S M D	0 1 2 3	_____	Monthly/Semimonthly

Gross Pay	FICA	Fed. Inc. Tax	State Inc. Tax	SDI	Medicare	Other	Total Deduc.	Net Pay

____/13   ____/13   ____/13

3. Prepare payroll for Kelley Jones, who is the office receptionist. She is single and claims herself only. She is paid $1,650 per month, and she elected not to enroll in the hospital insurance plan.

Status	Exemptions	Salary/hrs Worked	Frequency of Pay
S M D	0 1 2 3	_____	Monthly/Semimonthly

Gross Pay	FICA	Fed. Inc. Tax	State Inc. Tax	SDI	Medicare	Other	Total Deduc.	Net Pay

____/13   ____/13   ____/13

4. Prepare payroll for Maryjane Moran, who works part-time doing insurance. She is paid hourly and earns $12.50 per hour. She is married and claims no dependents because her husband claims her. She worked 80 hours this month.

Status	Exemptions	Salary/hrs Worked	Frequency of Pay
S M D	0 1 2 3	_____	Monthly/Semimonthly

Gross Pay	FICA	Fed. Inc. Tax	State Inc. Tax	SDI	Medicare	Other	Total Deduc.	Net Pay

____/13   ____/13   ____/13

5. Prepare payroll for Carla O'Hare, who is the administrative medical assistant. She is divorced and has three children. She claims herself and her children. She is paid $1,675 a month, and she is a member of the hospital insurance plan.

Status	Exemptions	Salary/hrs Worked	Frequency of Pay
S M D	0 1 2 3	_____	Monthly/Semimonthly

Gross Pay	FICA	Fed. Inc. Tax	State Inc. Tax	SDI	Medicare	Other	Total Deduc.	Net Pay

JOB SKILL 18-4 (*continued*)

___/13 ___/13 ___/13   6. Prepare payroll for Amy Seaforth, who is a part-time laboratory techni-
cian. She is married; her husband does not claim her, and she does not
wish to claim herself either. She joined the hospital insurance plan.
She is paid a salary of $145 per week plus car expense figured at $0.34
per mile. She drove 36 miles this month. Amy is a new employee hired
on May 1, 20XX. [You will be completing an employee earning record
card for her in a future Job Skill.] Her address is: 29926 West Ridgeway
Avenue, Woodland Hills, XY 12345; telephone 555-692-4408; Social
Security number 043-XX-1945; birth date 08-04-50.

Status	Exemptions	Salary/hrs Worked	Frequency of Pay
S M D	0 1 2 3	_____	Monthly/Semimonthly

Gross Pay	FICA	Fed. Inc. Tax	State Inc. Tax	SDI	Medicare	Other	Total Deduc.	Net Pay

___/13 ___/13 ___/13   7. Prepare payroll for Lisa Adams, who is the clinical medical assistant. She
is married and has one child, whom she claims along with herself as
deductions. She is paid $1,750 per month, and she joined the hospital
insurance plan.

Status	Exemptions	Salary/hrs Worked	Frequency of Pay
S M D	0 1 2 3	_____	Monthly/Semimonthly

Gross Pay	FICA	Fed. Inc. Tax	State Inc. Tax	SDI	Medicare	Other	Total Deduc.	Net Pay

_____ _____ _____   Complete within specified time.

___/93 ___/93 ___/93   **Total points earned** (To obtain a percentage score, divide the total points earned
by the number of points possible.)

Comments:

Evaluator's Signature: _____   **Need to Repeat:** _____

National Curriculum Competency: CAAHEP: III.C.3.a(2)   ABHES: VI.B.1.a.8(f)

JOB SKILL 18-4 *(continued)*

SINGLE Persons—SEMIMONTHLY Payroll Period   **FEDERAL**

(For Wages Paid in 2006)

At least	But less than	0	1	2	3	4	5	6	7	8	9	10
$0	$115	$0	$0	$0	$0	$0	$0	$0	$0	$0	$0	$0
115	120	1	0	0	0	0	0	0	0	0	0	0
120	125	1	0	0	0	0	0	0	0	0	0	0
125	130	2	0	0	0	0	0	0	0	0	0	0
130	135	2	0	0	0	0	0	0	0	0	0	0
135	140	3	0	0	0	0	0	0	0	0	0	0
140	145	3	0	0	0	0	0	0	0	0	0	0
145	150	4	0	0	0	0	0	0	0	0	0	0
150	155	4	0	0	0	0	0	0	0	0	0	0
155	160	5	0	0	0	0	0	0	0	0	0	0
160	165	5	0	0	0	0	0	0	0	0	0	0
165	170	6	0	0	0	0	0	0	0	0	0	0
170	175	6	0	0	0	0	0	0	0	0	0	0
175	180	7	0	0	0	0	0	0	0	0	0	0
180	185	7	0	0	0	0	0	0	0	0	0	0
185	190	8	0	0	0	0	0	0	0	0	0	0
190	195	8	0	0	0	0	0	0	0	0	0	0
195	200	9	0	0	0	0	0	0	0	0	0	0
200	205	9	0	0	0	0	0	0	0	0	0	0
205	210	10	0	0	0	0	0	0	0	0	0	0
210	215	10	0	0	0	0	0	0	0	0	0	0
215	220	11	0	0	0	0	0	0	0	0	0	0
220	225	11	0	0	0	0	0	0	0	0	0	0
225	230	12	0	0	0	0	0	0	0	0	0	0
230	235	12	0	0	0	0	0	0	0	0	0	0
235	240	13	0	0	0	0	0	0	0	0	0	0
240	245	13	0	0	0	0	0	0	0	0	0	0
245	250	14	0	0	0	0	0	0	0	0	0	0
250	260	14	1	0	0	0	0	0	0	0	0	0
260	270	15	2	0	0	0	0	0	0	0	0	0
270	280	16	3	0	0	0	0	0	0	0	0	0
280	290	17	4	0	0	0	0	0	0	0	0	0
290	300	18	5	0	0	0	0	0	0	0	0	0
300	310	19	6	0	0	0	0	0	0	0	0	0
310	320	20	7	0	0	0	0	0	0	0	0	0
320	330	21	8	0	0	0	0	0	0	0	0	0
330	340	22	9	0	0	0	0	0	0	0	0	0
340	350	23	10	0	0	0	0	0	0	0	0	0
350	360	24	11	0	0	0	0	0	0	0	0	0
360	370	25	12	0	0	0	0	0	0	0	0	0
370	380	26	13	0	0	0	0	0	0	0	0	0
380	390	27	14	0	0	0	0	0	0	0	0	0
390	400	28	15	1	0	0	0	0	0	0	0	0
400	410	29	16	2	0	0	0	0	0	0	0	0
410	420	30	17	3	0	0	0	0	0	0	0	0
420	430	32	18	4	0	0	0	0	0	0	0	0
430	440	33	19	5	0	0	0	0	0	0	0	0
440	450	35	20	6	0	0	0	0	0	0	0	0
450	460	36	21	7	0	0	0	0	0	0	0	0
460	470	38	22	8	0	0	0	0	0	0	0	0
470	480	39	23	9	0	0	0	0	0	0	0	0
480	490	41	24	10	0	0	0	0	0	0	0	0
490	500	42	25	11	0	0	0	0	0	0	0	0
500	520	45	26	12	0	0	0	0	0	0	0	0
520	540	48	28	14	1	0	0	0	0	0	0	0
540	560	51	30	16	3	0	0	0	0	0	0	0
560	580	54	33	18	5	0	0	0	0	0	0	0
580	600	57	36	20	7	0	0	0	0	0	0	0
600	620	60	39	22	9	0	0	0	0	0	0	0
620	640	63	42	24	11	0	0	0	0	0	0	0
640	660	66	45	26	13	0	0	0	0	0	0	0
660	680	69	48	28	15	1	0	0	0	0	0	0
680	700	72	51	30	17	3	0	0	0	0	0	0
700	720	75	54	33	19	5	0	0	0	0	0	0
720	740	78	57	36	21	7	0	0	0	0	0	0
740	760	81	60	39	23	9	0	0	0	0	0	0
760	780	84	63	42	25	11	0	0	0	0	0	0
780	800	87	66	45	27	13	0	0	0	0	0	0
800	820	90	69	48	29	15	1	0	0	0	0	0
820	840	93	72	51	31	17	3	0	0	0	0	0

Figure 18-3

JOB SKILL 18-4 *(continued)*

SINGLE Persons—MONTHLY Payroll Period   FEDERAL
(For Wages Paid in 2006)

| If the wages are— | | And the number of withholding allowances claimed is— | | | | | | | | | | |
At least	But less than	0	1	2	3	4	5	6	7	8	9	10
		The amount of income tax to be withheld is—										
$0	$220	$0	$0	$0	$0	$0	$0	$0	$0	$0	$0	$0
220	230	0	0	0	0	0	0	0	0	0	0	0
230	240	1	0	0	0	0	0	0	0	0	0	0
240	250	2	0	0	0	0	0	0	0	0	0	0
250	260	3	0	0	0	0	0	0	0	0	0	0
260	270	4	0	0	0	0	0	0	0	0	0	0
270	280	5	0	0	0	0	0	0	0	0	0	0
280	290	6	0	0	0	0	0	0	0	0	0	0
290	300	7	0	0	0	0	0	0	0	0	0	0
300	320	9	0	0	0	0	0	0	0	0	0	0
320	340	11	0	0	0	0	0	0	0	0	0	0
340	360	13	0	0	0	0	0	0	0	0	0	0
360	380	15	0	0	0	0	0	0	0	0	0	0
380	400	17	0	0	0	0	0	0	0	0	0	0
400	420	19	0	0	0	0	0	0	0	0	0	0
420	440	21	0	0	0	0	0	0	0	0	0	0
440	460	23	0	0	0	0	0	0	0	0	0	0
460	480	25	0	0	0	0	0	0	0	0	0	0
480	500	27	0	0	0	0	0	0	0	0	0	0
500	520	29	1	0	0	0	0	0	0	0	0	0
520	540	31	3	0	0	0	0	0	0	0	0	0
540	560	33	5	0	0	0	0	0	0	0	0	0
560	580	35	7	0	0	0	0	0	0	0	0	0
580	600	37	9	0	0	0	0	0	0	0	0	0
600	640	40	12	0	0	0	0	0	0	0	0	0
640	680	44	16	0	0	0	0	0	0	0	0	0
680	720	48	20	0	0	0	0	0	0	0	0	0
720	760	52	24	0	0	0	0	0	0	0	0	0
760	800	56	28	1	0	0	0	0	0	0	0	0
800	840	60	32	5	0	0	0	0	0	0	0	0
840	880	65	36	9	0	0	0	0	0	0	0	0
880	920	71	40	13	0	0	0	0	0	0	0	0
920	960	77	44	17	0	0	0	0	0	0	0	0
960	1,000	83	48	21	0	0	0	0	0	0	0	0
1,000	1,040	89	52	25	0	0	0	0	0	0	0	0
1,040	1,080	95	56	29	1	0	0	0	0	0	0	0
1,080	1,120	101	60	33	5	0	0	0	0	0	0	0
1,120	1,160	107	66	37	9	0	0	0	0	0	0	0
1,160	1,200	113	72	41	13	0	0	0	0	0	0	0
1,200	1,240	119	78	45	17	0	0	0	0	0	0	0
1,240	1,280	125	84	49	21	0	0	0	0	0	0	0
1,280	1,320	131	90	53	25	0	0	0	0	0	0	0
1,320	1,360	137	96	57	29	2	0	0	0	0	0	0
1,360	1,400	143	102	61	33	6	0	0	0	0	0	0
1,400	1,440	149	108	67	37	10	0	0	0	0	0	0
1,440	1,480	155	114	73	41	14	0	0	0	0	0	0
1,480	1,520	161	120	79	45	18	0	0	0	0	0	0
1,520	1,560	167	126	85	49	22	0	0	0	0	0	0
1,560	1,600	173	132	91	53	26	0	0	0	0	0	0
1,600	1,640	179	138	97	57	30	2	0	0	0	0	0
1,640	1,680	185	144	103	62	34	6	0	0	0	0	0
1,680	1,720	191	150	109	68	38	10	0	0	0	0	0
1,720	1,760	197	156	115	74	42	14	0	0	0	0	0
1,760	1,800	203	162	121	80	46	18	0	0	0	0	0
1,800	1,840	209	168	127	86	50	22	0	0	0	0	0
1,840	1,880	215	174	133	92	54	26	0	0	0	0	0
1,880	1,920	221	180	139	98	58	30	3	0	0	0	0
1,920	1,960	227	186	145	104	62	34	7	0	0	0	0
1,960	2,000	233	192	151	110	68	38	11	0	0	0	0
2,000	2,040	239	198	157	116	74	42	15	0	0	0	0
2,040	2,080	245	204	163	122	80	46	19	0	0	0	0
2,080	2,120	251	210	169	128	86	50	23	0	0	0	0
2,120	2,160	257	216	175	134	92	54	27	0	0	0	0
2,160	2,200	263	222	181	140	98	58	31	3	0	0	0
2,200	2,240	269	228	187	146	104	63	35	7	0	0	0
2,240	2,280	275	234	193	152	110	69	39	11	0	0	0
2,280	2,320	281	240	199	158	116	75	43	15	0	0	0
2,320	2,360	287	246	205	164	122	81	47	19	0	0	0
2,360	2,400	293	252	211	170	128	87	51	23	0	0	0
2,400	2,440	299	258	217	176	134	93	55	27	0	0	0

Figure 18-4

JOB SKILL 18-4 *(continued)*

MARRIED Persons—MONTHLY Payroll Period   FEDERAL
(For Wages Paid in 2006)

If the wages are—		And the number of withholding allowances claimed is—										
At least	But less than	0	1	2	3	4	5	6	7	8	9	10
		The amount of income tax to be withheld is—										
$0	$540	$0	$0	$0	$0	$0	$0	$0	$0	$0	$0	$0
540	560	0	0	0	0	0	0	0	0	0	0	0
560	580	0	0	0	0	0	0	0	0	0	0	0
580	600	0	0	0	0	0	0	0	0	0	0	0
600	640	0	0	0	0	0	0	0	0	0	0	0
640	680	0	0	0	0	0	0	0	0	0	0	0
680	720	3	0	0	0	0	0	0	0	0	0	0
720	760	7	0	0	0	0	0	0	0	0	0	0
760	800	11	0	0	0	0	0	0	0	0	0	0
800	840	15	0	0	0	0	0	0	0	0	0	0
840	880	19	0	0	0	0	0	0	0	0	0	0
880	920	23	0	0	0	0	0	0	0	0	0	0
920	960	27	0	0	0	0	0	0	0	0	0	0
960	1,000	31	4	0	0	0	0	0	0	0	0	0
1,000	1,040	35	8	0	0	0	0	0	0	0	0	0
1,040	1,080	39	12	0	0	0	0	0	0	0	0	0
1,080	1,120	43	16	0	0	0	0	0	0	0	0	0
1,120	1,160	47	20	0	0	0	0	0	0	0	0	0
1,160	1,200	51	24	0	0	0	0	0	0	0	0	0
1,200	1,240	55	28	0	0	0	0	0	0	0	0	0
1,240	1,280	59	32	4	0	0	0	0	0	0	0	0
1,280	1,320	63	36	8	0	0	0	0	0	0	0	0
1,320	1,360	67	40	12	0	0	0	0	0	0	0	0
1,360	1,400	71	44	16	0	0	0	0	0	0	0	0
1,400	1,440	75	48	20	0	0	0	0	0	0	0	0
1,440	1,480	79	52	24	0	0	0	0	0	0	0	0
1,480	1,520	83	56	28	1	0	0	0	0	0	0	0
1,520	1,560	87	60	32	5	0	0	0	0	0	0	0
1,560	1,600	91	64	36	9	0	0	0	0	0	0	0
1,600	1,640	95	68	40	13	0	0	0	0	0	0	0
1,640	1,680	99	72	44	17	0	0	0	0	0	0	0
1,680	1,720	103	76	48	21	0	0	0	0	0	0	0
1,720	1,760	107	80	52	25	0	0	0	0	0	0	0
1,760	1,800	111	84	56	29	1	0	0	0	0	0	0
1,800	1,840	115	88	60	33	5	0	0	0	0	0	0
1,840	1,880	119	92	64	37	9	0	0	0	0	0	0
1,880	1,920	123	96	68	41	13	0	0	0	0	0	0
1,920	1,960	129	100	72	45	17	0	0	0	0	0	0
1,960	2,000	135	104	76	49	21	0	0	0	0	0	0
2,000	2,040	141	108	80	53	25	0	0	0	0	0	0
2,040	2,080	147	112	84	57	29	2	0	0	0	0	0
2,080	2,120	153	116	88	61	33	6	0	0	0	0	0
2,120	2,160	159	120	92	65	37	10	0	0	0	0	0
2,160	2,200	165	124	96	69	41	14	0	0	0	0	0
2,200	2,240	171	130	100	73	45	18	0	0	0	0	0
2,240	2,280	177	136	104	77	49	22	0	0	0	0	0
2,280	2,320	183	142	108	81	53	26	0	0	0	0	0
2,320	2,360	189	148	112	85	57	30	2	0	0	0	0
2,360	2,400	195	154	116	89	61	34	6	0	0	0	0
2,400	2,440	201	160	120	93	65	38	10	0	0	0	0
2,440	2,480	207	166	124	97	69	42	14	0	0	0	0
2,480	2,520	213	172	130	101	73	46	18	0	0	0	0
2,520	2,560	219	178	136	105	77	50	22	0	0	0	0
2,560	2,600	225	184	142	109	81	54	26	0	0	0	0
2,600	2,640	231	190	148	113	85	58	30	3	0	0	0
2,640	2,680	237	196	154	117	89	62	34	7	0	0	0
2,680	2,720	243	202	160	121	93	66	38	11	0	0	0
2,720	2,760	249	208	166	125	97	70	42	15	0	0	0
2,760	2,800	255	214	172	131	101	74	46	19	0	0	0
2,800	2,840	261	220	178	137	105	78	50	23	0	0	0
2,840	2,880	267	226	184	143	109	82	54	27	0	0	0
2,880	2,920	273	232	190	149	113	86	58	31	3	0	0
2,920	2,960	279	238	196	155	117	90	62	35	7	0	0
2,960	3,000	285	244	202	161	121	94	66	39	11	0	0
3,000	3,040	291	250	208	167	126	98	70	43	15	0	0
3,040	3,080	297	256	214	173	132	102	74	47	19	0	0
3,080	3,120	303	262	220	179	138	106	78	51	23	0	0
3,120	3,160	309	268	226	185	144	110	82	55	27	0	0
3,160	3,200	315	274	232	191	150	114	86	59	31	4	0
3,200	3,240	321	280	238	197	156	118	90	63	35	8	0

Figure 18-5

JOB SKILL 18-4 (*continued*)

MARRIED Persons—SEMIMONTHLY Payroll Period **FEDERAL**

(For Wages Paid in 2006)

If the wages are—		And the number of withholding allowances claimed is—										
At least	But less than	0	1	2	3	4	5	6	7	8	9	10
		The amount of income tax to be withheld is—										
$0	$270	$0	$0	$0	$0	$0	$0	$0	$0	$0	$0	$0
270	280	0	0	0	0	0	0	0	0	0	0	0
280	290	0	0	0	0	0	0	0	0	0	0	0
290	300	0	0	0	0	0	0	0	0	0	0	0
300	310	0	0	0	0	0	0	0	0	0	0	0
310	320	0	0	0	0	0	0	0	0	0	0	0
320	330	0	0	0	0	0	0	0	0	0	0	0
330	340	0	0	0	0	0	0	0	0	0	0	0
340	350	1	0	0	0	0	0	0	0	0	0	0
350	360	2	0	0	0	0	0	0	0	0	0	0
360	370	3	0	0	0	0	0	0	0	0	0	0
370	380	4	0	0	0	0	0	0	0	0	0	0
380	390	5	0	0	0	0	0	0	0	0	0	0
390	400	6	0	0	0	0	0	0	0	0	0	0
400	410	7	0	0	0	0	0	0	0	0	0	0
410	420	8	0	0	0	0	0	0	0	0	0	0
420	430	9	0	0	0	0	0	0	0	0	0	0
430	440	10	0	0	0	0	0	0	0	0	0	0
440	450	11	0	0	0	0	0	0	0	0	0	0
450	460	12	0	0	0	0	0	0	0	0	0	0
460	470	13	0	0	0	0	0	0	0	0	0	0
470	480	14	0	0	0	0	0	0	0	0	0	0
480	490	15	1	0	0	0	0	0	0	0	0	0
490	500	16	2	0	0	0	0	0	0	0	0	0
500	520	18	4	0	0	0	0	0	0	0	0	0
520	540	20	6	0	0	0	0	0	0	0	0	0
540	560	22	8	0	0	0	0	0	0	0	0	0
560	580	24	10	0	0	0	0	0	0	0	0	0
580	600	26	12	0	0	0	0	0	0	0	0	0
600	620	28	14	0	0	0	0	0	0	0	0	0
620	640	30	16	2	0	0	0	0	0	0	0	0
640	660	32	18	4	0	0	0	0	0	0	0	0
660	680	34	20	6	0	0	0	0	0	0	0	0
680	700	36	22	8	0	0	0	0	0	0	0	0
700	720	38	24	10	0	0	0	0	0	0	0	0
720	740	40	26	12	0	0	0	0	0	0	0	0
740	760	42	28	14	0	0	0	0	0	0	0	0
760	780	44	30	16	2	0	0	0	0	0	0	0
780	800	46	32	18	4	0	0	0	0	0	0	0
800	820	48	34	20	6	0	0	0	0	0	0	0
820	840	50	36	22	8	0	0	0	0	0	0	0
840	860	52	38	24	10	0	0	0	0	0	0	0
860	880	54	40	26	12	0	0	0	0	0	0	0
880	900	56	42	28	14	1	0	0	0	0	0	0
900	920	58	44	30	16	3	0	0	0	0	0	0
920	940	60	46	32	18	5	0	0	0	0	0	0
940	960	62	48	34	20	7	0	0	0	0	0	0
960	980	64	50	36	22	9	0	0	0	0	0	0
980	1,000	67	52	38	24	11	0	0	0	0	0	0
1,000	1,020	70	54	40	26	13	0	0	0	0	0	0
1,020	1,040	73	56	42	28	15	1	0	0	0	0	0
1,040	1,060	76	58	44	30	17	3	0	0	0	0	0
1,060	1,080	79	60	46	32	19	5	0	0	0	0	0
1,080	1,100	82	62	48	34	21	7	0	0	0	0	0
1,100	1,120	85	65	50	36	23	9	0	0	0	0	0
1,120	1,140	88	68	52	38	25	11	0	0	0	0	0
1,140	1,160	91	71	54	40	27	13	0	0	0	0	0
1,160	1,180	94	74	56	42	29	15	1	0	0	0	0
1,180	1,200	97	77	58	44	31	17	3	0	0	0	0
1,200	1,220	100	80	60	46	33	19	5	0	0	0	0
1,220	1,240	103	83	62	48	35	21	7	0	0	0	0
1,240	1,260	106	86	65	50	37	23	9	0	0	0	0
1,260	1,280	109	89	68	52	39	25	11	0	0	0	0
1,280	1,300	112	92	71	54	41	27	13	0	0	0	0
1,300	1,320	115	95	74	56	43	29	15	1	0	0	0
1,320	1,340	118	98	77	58	45	31	17	3	0	0	0
1,340	1,360	121	101	80	60	47	33	19	5	0	0	0
1,360	1,380	124	104	83	63	49	35	21	7	0	0	0
1,380	1,400	127	107	86	66	51	37	23	9	0	0	0
1,400	1,420	130	110	89	69	53	39	25	11	0	0	0

Figure 18-6

JOB SKILL 18-4 (continued)

CALIFORNIA WITHHOLDING SCHEDULES FOR 2006

SINGLE PERSONS, DUAL INCOME MARRIED
OR MARRIED WITH MULTIPLE EMPLOYERS----SEMI-MONTHLY PAYROLL PERIOD

(FOR WAGES PAID IN 2006)

IF WAGES ARE...   AND THE NUMBER OF WITHHOLDING ALLOWANCES CLAIMED IS...   **STATE**

AT LEAST	BUT LESS THAN	0	1	2	3	4	5	6	7	8	9	10 OR MORE
		...THE AMOUNT OF INCOME TAX TO BE WITHHELD SHALL BE...										
$1	$300											
300	320	1.74										
320	340	1.94										
340	360	2.14										
360	380	2.34										
380	400	2.54										
400	420	2.86										
420	440	3.26										
440	460	3.66	0.03									
460	480	4.06	0.43									
480	500	4.46	0.83									
500	540	5.06	1.43									
540	580	5.86	2.23									
580	620	6.66	3.03									
620	660	7.46	3.83	0.20								
660	700	8.26	4.63	1.00								
700	740	9.06	5.43	1.80								
740	780	9.87	6.24	2.61								
780	820	11.47	7.84	4.21	0.58							
820	860	13.07	9.44	5.81	2.18							
860	900	14.67	11.04	7.41	3.78	0.15						
900	940	16.27	12.64	9.01	5.38	1.75						
940	980	17.87	14.24	10.61	6.98	3.35						
980	1020	19.47	15.84	12.21	8.58	4.95	1.32					
1020	1060	21.07	17.44	13.81	10.18	6.55	2.92					
1060	1100	22.67	19.04	15.41	11.78	8.15	4.52	0.89				
1100	1140	24.27	20.64	17.01	13.38	9.75	6.12	2.49				
1140	1180	26.66	23.03	19.40	15.77	12.14	8.51	4.88	1.25			
1180	1220	29.06	25.43	21.80	18.17	14.54	10.91	7.28	3.65	0.02		
1220	1260	31.46	27.83	24.20	20.57	16.94	13.31	9.68	6.05	2.42		
1260	1300	33.86	30.23	26.60	22.97	19.34	15.71	12.08	8.45	4.82	1.19	
1300	1340	36.26	32.63	29.00	25.37	21.74	18.11	14.48	10.85	7.22	3.59	
1340	1380	38.66	35.03	31.40	27.77	24.14	20.51	16.88	13.25	9.62	5.99	2.36
1380	1420	41.06	37.43	33.80	30.17	26.54	22.91	19.28	15.65	12.02	8.39	4.76
1420	1460	43.46	39.83	36.20	32.57	28.94	25.31	21.68	18.05	14.42	10.79	7.16
1460	1500	45.86	42.23	38.60	34.97	31.34	27.71	24.08	20.45	16.82	13.19	9.56
1500	1540	48.60	44.97	41.34	37.71	34.08	30.45	26.82	23.19	19.56	15.93	12.30
1540	1580	51.80	48.17	44.54	40.91	37.28	33.65	30.02	26.39	22.76	19.13	15.50
1580	1620	55.00	51.37	47.74	44.11	40.48	36.85	33.22	29.59	25.96	22.33	18.70
1620	1660	58.20	54.57	50.94	47.31	43.68	40.05	36.42	32.79	29.16	25.53	21.90
1660	1700	61.40	57.77	54.14	50.51	46.88	43.25	39.62	35.99	32.36	28.73	25.10
1700	1750	65.00	61.37	57.74	54.11	50.48	46.85	43.22	39.59	35.96	32.33	28.70
1750	1800	69.00	65.37	61.74	58.11	54.48	50.85	47.22	43.59	39.96	36.33	32.70
1800	1850	73.00	69.37	65.74	62.11	58.48	54.85	51.22	47.59	43.96	40.33	36.70
1850	1900	77.15	73.52	69.89	66.26	62.63	59.00	55.37	51.74	48.11	44.48	40.85
1900	1950	81.80	78.17	74.54	70.91	67.28	63.65	60.02	56.39	52.76	49.13	45.50
1950	2000	86.45	82.82	79.19	75.56	71.93	68.30	64.67	61.04	57.41	53.78	50.15
2000	2100	93.43	89.80	86.17	82.54	78.91	75.28	71.65	68.02	64.39	60.76	57.13
2100	2200	102.73	99.10	95.47	91.84	88.21	84.58	80.95	77.32	73.69	70.06	66.43
2200	2300	112.03	108.40	104.77	101.14	97.51	93.88	90.25	86.62	82.99	79.36	75.73
2300	2400	121.33	117.70	114.07	110.44	106.81	103.18	99.55	95.92	92.29	88.66	85.03

2400 and over   (Table Amount PLUS 9.3 Percent of the Amount Over 2350)

Figure 18-7

JOB SKILL 18-4 *(continued)*

MARRIED PERSONS----SEMI-MONTHLY PAYROLL PERIOD

(FOR WAGES PAID IN 2006)

IF WAGES ARE...　　　　AND THE NUMBER OF WITHHOLDING ALLOWANCES CLAIMED IS...　**STATE**

AT LEAST	BUT LESS THAN	0	1	2	3	4	5	6	7	8	9	10 OR MORE
		...THE AMOUNT OF INCOME TAX TO BE WITHHELD SHALL BE...										
$1	$300											
300	320	1.74										
320	340	1.94										
340	360	2.14										
360	380	2.34										
380	400	2.54										
400	420	2.74										
420	440	2.94										
440	460	3.14										
460	480	3.34										
480	500	3.54										
500	520	3.74	0.11									
520	540	3.94	0.31									
540	560	4.14	0.51									
560	580	4.34	0.71									
580	600	4.54	0.91									
600	620	4.74	1.11									
620	640	4.94	1.31									
640	660	5.14	1.51									
660	680	5.43	1.80									
680	700	5.83	2.20									
700	720	6.23	2.60									
720	740	6.63	3.00									
740	760	7.03	3.40									
760	780	7.43	3.80									
780	800	7.83	4.20									
800	820	8.23	4.60									
820	840	8.63	5.00									
840	860	9.03	5.40									
860	880	9.43	5.80									
880	900	9.83	6.20									
900	920	10.23	6.60	0.26								
920	940	10.63	7.00	0.66								
940	960	11.03	7.40	1.06								
960	980	11.43	7.80	1.46								
980	1000	11.83	8.20	1.86								
1000	1040	12.43	8.80	2.46								
1040	1080	13.23	9.60	3.26								
1080	1120	14.03	10.40	4.06	0.43							
1120	1160	14.83	11.20	4.86	1.23							
1160	1200	15.63	12.00	5.66	2.03							
1200	1240	16.43	12.80	6.46	2.83							
1240	1280	17.23	13.60	7.26	3.63							
1280	1320	18.03	14.40	8.06	4.43	0.80						
1320	1360	18.83	15.20	8.86	5.23	1.60						
1360	1400	19.63	16.00	9.66	6.03	2.40						
1400	1440	21.16	17.53	10.46	6.83	3.20						
1440	1480	22.76	19.13	11.26	7.63	4.00	0.37					
1480	1520	24.36	20.73	12.06	8.43	4.80	1.17					
1520	1560	25.96	22.33	13.27	9.64	6.01	2.38					
1560	1600	27.56	23.93	14.87	11.24	7.61	3.98	0.35				

Figure 18-8

JOB SKILL 18-4 *(continued)*

CALIFORNIA WITHHOLDING SCHEDULES FOR 2006

UNMARRIED HEAD OF HOUSEHOLD----SEMI-MONTHLY PAYROLL PERIOD

(FOR WAGES PAID IN 2006)

IF WAGES ARE...   AND THE NUMBER OF WITHHOLDING ALLOWANCES CLAIMED IS...   **STATE**

AT LEAST	BUT LESS THAN	0	1	2	3	4	5	6	7	8	9	10 OR MORE
				...THE AMOUNT OF INCOME TAX TO BE WITHHELD SHALL BE...								
$1	$600											
600	620	3.39										
620	640	3.59										
640	660	3.79	0.16									
660	680	3.99	0.36									
680	700	4.19	0.56									
700	720	4.39	0.76									
720	740	4.59	0.96									
740	760	4.79	1.16									
760	780	4.99	1.36									
780	800	5.19	1.56									
800	820	5.51	1.88									
820	840	5.91	2.28									
840	860	6.31	2.68									
860	880	6.71	3.08									
880	900	7.11	3.48									
900	920	7.51	3.88	0.25								
920	940	7.91	4.28	0.65								
940	960	8.31	4.68	1.05								
960	980	8.71	5.08	1.45								
980	1000	9.11	5.48	1.85								
1000	1025	9.56	5.93	2.30								
1025	1050	10.06	6.43	2.80								
1050	1075	10.56	6.93	3.30								
1075	1100	11.06	7.43	3.80	0.17							
1100	1125	11.56	7.93	4.30	0.67							
1125	1150	12.06	8.43	4.80	1.17							
1150	1175	12.56	8.93	5.30	1.67							
1175	1200	13.06	9.43	5.80	2.17							
1200	1225	13.56	9.93	6.30	2.67							
1225	1250	14.06	10.43	6.80	3.17							
1250	1275	14.56	10.93	7.30	3.67	0.04						
1275	1300	15.06	11.43	7.80	4.17	0.54						
1300	1325	15.56	11.93	8.30	4.67	1.04						
1325	1350	16.06	12.43	8.80	5.17	1.54						
1350	1375	16.56	12.93	9.30	5.67	2.04						
1375	1400	17.06	13.43	9.80	6.17	2.54						
1400	1450	17.81	14.18	10.55	6.92	3.29						
1450	1500	18.81	15.18	11.55	7.92	4.29	0.66					
1500	1550	19.92	16.29	12.66	9.03	5.40	1.77					
1550	1600	21.92	18.29	14.66	11.03	7.40	3.77	0.14				
1600	1650	23.92	20.29	16.66	13.03	9.40	5.77	2.14				
1650	1700	25.92	22.29	18.66	15.03	11.40	7.77	4.14	0.51			
1700	1750	27.92	24.29	20.66	17.03	13.40	9.77	6.14	2.51			
1750	1800	29.92	26.29	22.66	19.03	15.40	11.77	8.14	4.51	0.88		
1800	1850	31.92	28.29	24.66	21.03	17.40	13.77	10.14	6.51	2.88		
1850	1900	33.92	30.29	26.66	23.03	19.40	15.77	12.14	8.51	4.88	1.25	
1900	2000	38.32	34.69	31.06	27.43	23.80	20.17	16.54	12.91	9.28	5.65	2.02
2000	2100	44.32	40.69	37.06	33.43	29.80	26.17	22.54	18.91	15.28	11.65	8.02
2100	2200	50.32	46.69	43.06	39.43	35.80	32.17	28.54	24.91	21.28	17.65	14.02
2200	2300	56.32	52.69	49.06	45.43	41.80	38.17	34.54	30.91	27.28	23.65	20.02

2300 and over   (Table Amount PLUS 9.3 Percent of the Amount Over 2250)

Figure 18-9

JOB SKILL 18-4 *(continued)*

MARRIED PERSONS----MONTHLY PAYROLL PERIOD

(FOR WAGES PAID IN 2006)

IF WAGES ARE...   AND THE NUMBER OF WITHHOLDING ALLOWANCES CLAIMED IS...   **STATE**

AT LEAST	BUT LESS THAN	0	1	2	3	4	5	6	7	8	9	10 OR MORE
		...THE AMOUNT OF INCOME TAX TO BE WITHHELD SHALL BE...										
$1	$600											
600	640	3.49										
640	680	3.89										
680	720	4.29										
720	760	4.69										
760	800	5.09										
800	840	5.49										
840	880	5.89										
880	920	6.29										
920	960	6.69										
960	1000	7.09										
1000	1040	7.49	0.23									
1040	1080	7.89	0.63									
1080	1120	8.29	1.03									
1120	1160	8.69	1.43									
1160	1200	9.09	1.83									
1200	1240	9.49	2.23									
1240	1280	9.89	2.63									
1280	1320	10.29	3.03									
1320	1360	10.86	3.60									
1360	1400	11.66	4.40									
1400	1440	12.46	5.20									
1440	1480	13.26	6.00									
1480	1520	14.06	6.80									
1520	1560	14.86	7.60									
1560	1600	15.66	8.40									
1600	1640	16.46	9.20									
1640	1680	17.26	10.00									
1680	1720	18.06	10.80									
1720	1760	18.86	11.60									
1760	1800	19.66	12.40									
1800	1840	20.46	13.20	0.51								
1840	1880	21.26	14.00	1.31								
1880	1920	22.06	14.80	2.11								
1920	1960	22.86	15.60	2.91								
1960	2000	23.66	16.40	3.71								
2000	2040	24.46	17.20	4.51								
2040	2080	25.26	18.00	5.31								
2080	2140	26.26	19.00	6.31								
2140	2200	27.46	20.20	7.51	0.25							
2200	2260	28.66	21.40	8.71	1.45							
2260	2320	29.86	22.60	9.91	2.65							
2320	2380	31.06	23.80	11.11	3.85							
2380	2440	32.26	25.00	12.31	5.05							
2440	2500	33.46	26.20	13.51	6.25							
2500	2560	34.66	27.40	14.71	7.45	0.19						
2560	2620	35.86	28.60	15.91	8.65	1.39						
2620	2680	37.06	29.80	17.11	9.85	2.59						
2680	2740	38.26	31.00	18.31	11.05	3.79						
2740	2800	39.51	32.25	19.51	12.25	4.99						
2800	2860	41.91	34.65	20.71	13.45	6.19						

Figure 18-10

JOB SKILL 18-4 *(continued)*

UNMARRIED HEAD OF HOUSEHOLD----MONTHLY PAYROLL PERIOD

(FOR WAGES PAID IN 2006)

IF WAGES ARE...   AND THE NUMBER OF WITHHOLDING ALLOWANCES CLAIMED IS...   **STATE**

AT LEAST	BUT LESS THAN	0	1	2	3	4	5	6	7	8	9	10 OR MORE
				...THE AMOUNT OF INCOME TAX TO BE WITHHELD SHALL BE...								
$1	1400											
1400	1420	8.68	1.42									
1420	1440	8.88	1.62									
1440	1460	9.08	1.82									
1460	1480	9.28	2.02									
1480	1500	9.48	2.22									
1500	1520	9.68	2.42									
1520	1540	9.88	2.62									
1540	1560	10.08	2.82									
1560	1580	10.28	3.02									
1580	1600	10.48	3.22									
1600	1620	10.81	3.55									
1620	1640	11.21	3.95									
1640	1660	11.61	4.35									
1660	1680	12.01	4.75									
1680	1720	12.61	5.35									
1720	1760	13.41	6.15									
1760	1800	14.21	6.95									
1800	1840	15.01	7.75	0.49								
1840	1880	15.81	8.55	1.29								
1880	1920	16.61	9.35	2.09								
1920	1960	17.41	10.15	2.89								
1960	2000	18.21	10.95	3.69								
2000	2040	19.01	11.75	4.49								
2040	2080	19.81	12.55	5.29								
2080	2120	20.61	13.35	6.09								
2120	2160	21.41	14.15	6.89								
2160	2200	22.21	14.95	7.69	0.43							
2200	2250	23.11	15.85	8.59	1.33							
2250	2300	24.11	16.85	9.59	2.33							
2300	2350	25.11	17.85	10.59	3.33							
2350	2400	26.11	18.85	11.59	4.33							
2400	2450	27.11	19.85	12.59	5.33							
2450	2500	28.11	20.85	13.59	6.33							
2500	2550	29.11	21.85	14.59	7.33	0.07						
2550	2600	30.11	22.85	15.59	8.33	1.07						
2600	2650	31.11	23.85	16.59	9.33	2.07						
2650	2700	32.11	24.85	17.59	10.33	3.07						
2700	2800	33.61	26.35	19.09	11.83	4.57						
2800	2900	35.61	28.35	21.09	13.83	6.57						
2900	3000	37.61	30.35	23.09	15.83	8.57	1.31					
3000	3100	39.85	32.59	25.33	18.07	10.81	3.55					
3100	3200	43.85	36.59	29.33	22.07	14.81	7.55	0.29				
3200	3300	47.85	40.59	33.33	26.07	18.81	11.55	4.29				
3300	3400	51.85	44.59	37.33	30.07	22.81	15.55	8.29	1.03			
3400	3500	55.85	48.59	41.33	34.07	26.81	19.55	12.29	5.03			
3500	3600	59.85	52.59	45.33	38.07	30.81	23.55	16.29	9.03	1.77		
3600	3800	65.85	58.59	51.33	44.07	36.81	29.55	22.29	15.03	7.77	0.51	
3800	4000	76.64	69.38	62.12	54.86	47.60	40.34	33.08	25.82	18.56	11.30	4.04
4000	4200	88.64	81.38	74.12	66.86	59.60	52.34	45.08	37.82	30.56	23.30	16.04
4200	4400	100.64	93.38	86.12	78.86	71.60	64.34	57.08	49.82	42.56	35.30	28.04

4400 and over   (Table Amount PLUS 9.3 Percent of the Amount Over 4300)

Figure 18-11

JOB SKILL 18-5
Complete a Payroll Register

Name _____ Date _____ Score _____

Performance Objective

Task:　　　　Complete a payroll register.

Conditions:　Use the payroll information obtained for seven employees from Job Skill 18-4, one payroll register (Form 103), and typewriter, pen, or pencil. Refer to Procedure 18-2 in the textbook for step-by-step directions and textbook Figure 18-19 for a visual example.

Standards:　Complete all steps listed in this skill in _____ minutes with a minimum score of _____. (Time element and accuracy criteria may be given by instructor.)

Time:　　　**Start:** _____ **Completed:** _____ **Total:** _____ minutes

Scoring:　　One point for each step performed satisfactorily unless otherwise listed or weighted by instructor.

Directions with Performance Evaluation Checklist

Refer to the employees in Job Skill 18-4. Alphabetize their names (last name first), and record the information in the payroll register.

1st Attempt	2nd Attempt	3rd Attempt	
_____	_____	_____	Gather materials (equipment and supplies) listed under "Conditions."
____/14	____/14	____/14	1. Complete payroll register information for employee Lisa Adams.
____/13	____/13	____/13	2. Complete payroll register information for employee Kelley Jones.
____/13	____/13	____/13	3. Complete payroll register information for employee Maryjane Moran.
____/13	____/13	____/13	4. Complete payroll register information for employee Carla O'Hare.
____/14	____/14	____/14	5. Complete payroll register information for employee Amy Seaforth.
____/13	____/13	____/13	6. Complete payroll register information for employee Hillary Sheehan.
____/11	____/11	____/11	7. Complete payroll register information for employee Roger Young.
_____	_____	_____	Complete within specified time.
____/93	____/93	____/93	**Total points earned** (To obtain a percentage score, divide the total points earned by the number of points possible.)

Comments:

Evaluator's Signature: _____ **Need to Repeat:** _____

JOB SKILL 18-6
Complete an Employee Earning Record

Name _____ Date _____ Score _____

Performance Objective

Task: Complete an employee earning record.

Conditions: Use information from Job Skill 18-4, one employee earning record (Form 104), and typewriter, pen, or pencil.

Standards: Complete all steps listed in this skill in _____ minutes with a minimum score of _____.
(Time element and accuracy criteria may be given by instructor.)

Time: Start: _____ **Completed:** _____ **Total:** _____ minutes

Scoring: One point for each step performed satisfactorily unless otherwise listed or weighted by instructor.

Directions with Performance Evaluation Checklist

Refer to Amy Seaforth's employment information in Job Skill 18-4 and complete an employee earning record; she is a new employee.

1st Attempt	2nd Attempt	3rd Attempt	
_____	_____	_____	Gather materials (equipment and supplies) listed under "Conditions."
_____/5	_____/5	_____/5	1. Fill in the employee's name, address, telephone number, and Social Security number.
_____/8	_____/8	_____/8	2. Fill in the employee's date of hire, birth date, position, number of exemptions, and rate of pay indicating (with a circle) whether she is part-time or full-time; single or married; and is paid hourly, weekly, or monthly.
____/12	____/12	____/12	3. Complete all line items in the earning's record that are applicable to Amy Seaforth for June 28, 20XX.
_____	_____	_____	Complete within specified time.
____/27	____/27	____/27	**Total points earned** (To obtain a percentage score, divide the total points earned by the number of points possible.)

Comments:

Evaluator's Signature: _____ **Need to Repeat:** _____

National Curriculum Competency: CAAHEP: III.C.3.a(2)	ABHES: VI.B.1.a.8(f)

JOB SKILL 18-7
Complete an Employee's Withholding Allowance Certificate

Name _____ Date _____ Score _____

Performance Objective

Task: Complete an employee's withholding allowance certificate.

Conditions: One Employee's Withholding Allowance Certificate (Form 105), and typewriter, pen, or pencil. Refer to Part IV of the *Workbook* for physician information.

Standards: Complete all steps listed in this skill in _____ minutes with a minimum score of _____. (Time element and accuracy criteria may be given by instructor.)

Time: **Start:** _____ **Completed:** _____ **Total:** _____ minutes

Scoring: One point for each step performed satisfactorily unless otherwise listed or weighted by instructor.

Directions with Performance Evaluation Checklist

Complete an Employee's Withholding Allowance Certificate for yourself as if you were being hired by Drs. Gerald and Fran Practon.

1st Attempt	2nd Attempt	3rd Attempt	
_____	_____	_____	Gather materials (equipment and supplies) listed under "Conditions."
_____/5	_____/5	_____/5	1. Read through Items A through G, and mark which allowances you would like to claim.
_____	_____	_____	2. Total all deductions and enter in Line H.
_____/4	_____/4	_____/4	3. Fill in your last name, first name, and address.
_____	_____	_____	4. Fill in your Social Security number.
_____	_____	_____	5. Indicate whether you are single, married, or married and withholding at a higher single rate.
_____	_____	_____	6. Verify your last name with that appearing on your Social Security card and indicate if it is different.
_____	_____	_____	7. Indicate the number of allowances in Item 5.
_____	_____	_____	8. Read Items 6 and 7 and mark if applicable.
_____/2	_____/2	_____/2	9. Sign and date the form.
_____/3	_____/3	_____/3	10. Complete the employer's name and address in Item 8.
_____	_____	_____	11. Fill in the Tax Identification Number for Practon Medical Group, Inc.
_____	_____	_____	Complete within specified time.
_____/23	_____/23	_____/23	**Total points earned** (To obtain a percentage score, divide the total points earned by the number of points possible.)

Comments:

Evaluator's Signature: _____ **Need to Repeat:** _____

National Curriculum Competency: CAAHEP: III.C.3.a(2)   ABHES: VI.B.1.a.8(f)

JOB SKILL 18-8
Complete an Employee Benefit Form

Name _____ Date _____ Score _____

Performance Objective

Task: Extract information from the case scenario, calculate employee benefits, and complete an Employee Benefit form.

Conditions: Employee Benefit form (Form 106); calculator; and computer, typewriter, pen, or pencil.

Standards: Complete all steps listed in this skill in _____ minutes with a minimum score of _____.
                (Time element and accuracy criteria may be given by instructor.)

Time: **Start:** _____ **Completed:** _____ **Total:** _____ minutes

Scoring: One point for each step performed satisfactorily unless otherwise listed or weighted by instructor.

Directions with Performance Evaluation Checklist

Extract information for the following case scenario and complete an employee benefit form.

Scenario: You have just been hired by Drs. Gerald and Fran Practon as a full-time administrative medical assistant, and they have agreed to pay you $1,760 per month, which amounts to approximately $10 per hour. You receive six paid holidays per year and one week paid vacation after the first year. You have 10 sick days per year and $150 yearly uniform allowance. There are no retirement benefits; there may be an incentive bonus if the practice does well. The practice pays for your medical insurance, which costs $60 per month, and you elect to get life insurance at your own expense, at $12 per month for $100,000 coverage. You also elect to get accident insurance at an additional $4.60 per month for $200,000 coverage. Drs. Practon pay $15.35 per month for your workers' compensation insurance and an additional $17.60 per month for your disability insurance. They pay for your dues to the American Association of Medical Assistants, which are $90 per year.

1st Attempt	2nd Attempt	3rd Attempt	
_____	_____	_____	Gather materials (equipment and supplies) listed under "Conditions."
_____	_____	_____	1. Calculate the employer/employee benefits for medical insurance.
_____	_____	_____	2. Calculate the employer/employee benefits for life insurance.
_____	_____	_____	3. Calculate the employer/employee benefits for accident insurance.
_____	_____	_____	4. Calculate the employer/employee benefits for disability insurance.
_____	_____	_____	5. Calculate the employer/employee benefits for workers' compensation
_____	_____	_____	6. Calculate the employer/employee benefits for holidays.
_____	_____	_____	7. Calculate the employer/employee benefits for vacation.
_____	_____	_____	8. Calculate the employer/employee benefits for sick leave.
_____	_____	_____	9. Complete the employer/employee benefits for personal leave.
_____	_____	_____	10. Complete the employer/employee benefits for education.
_____	_____	_____	11. Complete the employer/employee benefits for incentive bonus.
_____	_____	_____	12. Complete the employer/employee benefits for retirement.
_____	_____	_____	13. Complete the employer/employee benefits for uniforms.
_____	_____	_____	14. Complete other employer/employee benefits.
_____	_____	_____	15. Total all employer-paid benefits.
_____	_____	_____	16. Total all employee-paid benefits.
_____	_____	_____	17. Fill in the wage of the employee.
_____/5	_____/5	_____/5	18. Calculate the gross wage for the year.
_____	_____	_____	19. Calculate the amount for the total employee package paid by the employer.

JOB SKILL 18-8 *(continued)*

_____ _____ _____ Complete within specified time.

____/25 ____/25 ____/25 **Total points earned** (To obtain a percentage score, divide the total points earned by the number of points possible.)

Comments:

Evaluator's Signature: _____ **Need to Repeat:** _____

National Curriculum Competency: CAAHEP: III.C.3.a(1)   ABHES: VI.B.1.a.6

C H A P T E R **19**

Seeking a Position As an Administrative Medical Assistant

OBJECTIVES

After completing the exercises, the student will be able to:

1. Enhance knowledge of medical terminology, interpret abbreviations, and accurately spell medical words.

2. Complete a job application form.

3. Compose a letter of introduction.

4. Key a resumé.

5. Prepare a follow-up thank-you letter.

FOCUS ON CERTIFICATION*

CMA Content Summary

- Accept responsibility for own actions
- Resumé and cover letter
- Methods of job searching
- Interviewing
- Professional presentation
- Work as team member
- Adapt communication to level of understanding
- Verbal and nonverbal communication
- Using tact, diplomacy, courtesy, and responsibility
- Interviewing
- Fundamental writing skills
- Keyboard, format, proofread data entry
- Word processing

*This *Workbook* and accompanying textbook meet the entry-level administrative and general competencies for the CMA outlined by the AAMA Examination Content Outline and Role Delineation Study and for the RMA and CMAS outlined by the AMT Competencies and Examination Specifications (see Competency Grid in textbook Appendix B).

RMA Content Summary

- Medical terminology definitions
- Interpersonal skills
- Oral and written communication

- Business format
- Listening skills

CMAS Content Summary

- Spell medical terms
- Professionalism
- Written and oral communication

- Format business correspondence
- PC-based environment; word processing
- Performance reviews

Abbreviation and Spelling Review

Read the following patient's chart note and write the meanings for the abbreviations listed below the note. To decode any abbreviations you do not understand or that appear unfamiliar to you, refer to the list of abbreviations in Part V of this *Workbook*. Step-by-step directions for this exercise are found in Procedure 1-1 of Chapter 1 in the textbook. Medical terms in the chart note are italicized; study them for spelling. Use your medical dictionary to look up their definitions. Your instructor may give a spelling and definition test that includes these words and abbreviations.

Mary Lee Brau

August 24, 20XX Pt comes in complaining of *postmenopausal* bleeding with known *cystic endometrial hyperplasia* associated with *fibroid* uterus and *uterine prolapse.* PH: I&D L breast, *abscess.* Pelvic done two months ago revealed Pap smr Class II. *Menstrual:* The pt is a G–3 Para 3, 2-0-1-2, Rh-, unsensitized. Scheduled for *hysterectomy* in two weeks. Pt to have preop HX and PX day before surg.

Gerald Practon, MD
Gerald Practon, MD

Pt	_____	Para 3	_____
PH	_____	Rh-	_____
I&D	_____	preop	_____
L	_____	HX	_____
Pap smr	_____	PX	_____
G–3	_____	surg.	_____

Note: Translation for 2-0-1-2 = 2 term infants, 0 premature, 1 abortion, 2 living children. What would be the translation for 3-1-0-3?

Review Questions

Review the objectives, glossary, and chapter information before completing the following review questions.

1. What are some of the reasons employers reject job applicants?

   a. _____

   b. _____

   c. _____

d. _____

e. _____

f. _____

g. _____

h. _____

2. Name at least three steps you would take to find medical job openings.

   a. _____

   b. _____

   c. _____

3. Why should you read the fine print in any contract an employment agency asks you to sign? _____

   _____

   _____

4. What should a job seeker do to make filling out numerous application forms easier? _____

   _____

   _____

5. A customized letter accompanying a resumé is called a/an _____ letter,

   or a/an _____ .

6. Define resumé. _____

   _____

7. A resumé style that stresses work experience dates is the _____ format;

   the _____ format highlights job skills.

8. Name three categories of people who might be listed on a reference sheet.

   a. _____

   b. _____

   c. _____

9. What is the purpose of a portfolio? _____

   _____

10. Name the five stages of an interview.

    a. _____

    b. _____

    c. _____

    d. _____

    e. _____

11. Name at least three personal items that legally do not have to be included on a resumé or discussed at a job interview.

    a. _____

    b. _____

    c. _____

12. If three days have elapsed since your interview and you have had no word from the potential employer, what two follow-up steps could you take?

    a. _____

    b. _____

13. In addition to the performance evaluation, list some items that might be included in a medical assistant's personnel file.

    a. _____

    b. _____

    c. _____

    d. _____

    e. _____

    f. _____

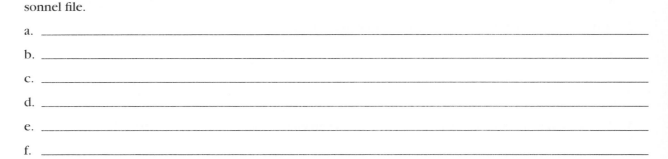

Critical Thinking Exercises

1. How would you handle an illegal question asked during a personal job interview?_____
   _____
   _____
   _____

2. State how you would you answer the following interview question: Why should I hire you? _____
   _____
   _____
   _____

3. Read the following questions and select the section on the resumé where the information is found. Write the corresponding letter for your choice in the space provided.

   a. personal information section

   b. work experience section

   c. education section

   d. job skill section

   e. reference section

   _____ 1. What is your career objective?

   _____ 2. What is your business telephone number?

   _____ 3. What is your name?

   _____ 4. Where did you go to school?

   _____ 5. What companies have you worked for?

   _____ 6. What is your e-mail address?

   _____ 7. How many references do you have listed?

   _____ 8. What is the address of your previous employer?

   _____ 9. What have been your previous job titles?

_____ 10. What is your address?

_____ 11. What courses have you taken that are related to the job you are applying for?

_____ 12. What school-related activities did you participate in?

_____ 13. What special skills do you have?

_____ 14. What are the starting and ending dates of your previous employment?

_____ 15. What degrees have you received?

_____ 16. What have been some of your job responsibilities?

_____ 17. What is your home telephone number?

_____ 18. What was your major in school?

_____ 19. What special awards or recognitions have you received?

_____ 20. What is your Social Security number?

JOB SKILL 19-1
Complete a Job Application Form

Name _____ Date _____ Score _____

Performance Objective

Task: Locate and research information and complete a mock job application form and preemployment worksheet in preparation for completing job applications and composing a resumé.

Conditions: Employment Application Form (Form 107), Preemployment Worksheet (Form 108), and pen or pencil. Refer to textbook Procedure 19-2 for step-by-step directions and Figure 19-3 for an example of a completed application form.

Standards: Complete all steps listed in this skill in _____ minutes with a minimum score of _____. (Time element and accuracy criteria may be given by instructor.)

Time: **Start:** _____ **Completed:** _____ **Total:** _____ minutes

Scoring: One point for each step performed satisfactorily unless otherwise listed or weighted by instructor.

Directions with Performance Evaluation Checklist

You will be gathering information and researching unknown details to complete a mock job application form and preemployment worksheet. These information sheets can be taken with you to potential places of employment and used to assist you when completing employment applications. Similar questions may appear on employment applications, and this information may be referred to when composing a resumé.

1st Attempt	2nd Attempt	3rd Attempt	
_____	_____	_____	Gather materials (equipment and supplies) listed under "Conditions."

Employment Application Form

1st Attempt	2nd Attempt	3rd Attempt	
_____	_____	_____	1. Make a copy of the Employment Application Form; you will be completing the first copy in pencil and the final copy in ink.
___/10	___/10	___/10	2. Fill in personal information.
___/10	___/10	___/10	3. Complete education history.
___/10	___/10	___/10	4. Record work experience.
___/9	___/9	___/9	5. List three references, other than relatives, who have known you for at least 2 years; notify each person and ask for their permission prior to listing.
___/2	___/2	___/2	6. Sign and date the application form.
___/5	___/5	___/5	7. Review the completed application form, and if everything looks satisfactory, copy the information on a clean form using ink.

Preemployment Worksheet

1st Attempt	2nd Attempt	3rd Attempt	
_____	_____	_____	8. Copy the Preemployment Worksheet and fill in the following information in pencil.
___/2	___/2	___/2	9. Compose a brief employment objective and write it on the first line.
_____	_____	_____	10. Record your driver's license number.
___/2	___/2	___/2	11. List your birthdate and indicate whether you are a United States citizen.
_____	_____	_____	12. Disclose any physical disabilities that may relate to the job applied for.
_____	_____	_____	13. Note volunteer activities; these may be related to the job and taken into consideration as work experience, or noted for freely giving of your time and energy.
___/2	___/2	___/2	14. List professional organization memberships.
_____	_____	_____	15. Note personal interests that occupy your free time.
___/25	___/25	___/25	16. List the top 25 job skills you have acquired that are related to the job you are seeking.

JOB SKILL 19-1 (*continued*)

_____/5   _____/5   _____/5   17. Review the completed worksheet, and if everything seems satisfactory, copy
the information on a clean form using ink.

_____   _____   _____   Complete within specified time.

____/90   ____/90   ____/90   **Total points earned** (To obtain a percentage score, divide the total points earned
by the number of points possible.)

Comments:

Evaluator's Signature: _____   **Need to Repeat:** _____

| National Curriculum Competency: CAAHEP: III.C.3.a(1) | ABHES: VI.B.1.a.2(j), VI.B.1.a.2(o), VI.B.1.a.3(a) |

JOB SKILL 19-2
Compose a Letter of Introduction

Name _____ Date _____ Score _____

Performance Objective

Task: Compose and key a letter of introduction to accompany a resumé and place in prepared envelope.

Conditions: Two sheets of white paper (rough and final drafts), number 10 envelope (Form 109), *Workbook* Figure 19-1, and computer or typewriter. Refer to textbook Figure 19-4 for a sample letter of introduction. Review Procedure 11-2 and instructions under "Parts of a Letter" in Chapter 11 of the textbook for format and style.

Standards: Complete all steps listed in this skill in _____ minutes with a minimum score of _____. (Time element and accuracy criteria may be given by instructor.)

Time: **Start:** _____ **Completed:** _____ **Total:** _____ minutes

Scoring: One point for each step performed satisfactorily unless otherwise listed or weighted by instructor.

Directions with Performance Evaluation Checklist

Read the job advertisements in *Workbook* Figure 19-1 and select one you wish to respond to. Compose a letter of introduction following the basic letter format and style in Chapter 11.

1st Attempt	2nd Attempt	3rd Attempt	
_____	_____	_____	Gather materials (equipment and supplies) listed under "Conditions."
___/10	___/10	___/10	1. Compose a letter of introduction in rough draft form and show to instructor for suggestions.
___/5	___/5	___/5	2. Key final draft, centering the letter with even margins; incorporate all suggestions.
_____	_____	_____	3. Date the letter using current date.
_____	_____	_____	4. Include inside address.
_____	_____	_____	5. Key appropriate salutation.
_____	_____	_____	6. Insert proper paragraphing.
_____	_____	_____	7. Use proper punctuation.
_____	_____	_____	8. Key closing line in correct position.
_____	_____	_____	9. Include enclosure notation; you will be including a resumé that will be completed in the next Job Skill.
_____	_____	_____	10. Proofread letter for typographical, spelling, punctuation, and capitalization errors while letter remains on screen or in typewriter.
_____	_____	_____	11. Correct all errors.
_____	_____	_____	12. Print letter and sign.
___/5	___/5	___/5	13. Address large envelope and key return address.
_____	_____	_____	14. Fold letter neatly and place in envelope; you will include a resumé that will be completed in the next Job Skill.
_____	_____	_____	Complete within specified time.
___/33	___/33	___/33	**Total points earned** (To obtain a percentage score, divide the total points earned by the number of points possible.)

JOB SKILL 19-2 *(continued)*

ADMINISTRATIVE MEDICAL ASSISTANT—Challenging, full-time opportunity for take-charge person with mature personality to use skills at a multiphysician practice in a pleasant work environment. Computer literate, typing/keying speed of 45 wpm, knowledge of grammar, spelling, and medical terminology essential. We offer top salary with excellent fringe benefits; outstanding potential for right person. Send resumé and salary history with your application letter telling us why you think you are the best candidate for the position. Reply to: Office Manager, Butler Medical Group, Salisbury, MD 21801.

RECEPTIONIST FOR A MEDICAL OFFICE—Rural pediatric clinic is looking for a person who has PR skills with children. Duties: Make appointments, assist and direct patients, become involved in general health care. Computer skills and some filing required. High school education, business math courses, and previous medical office experience preferred; however, right person will be considered. Salary based on experience. Excellent benefits with opportunity for swift advancement. Pleasant working environment for candidate interested in joining our team. Reply with handwritten letter; attach resumé. Include salary history and references. All information confidential. Reply to: Personnel Office, Lasalle Pediatric Clinic, 145 Hobart Ave., Dade City, FL 33425.

MEDICAL ASSISTANT/BILLER—Busy midtown general family practice physician is accepting applications from persons wishing to work in stimulating environment. Medical terminology and health insurance background are essential; experience in medical software, Medicare, and coding desired. Competitive salary, excellent fringe benefits, flexible hours, and pleasant working conditions. Outstanding potential for right person. Send resumé and salary history with your letter telling us why you think you are qualified for this position. K. Cain, CMA, 44901 Valley View Blvd., 2215 West University Dr., Suite F1088, Rochester, MN 55904.

Figure 19-1

Comments:

Evaluator's Signature: _____ **Need to Repeat:** _____

National Curriculum Competency: CAAHEP: III.C.3.a(1)	ABHES: VI.B.1.a.2(j), VI.B.1.a.2(o)

JOB SKILL 19-3
Key a Resumé

Name _____ Date _____ Score _____

Performance Objective

Task: Key a resumé in an attractive format that includes all essential information.

Conditions: Two sheets of white paper (rough draft and final copy) and computer or typewriter. Refer to the advertisements shown in *Workbook* Figure 19-1. See Job Skill 19-3 in the textbook for step-by-step directions and textbook Figures 19-5, 19-6, and 19-7 for visual examples of resumé styles.

Standards: Complete all steps listed in this skill in _____ minutes with a minimum score of _____. (Time element and accuracy criteria may be given by instructor.)

Time: Start: _____ **Completed:** _____ **Total:** _____ minutes

Scoring: One point for each step performed satisfactorily unless otherwise listed or weighted by instructor.

Directions with Performance Evaluation Checklist

Use the information gathered in Job Skill 19-1 on the job application form and preemployment worksheet to prepare a resumé in response to an advertisement.

1st Attempt	2nd Attempt	3rd Attempt	
_____	_____	_____	Gather materials (equipment and supplies) listed under "Conditions."
_____	_____	_____	1. Refer to resumé formats listed in Chapter 19 of the textbook (chronological, functional, combination, and results-oriented) to help you determine which type of resumé bests suits your work history, background, and skills. State which format you will use:
			_____
____/5	____/5	____/5	2. Abstract all necessary data.
____/5	____/5	____/5	3. Organize data according to the chosen format.
____/5	____/5	____/5	4. Key a rough draft of your resumé and have it reviewed by your instructor.
____/15	____/15	____/15	5. Key a final copy in an attractive format incorporating all suggestions.
_____	_____	_____	6. Use proper heading.
_____	_____	_____	7. Center resumé with well balanced margins.
_____	_____	_____	8. Include contact information.
____/2	____/2	____/2	9. Make sure format is easy to read and attracts attention to the areas you would like to highlight.
____/4	____/4	____/4	10. Proofread resumé for typographical, spelling, punctuation, and capitalization errors while resumé remains on screen or in typewriter.
_____	_____	_____	11. Correct all errors.
____/5	____/5	____/5	12. Print final copy of resumé and proofread hard copy.
_____	_____	_____	13. Verify a perfect copy has been produced.
_____	_____	_____	14. Fold resumé and place in envelope prepared in Job Skill 19-2.
_____	_____	_____	Complete within specified time.
____/50	____/50	____/50	**Total points earned** (To obtain a percentage score, divide the total points earned by the number of points possible.)

JOB SKILL 19-3 *(continued)*

Comments:

Evaluator's Signature: _____ **Need to Repeat:** _____

| National Curriculum Competency: CAAHEP: III.C.3.a(1) | ABHES: VI.B.1.a.2(j), VI.B.1.a.2(o), VI.B.1.a.3(a) |

JOB SKILL 19-4
Prepare a Follow-Up Thank-You Letter

Name _____ Date _____ Score _____

Performance Objective

Task: Compose and key a follow-up thank-you letter and address a small envelope.

Conditions: Two sheets of white paper (for rough draft and final copy) and one number 6 envelope (or Form 110). Refer to Procedure 19-6 in the textbook for step-by-step directions and textbook Figure 19-10 for an example of a thank-you letter written to follow up after an interview.

Standards: Complete all steps listed in this skill in _____ minutes with a minimum score of _____. (Time element and accuracy criteria may be given by instructor.)

Time: **Start:** _____ **Completed:** _____ **Total:** _____ minutes

Scoring: One point for each step performed satisfactorily unless otherwise listed or weighted by instructor.

Directions with Performance Evaluation Checklist

It has been two days since you had an interview for one of the three positions advertised in the local newspaper, and you have decided to send a follow-up thank-you letter to the person who interviewed you. Compose and key a letter using the same information you used for your letter of introduction and resumé.

1st Attempt	2nd Attempt	3rd Attempt	
_____	_____	_____	Gather materials (equipment and supplies) listed under "Conditions."
_____/5	_____/5	_____/5	1. Compose a thank-you letter.
_____/5	_____/5	_____/5	2. Key a rough draft of the letter for instructor's comments.
_____	_____	_____	3. Date letter using the current date.
_____	_____	_____	4. Center letter with even margins.
_____	_____	_____	5. Key inside address.
_____	_____	_____	6. Use appropriate salutation.
_____	_____	_____	7. Insert proper paragraphing.
_____	_____	_____	8. Key closing line in correct position.
_____/4	_____/4	_____/4	9. Proofread letter on screen or prior to removing it from typewriter for typographical, spelling, punctuation, and capitalization errors.
_____	_____	_____	10. Give to instructor for suggestions.
_____/2	_____/2	_____/2	11. Correct all errors and follow any suggestions given.
_____/2	_____/2	_____/2	12. Print a final copy of the letter and sign it.
_____	_____	_____	13. Proofread the letter again.
_____/5	_____/5	_____/5	14. Address a small envelope and key return address.
_____	_____	_____	15. Fold letter neatly and place in envelope.
_____	_____	_____	Complete within specified time.
_____/34	_____/34	_____/34	**Total points earned** (To obtain a percentage score, divide the total points earned by the number of points possible.)

JOB SKILL 19-4 *(continued)*

Comments:

Blank Forms

LIST OF FORMS

Number	Name	Number	Name
1	Patient Registration Information Form	36	Number 6 Envelope
2	Disabled Person Parking Placard Application	37	Number 6 Envelope
3	Telephone Message Forms	38	U.S. Postal Service Stamps by Mail Order Form
4	Telephone Message Forms	39	Letterhead
5	Telephone Message Forms	40	Number 10 Envelope
6	Telephone Message Forms	41	U.S. Postal Service Certified Mail Receipt Form
7	Telephone Message Forms	42	Fax Transmittal Sheet
8	Telephone Message Forms	43	Letterhead
9	Appointment Record	44	Number 6 Envelope
10	Appointment Record	45	U.S. Postal Service Certified Mail Receipt
11	Appointment Record	46	Letterhead
12	Appointment Cards	47	Number 10 Envelope
13	Hospital/Surgery Scheduling Form	48	U.S. Postal Service Certified Mail Receipt
14	Surgical Form Letter	49	Ledger/Statement (with dates and figures inserted)
15	Laboratory Requisition Form	50	Ledger/Statement
16	X-Ray Request Form	51	Cash Receipt Forms
17	File Labels	52	Letterhead
18	File Labels	53	Number 10 Envelope
19	File Labels	54	Ledger/Statement
20	Patient Record	55	Authorization to Charge Credit Card Form
21	Patient Record	56	Financial Agreement Form
22	Medical Record Abstract Form	57	Deposit Slip
23	Patient Record	58	Invoices and Blank Checks
24	Prescription Labels	59	Bank Statement Reconciliation
25	Prescription Form	60	Ledger Card
26	Medication Schedule	61	Ledger Card
27	Letterhead	62	Ledger Card
28	Letterhead	63	Ledger Card
29	Letterhead	64	Ledger Card
30	Letterhead	65	Ledger Card
31	Letterhead	66	Ledger Card
32	Interoffice Memo	67	Ledger Card
33	Interoffice Memo	68	Ledger Card
34	Letterhead	69	Ledger Card
35	Letterhead		

Number	Name	Number	Name
70	Ledger Card	90	Order Form
71	Ledger Card	91	Travel Expense Report
72	Ledger Card	92	Check Register Form
73	Ledger Card	93	Check Register Form
74	Checks	94	Check Register Form
75	Checks	95	Checks
76	Cash Receipts	96	Checks
77	Daily Journal—Day 1	97	Checks
78	Daily Journal—Day 2	98	Checks
79	Checks	99	Checks
80	Daily Journal—Day 3	100	Checks
81	Checks	101	Petty Cash Receipt Envelope
82	Daily Journal Heading and Bottom Section	102	Bank Account Reconciliation Form
83	Managed Care Plan Treatment Authorization Request	103	Payroll Register
84	Health Insurance Claim Form CMS-1500 (08/05)	104	Employee Earning Record
85	Health Insurance Claim Form CMS-1500 (08/05)	105	Employee's Withholding Allowance Certificate
86	Health Insurance Claim Form CMS-1500 (08/05)	106	Employee Benefit Form
87	Order Form	107	Employment Application Form
88	Order Form	108	Preemployment Worksheet
89	Order Form	109	Number 10 Envelope
		110	Number 6 Envelope

Insurance cards copied ☐
Date: _____

Patient Registration
Information

Please PRINT AND complete ALL sections below!

Account # : _____
Insurance # : _____
Co-Payment: $ _____

Is your condition a result of a work injury? YES NO   An auto accident? YES NO   Date of injury: _____

PATIENT'S PERSONAL INFORMATION   Marital Status: ☐ Single ☐ Married ☐ Divorced ☐ Widowed Sex: ☐ Male ☐ Female

Name: _____ _____ _____
　　　　　last name　　　　　　　　　　　　　　　first name　　　　　　　　　initial

Street address: _____ (Apt # _____) City: _____ State: _____ Zip: _____

Home phone: (___) _____ Work phone: (___) _____ Social Security # _____ - _____ - _____

Date of Birth: _____ / _____ / _____ Driver's License: (State & Number) _____
　　　　　month　　day　　　year

Employer / Name of School _____ ☐ Full Time ☐ Part Time

Spouse's Name: _____ _____ _____ Spouse's Work phone: (___) _____
　　　　　　　last name　　　first name　　initial

How do you wish to be addressed? _____ Social Security # _____ - _____ - _____

PATIENT'S / RESPONSIBLE PARTY INFORMATION

Responsible party: _____ Date of Birth: _____

Relationship to Patient: ☐ Self ☐ Spouse ☐ Other _____ Social Security # _____ - _____ - _____

Responsible party's home phone: (_____) _____ Work phone: (_____) _____

　　Address: _____ (Apt # _____) City: _____ State: _____ Zip: _____

Employer's name: _____ Phone number: (_____) _____

　　Address: _____ City: _____ State: _____ Zip: _____

　　Your occupation: _____

Spouse's Employer's name: _____ Spouse's Work phone: (___) _____

　　Address: _____ City: _____ State: _____ Zip: _____

PATIENT'S INSURANCE INFORMATION   Please present insurance cards to receptionist.

PRIMARY insurance company's name: _____

Insurance address: _____ City: _____ State: _____ Zip: _____

Name of insured: _____ Date of Birth: _____ Relationship to insured: ☐ Self ☐ Other ☐ Spouse ☐ Child

Insurance ID number: _____ Group number: _____

SECONDARY insurance company's name: _____

Insurance address: _____ City: _____ State: _____ Zip: _____

Name of insured: _____ Date of Birth: _____ Relationship to insured: ☐ Self ☐ Other ☐ Spouse ☐ Child

Insurance ID number: _____ Group number: _____

Check if appropriate: ☐ Medigap policy ☐ Retiree coverage

PATIENT'S REFERRAL INFORMATION   (please circle one)

Referred by: _____ If referred by a friend, may we thank her or him? YES NO

Name(s) of other physician(s) who care for you: _____
_____

EMERGENCY CONTACT

Name of person not living with you: _____ Relationship: _____

Address: _____ City: _____ State: _____ Zip: _____

Phone number (home): (_____) _____ Phone number (work): (_____) _____

Assignment of Benefits • Financial Agreement

I hereby give lifetime authorization for payment of insurance benefits to be made directly to _____ , and any assisting physicians, for services rendered. I understand that I am financially responsible for all charges whether or not they are covered by insurance. In the event of default, I agree to pay all costs of collection, and reasonable attorney's fees. I hereby authorize this healthcare provider to release all information necessary to secure the payment of benefits.

I further agree that a photocopy of this agreement shall be as valid as the original.

Date: _____ Your Signature: _____

Method of Payment: ☐ Cash ☐ Check ☐ Credit Card

PATIENT REGISTRATION

Form 1

DMV
Nevada Department of Motor Vehicles

555 Wright Way
Carson City, NV 89711
Reno/Sparks/Carson City (775) 684-4DMV (4368)
Las Vegas area (702) 486-4DMV (4368)
Rural Nevada or Out of State (877) 368-7828
www.dmvnv.com

APPLICATION FOR DISABLED PERSONS LICENSE PLATES AND/OR PLACARDS
NRS 482.384

☐ Disabled Plates *(permanent disability only)*   Disabled Placard(s) ☐ One ☐ Two

You may select either plates and one (1) placard, or two (2) placards.

Disabled Motorcycle Sticker ☐ One ☐ Other _____

First time applications for a Disabled Persons license plate or motorcycle sticker must be made in person.

In order to apply for disabled persons license plates or disabled motorcycle stickers(s) your name must appear on the vehicle registration certificate. If your vehicle is currently registered, you have the option of maintaining your current vehicle registration expiration date, or renewing for a full twelve (12) month period. Credit for any unused portion of your current registration is transferable to your disabled license plate registration. In applicable counties, if you are renewing for a full 12-month period, and your previous evidence of compliance with emissions standards was obtained more than 90 days ago, the vehicle must be re-inspected prior to registration. **You must have a permanent disability to qualify for Disabled Persons license plates** *(see description below).*

Please Print or Type

Applicant's Name _____   ____/____/____
(Disabled Person)   First   Middle   Last   Date of Birth

Address_____
                            Address   City   State   Zip Code

County of Residence _____ Nevada DL or ID No. _____ Daytime Telephone No. (____)_____

Signature of Applicant _____ Date _____

A LICENSED PHYSICIAN MUST COMPLETE THIS PORTION*
As a Physician for the above-named patient, I hereby certify that the applicant:

1. _____   Cannot walk two hundred feet without stopping to rest.

2. _____   Cannot walk without the use of a brace, cane, crutch, wheelchair, or other device or another person.

3. _____   Has a cardiac condition to the extent that functional limitations are classified as a Class III or Class IV according to standards adopted by the American Heart Association.

4. _____   Is restricted by a lung disease.

5. _____   Is severely limited in his/her ability to walk because of an arthritic, neurological, or orthopedic condition.

6. _____   Is visually handicapped.

7. _____   Uses portable oxygen.

I further certify that my patient's condition is a:

☐ **Temporary Disability** (6 months or less) Must indicate length of time not to exceed 6 months *beginning* _____
ending _____

☐ **Moderate Disability** (reversible but disabled longer than 6 months)
Must indicate length of time not to exceed 2 years *beginning* _____ *ending* _____

☐ **Permanent Disability** (irreversible, permanently disabled in his/her ability to walk, certification is valid indefinitely)

Please Print or Type

Physician's Name_____

Mailing Address _____
                            Address   City   State   Zip Code

Physician's License Number _____ Telephone No. (_____)_____

Physician's Signature _____ Date _____
          * Physicians Assistant Certified (PA-C) or Advanced Practice Nurse (APN) are not authorized to complete this document.
SP27 (Rev 4/2007)

Form 2

72623

PRIORITY ☐

PATIENT   AGE

CALLER

TELEPHONE

REFERRED TO

CHART #

CHART ATTACHED ☐ YES   ☐ NO

DATE   /   /   TIME   REC'D BY

Copyright © 1978 Bibbero Systems, Inc.
Printed in the U.S.A.

TELEPHONE RECORD ☎

MESSAGE

	TEMP	ALLERGIES

RESPONSE

PHY/RN INITIALS	DATE / /	TIME	HANDLED BY

PRIORITY ☐

PATIENT   AGE

CALLER

TELEPHONE

REFERRED TO

CHART #

CHART ATTACHED ☐ YES   ☐ NO

DATE   /   /   TIME   REC'D BY

Copyright © 1978 Bibbero Systems, Inc.
Printed in the U.S.A.

TELEPHONE RECORD ☎

MESSAGE

	TEMP	ALLERGIES

RESPONSE

PHY/RN INITIALS	DATE / /	TIME	HANDLED BY

PRIORITY ☐

PATIENT   AGE

CALLER

TELEPHONE

REFERRED TO

CHART #

CHART ATTACHED ☐ YES   ☐ NO

DATE   /   /   TIME   REC'D BY

Copyright © 1978 Bibbero Systems, Inc.
Printed in the U.S.A.

TELEPHONE RECORD ☎

MESSAGE

	TEMP	ALLERGIES

RESPONSE

PHY/RN INITIALS	DATE / /	TIME	HANDLED BY

PRIORITY ☐

PATIENT   AGE

CALLER

TELEPHONE

REFERRED TO

CHART #

CHART ATTACHED ☐ YES   ☐ NO

DATE   /   /   TIME   REC'D BY

Copyright © 1978 Bibbero Systems, Inc.
Printed in the U.S.A.

TELEPHONE RECORD ☎

MESSAGE

	TEMP	ALLERGIES

RESPONSE

PHY/RN INITIALS	DATE / /	TIME	HANDLED BY

Form 3

72623

PRIORITY ☐

PATIENT AGE

CALLER

TELEPHONE

REFERRED TO

CHART #

CHART ATTACHED ☐ YES ☐ NO

DATE / / TIME REC'D BY

TELEPHONE RECORD

MESSAGE

TEMP ALLERGIES

RESPONSE

PHY/RN INITIALS DATE / / TIME HANDLED BY

PRIORITY ☐

PATIENT AGE

CALLER

TELEPHONE

REFERRED TO

CHART #

CHART ATTACHED ☐ YES ☐ NO

DATE / / TIME REC'D BY

Copyright © 1978 Bibbero Systems, Inc.
Printed in the U.S.A.

TELEPHONE RECORD

MESSAGE

TEMP ALLERGIES

RESPONSE

PHY/RN INITIALS DATE / / TIME HANDLED BY

PRIORITY ☐

PATIENT AGE

CALLER

TELEPHONE

REFERRED TO

CHART #

CHART ATTACHED ☐ YES ☐ NO

DATE / / TIME REC'D BY

Copyright © 1978 Bibbero Systems, Inc.
Printed in the U.S.A.

TELEPHONE RECORD

MESSAGE

TEMP ALLERGIES

RESPONSE

PHY/RN INITIALS DATE / / TIME HANDLED BY

PRIORITY ☐

PATIENT AGE

CALLER

TELEPHONE

REFERRED TO

CHART #

CHART ATTACHED ☐ YES ☐ NO

DATE / / TIME REC'D BY

Copyright © 1978 Bibbero Systems, Inc.
Printed in the U.S.A.

TELEPHONE RECORD

MESSAGE

TEMP ALLERGIES

RESPONSE

PHY/RN INITIALS DATE / / TIME HANDLED BY

Form 4

72623

PRIORITY ☐

TELEPHONE RECORD 📞

PATIENT   AGE

MESSAGE

CALLER

TELEPHONE

REFERRED TO

TEMP   ALLERGIES

CHART #

RESPONSE

CHART ATTACHED ☐ YES ☐ NO

DATE   /   /   TIME   REC'D BY

Copyright © 1978 Bibbero Systems, Inc.
Printed in the U.S.A.

PHY/RN INITIALS   DATE   /   /   TIME   HANDLED BY

PRIORITY ☐

TELEPHONE RECORD 📞

PATIENT   AGE

MESSAGE

CALLER

TELEPHONE

REFERRED TO

TEMP   ALLERGIES

CHART #

RESPONSE

CHART ATTACHED ☐ YES ☐ NO

DATE   /   /   TIME   REC'D BY

Copyright © 1978 Bibbero Systems, Inc.
Printed in the U.S.A.

PHY/RN INITIALS   DATE   /   /   TIME   HANDLED BY

PRIORITY ☐

TELEPHONE RECORD 📞

PATIENT   AGE

MESSAGE

CALLER

TELEPHONE

REFERRED TO

TEMP   ALLERGIES

CHART #

RESPONSE

CHART ATTACHED ☐ YES ☐ NO

DATE   /   /   TIME   REC'D BY

Copyright © 1978 Bibbero Systems, Inc.
Printed in the U.S.A.

PHY/RN INITIALS   DATE   /   /   TIME   HANDLED BY

PRIORITY ☐

TELEPHONE RECORD 📞

PATIENT   AGE

MESSAGE

CALLER

TELEPHONE

REFERRED TO

TEMP   ALLERGIES

CHART #

RESPONSE

CHART ATTACHED ☐ YES ☐ NO

DATE   /   /   TIME   REC'D BY

Copyright © 1978 Bibbero Systems, Inc.
Printed in the U.S.A.

PHY/RN INITIALS   DATE   /   /   TIME   HANDLED BY

Form 5

72623

PRIORITY ☐ | **TELEPHONE RECORD** ☎

PATIENT   AGE
CALLER
TELEPHONE
REFERRED TO
CHART #
CHART ATTACHED ☐ YES ☐ NO
DATE / /   TIME   REC'D BY
Copyright © 1978 Bibbero Systems, Inc.
Printed in the U.S.A.

MESSAGE
TEMP   ALLERGIES
RESPONSE
PHY/RN INITIALS   DATE / /   TIME   HANDLED BY

PRIORITY ☐ | **TELEPHONE RECORD** ☎

PATIENT   AGE
CALLER
TELEPHONE
REFERRED TO
CHART #
CHART ATTACHED ☐ YES ☐ NO
DATE / /   TIME   REC'D BY
Copyright © 1978 Bibbero Systems, Inc.
Printed in the U.S.A.

MESSAGE
TEMP   ALLERGIES
RESPONSE
PHY/RN INITIALS   DATE / /   TIME   HANDLED BY

PRIORITY ☐ | **TELEPHONE RECORD** ☎

PATIENT   AGE
CALLER
TELEPHONE
REFERRED TO
CHART #
CHART ATTACHED ☐ YES ☐ NO
DATE / /   TIME   REC'D BY
Copyright © 1978 Bibbero Systems, Inc.
Printed in the U.S.A.

MESSAGE
TEMP   ALLERGIES
RESPONSE
PHY/RN INITIALS   DATE / /   TIME   HANDLED BY

PRIORITY ☐ | **TELEPHONE RECORD** ☎

PATIENT   AGE
CALLER
TELEPHONE
REFERRED TO
CHART #
CHART ATTACHED ☐ YES ☐ NO
DATE / /   TIME   REC'D BY
Copyright © 1978 Bibbero Systems, Inc.
Printed in the U.S.A.

MESSAGE
TEMP   ALLERGIES
RESPONSE
PHY/RN INITIALS   DATE / /   TIME   HANDLED BY

Form 6

MESSAGE FROM

For Dr.	Name of Caller	Rel. to Pt.	Patient	Pt. Age	Pt. Temp.	Message Date / /	Message Time AM PM	Urgent ❑ Yes ❑ No

Message:

Allergies

Respond to Phone #	Best Time to Call AM PM	Pharmacy Name / #	Patient's Chart Attached ❑ Yes ❑ No	Patient's Chart #	Initials

DOCTOR - STAFF RESPONSE

Doctor's / Staff Orders / Follow-Up Action

	Call Back ❑ Yes ❑ No	Chart Mess. ❑ Yes ❑ No	Follow-Up Date / /	Follow-Up Completed-Date/Time / / AM PM	Response by

Product #78-9156 Pkg., #78-9157 Pads, Bibbero Systems, Inc., Petaluma, CA. To order, call toll free 800-Bibbero (800-242-2376) or Fax 800-242-9330.

MESSAGE FROM

For Dr.	Name of Caller	Rel. to Pt.	Patient	Pt. Age	Pt. Temp.	Message Date / /	Message Time AM PM	Urgent ❑ Yes ❑ No

Message:

Allergies

Respond to Phone #	Best Time to Call AM PM	Pharmacy Name / #	Patient's Chart Attached ❑ Yes ❑ No	Patient's Chart #	Initials

DOCTOR - STAFF RESPONSE

Doctor's / Staff Orders / Follow-Up Action

	Call Back ❑ Yes ❑ No	Chart Mess. ❑ Yes ❑ No	Follow-Up Date / /	Follow-Up Completed-Date/Time / / AM PM	Response by

Product #78-9156 Pkg., #78-9157 Pads, Bibbero Systems, Inc., Petaluma, CA. To order, call toll free 800-Bibbero (800-242-2376) or Fax 800-242-9330.

Form 7

MESSAGE FROM

For Dr.	Name of Caller	Rel. to Pt.	Patient	Pt. Age	Pt. Temp.	Message Date / /	Message Time AM PM	Urgent ☐ Yes ☐ No

Message:

Allergies

Respond to Phone #	Best Time to Call AM PM	Pharmacy Name / #	Patient's Chart Attached ☐ Yes ☐ No	Patient's Chart #	Initials

DOCTOR - STAFF RESPONSE

Doctor's / Staff Orders / Follow-Up Action

Call Back ☐ Yes ☐ No	Chart Mess. ☐ Yes ☐ No	Follow-Up Date / /	Follow-Up Completed-Date/Time / / AM PM	Response by

Product #78-9156 Pkg., #78-9157 Pads, Bibbero Systems, Inc., Petaluma, CA. To order, call toll free 800-Bibbero (800-242-2376) or Fax 800-242-9330.

MESSAGE FROM

For Dr.	Name of Caller	Rel. to Pt.	Patient	Pt. Age	Pt. Temp.	Message Date / /	Message Time AM PM	Urgent ☐ Yes ☐ No

Message:

Allergies

Respond to Phone #	Best Time to Call AM PM	Pharmacy Name / #	Patient's Chart Attached ☐ Yes ☐ No	Patient's Chart #	Initials

DOCTOR - STAFF RESPONSE

Doctor's / Staff Orders / Follow-Up Action

Call Back ☐ Yes ☐ No	Chart Mess. ☐ Yes ☐ No	Follow-Up Date / /	Follow-Up Completed-Date/Time / / AM PM	Response by

Product #78-9156 Pkg., #78-9157 Pads, Bibbero Systems, Inc., Petaluma, CA. To order, call toll free 800-Bibbero (800-242-2376) or Fax 800-242-9330.

Form 8

APPOINTMENT RECORD

		DOCTOR		
		DATE		
		DAY		

		AM	00		
		8	15		
			30		
			45		
		9	00		
			15		
			30		
			45		
		10	00		
			15		
			30		
			45		
		11	00		
			15		
			30		
			45		
		12	00		
			15		
			30		
			45		
		PM	00		
		1	15		
			30		
			45		
		2	00		
			15		
			30		
			45		
		3	00		
			15		
			30		
			45		
		4	00		
			15		
			30		
			45		
		5	00		
			15		
			30		
			45		

REMARKS & NOTES

FORM # 56-0315 ©1965 BIBBERO SYSTEMS, INC., PETALUMA, CA.   To order call TOLL FREE: 800-BIBBERO (CA) or 800-358-8240 (U.S.)

Form 9

APPOINTMENT RECORD

		DOCTOR			
		DATE			
		DAY			
		AM	00		
		8	15		
			30		
			45		
			00		
		9	15		
			30		
			45		
			00		
		10	15		
			30		
			45		
			00		
		11	15		
			30		
			45		
			00		
		12	15		
			30		
			45		
		PM	00		
		1	15		
			30		
			45		
		2	00		
			15		
			30		
			45		
		3	00		
			15		
			30		
			45		
		4	00		
			15		
			30		
			45		
		5	00		
			15		
			30		
			45		

REMARKS & NOTES

FORM # 56-0315 ©1965 BIBBERO SYSTEMS, INC., PETALUMA, CA.   To order call TOLL FREE: 800-BIBBERO (CA) or 800-358-8240 (U.S.)

Form 10

APPOINTMENT RECORD

		DOCTOR		
		DATE		
		DAY		
		AM	00		
			15		
		8	30		
			45		
			00		
			15		
		9	30		
			45		
			00		
			15		
		10	30		
			45		
			00		
			15		
		11	30		
			45		
			00		
			15		
		12	30		
			45		
		PM	00		
			15		
		1	30		
			45		
			00		
			15		
		2	30		
			45		
			00		
			15		
		3	30		
			45		
			00		
			15		
		4	30		
			45		
			00		
			15		
		5	30		
			45		

REMARKS & NOTES

Form 11

M_____

has an appointment with:
☐ Fran Practon MD   ☐ Gerald Practon MD
PRACTON MEDICAL GROUP, INC.
4567 Broad Avenue
Woodland Hills, XY 12345
Tel. 555/486-9002

for

Mon. _____at_____

Tues. _____at_____

Wed. _____at_____

Thurs._____at_____

Fri. _____at_____

Sat. _____at_____

If unable to keep this appointment
kindly give 24 hours notice.

M_____

has an appointment with:
☐ Fran Practon MD   ☐ Gerald Practon MD
PRACTON MEDICAL GROUP, INC.
4567 Broad Avenue
Woodland Hills, XY 12345
Tel. 555/486-9002

for

Mon. _____at_____

Tues. _____at_____

Wed. _____at_____

Thurs._____at_____

Fri. _____at_____

Sat. _____at_____

If unable to keep this appointment
kindly give 24 hours notice.

M_____

has an appointment with:
☐ Fran Practon MD   ☐ Gerald Practon MD
PRACTON MEDICAL GROUP, INC.
4567 Broad Avenue
Woodland Hills, XY 12345
Tel. 555/486-9002

for

Mon. _____at_____

Tues. _____at_____

Wed. _____at_____

Thurs._____at_____

Fri. _____at_____

Sat. _____at_____

If unable to keep this appointment
kindly give 24 hours notice.

M_____

has an appointment with:
☐ Fran Practon MD   ☐ Gerald Practon MD
PRACTON MEDICAL GROUP, INC.
4567 Broad Avenue
Woodland Hills, XY 12345
Tel. 555/486-9002

for

Mon. _____at_____

Tues. _____at_____

Wed. _____at_____

Thurs._____at_____

Fri. _____at_____

Sat. _____at_____

If unable to keep this appointment
kindly give 24 hours notice.

Form 12

HOSPITAL/SURGERY SCHEDULING FORM

Section 1   **Completed by physician**

1. _____   Patient's name_____

2. _____   Procedure_____

3. _____   Emergency: Urgent_____   Elective_____

4. _____   Diagnoses 1. _____

                               2. _____

5. _____   Hospital/Facility name_____

6. _____   Inpatient_____   Outpatient_____   Day Surgery_____

7. _____   Surgical assistant required?   Yes_____   No_____

                 Who preferred?_____

8. _____   Anesthesia required?   Yes_____   No_____   General_____   Local_____

                 Who preferred?_____

9. _____   Referring physician_____

Section 2   **Completed by patient**

10. _____   Age of patient_____   Date of birth _____   Smoker_____Nonsmoker_____

11. _____   Room accommodations: Private_____   Semi-private_____   Ward_____

12. _____   Telephone numbers: Home (_____)_____ Work (_____)_____

13. _____   Insurance company_____ Policy number_____

                 Secondary insurance_____ Policy number_____

14. _____   Second surgical opinion needed for insurance?   Yes_____   No_____

15. _____   Name of nearest relative_____

                 Address_____Phone number_____

16. _____   Admitted to this facility previous?   Yes_____   No_____

                 Date_____ Type of procedure_____

17. _____   Patient has had preadmission testing of CBC_____, EKG_____,

                 Chest x-ray_____within _____ weeks.

18. _____   Admission and procedures reported to patient on   Date:_____

19. _____   Preadmission and operation instructions given to me?   Yes_____   No_____

20. _____   Insurance and financial arrangements discussed with me? Yes_____   No_____

Section 3   **Completed by medical assistant**

21. _____   Operation room reserved for surgery on this date_____and time_____

22. _____   Name of hospital employee who scheduled surgery_____

23. _____   Name of surgical assistant scheduled and called_____

24. _____   Name of anesthesiologist scheduled and called_____

25. _____   Reported to referring physician's office and talked to_____

26. _____   Hospital/Facility admission confirmed/preadmission test scheduled

27. _____   Prior authorizations/second opinions obtained

                 Authorization/precertification #_____Date provided_____

                 Who provided number?_____

28. _____   Admitting date and surgical procedure entered in appointment book

29. _____   Arrangements confirmed with patient

30. _____   History and physical report ready

                 Name of office employee who scheduled surgery_____Date_____

Form 13

FRAN T. PRACTON, MD
Family Practice

GERALD M. PRACTON, MD
General Practice

PRACTON MEDICAL GROUP, INC.
4567 Broad Avenue
Woodland Hills, XY 12345-4700
Tel 555/486-9002
Fax No.555/488-7815

_____
_____
_____
_____

The following arrangements have been made for your hospitalization under the care of

_____. You are to enter _____ on _____,

_____ at _____.

Your procedure, _____, is scheduled for _____, _____

at _____ (subject to change in time). A _____ room has been reserved for you as requested.

You should take robe, slippers, and personal grooming articles with you. Please leave valuables

at home. If it should become necessary for you to cancel these arrangements, please notify

me immediately.

Sincerely,

_____, Medical Assistant

Surgeon: _____

Assistant Surgeon: _____

Anesthetist: _____

SPECIAL NOTE to patients covered by Medicare. Medicare will only pay for a semiprivate room;

therefore, patients requesting private rooms will be required to pay the difference in cost.

Form 14

LABORATORY REQUISITION

I.D.#	PATIENT LAST NAME		FIRST		M.I.	REFERRING PHYSICIAN

| REFERRED BY | SS #: | BILL: ☐ PHYSICIAN ☐ MEDI-CAL ☐ HMO ☐ CHDP ☐ MEDICARE ☐ INSURANCE ☐ PATIENT PLEASE COMPLETE BILLING INFORMATION AT BOTTOM | D.O.B. | AGE | SEX |

ADDRESS	PHONE NUMBER ( )	DATE COLLECTED	TIME COLLECTED

| CITY | STATE | ZIP CODE | FASTING YES \| NO | STAT | CALL RESULT |

| MEDICARE # | MEDICAL # | INFO. BELOW WILL APPEAR ON REPORT |

CUSTOM PROFILES & ADDITIONAL TESTS

```
  173    [ ] CHEMISTRY PANEL, COMPLETE BLOOD COUNT (ZPP), LIPID PROFILE, T4
  05050  [ ] CHOL, TRIG, HDL CHOL, VLDL CHOL, LDL CHOL, RISK FACTOR
```

PROFILES

00011 ☐ SPECIAL COMPREHENSIVE	2 SS,L	03536 ☐ HYPERTHYROID PROFILE				SS
00001 ☐ COMPREHENSIVE HEALTH SURVEY	SS,L	05037 ☐ HYPOTHYROID PROFILE				SS
00002 ☐ GENERAL SURVEY	SS,L	05051 ☐ LIPID PROFILE				SS
00003 ☐ CHEMISTRY PANEL	SS	05021 ☐ LIVER PROFILE				SS
CH7 ☐ CHEM 7 PANEL	SS	03350 ☐ LUPUS PROFILE				SS
03280 ☐ ANEMIA PROFILE	SS,L	03959 ☐ MENOPAUSAL PROFILE	SS /	03960 ☐ POST MENOPAUSAL	SS
05016 ☐ ARTHRITIS PROFILE	SS,L	02280 ☐ OVARIAN FUNCTION PROFILE	SS /	02281 ☐ TESTICULAR FUNC. PROF.	SS
05726 ☐ COMPREHENSIVE THYROID SURVEY	SS	02808 ☐ PRENATAL PROFILE				L,R
02691 ☐ EPSTEIN BARR PROFILE	SS	05006 ☐ THYROID PROFILE				SS
05010 ☐ ELECTROLYTES	SS	03191 ☐ TORCH PANEL				SS
06826 ☐ HEPATITIS PROFILE	SS	5756 ☐ URINE DRUG SCREEN	U /	☐ VENIPUNCTURE	

TESTS

0361 ☐ ABO & Rh TYPE	R, L	0141 ☐ C-REACTIVE PROTEIN	SS	0673 ☐ HEPATITIS B SURFACE ANTIGEN	SS	0237 ☐ PTT	B
0302 ☐ ALKALINE PHOSPHATASE	SS	1341 ☐ DHEA-S	SS	0245 ☐ HEPATITIS C ANTIBODY	SS	0317 ☐ RA FACTOR	SS
0109 ☐ AMYLASE	SS	0119 ☐ DIGOXIN	SS	0257 ☐ IRON	SS	0321 ☐ RUBELLA	SS
0613 ☐ ANA	SS	0224 ☐ DILANTIN	SS	LDL-A ☐ LDL CHOLESTEROL	SS	0381 ☐ RPR	SS
0366 ☐ ANTIBODY SCREEN	R	0835 ☐ ESTRADIOL	SS	0283 ☐ LEAD BLOOD	RB	0335 ☐ SEMEN ANALYSIS	SEMEN
0110 ☐ ASO (STREPTOZYME)	SS	0833 ☐ FERRITIN	SS	0281 ☐ LIPASE	SS	0328 ☐ SEDIMENTATION RATE (ESR)	L
0126 ☐ BILIRUBIN TOTAL	SS	0003 ☐ FOLIC ACID & VITAMIN B12	SS	8225 ☐ LH	SS	0349 ☐ SGOT (AST)	SS
0132 ☐ BUN	SS	0651 ☐ FSH	SS	0247 ☐ MONONUCLEOSIS	SS	0348 ☐ SGPT (ALT)	SS
8728 ☐ CA125	SS	0140 ☐ FTA-ABS	SS	0778 ☐ PHENOBARBITAL	SS	0330 ☐ SICKLE CELL SCREEN	L
0142 ☐ CALCIUM	SS	0210 ☐ GGTP	SS	0307 ☐ POTASSIUM	SS	0354 ☐ T4 (THYROXINE)	SS
0130 ☐ CBC	L	0536 ☐ GLUCOSE, FASTING	GY	0557 ☐ PREGNANCY (SERUM)	SS	1358 ☐ T4 FREE	SS
0388 ☐ CEA-ROCHE	SS	☐ GLUCOSE, ____ HR PP	GY	0308 ☐ PREGNANCY (URINE)	U	8456 ☐ TESTOSTERONE	SS
0152 ☐ CHOLESTEROL	SS	0771 ☐ GLYCOHEMOGLOBIN	L	0859 ☐ PROGESTERONE	SS	0824 ☐ THEOPHYLLINE	SS
0786 ☐ CORTISOL	SS	0534 ☐ H. PYLORI	SS	8041 ☐ PROLACTIN	SS	0360 ☐ TRIGLYCERIDE	SS
0162 ☐ CPK	SS	0823 ☐ HCG QUANTITATIVE	SS	0103 ☐ PROTEIN, TOTAL	SS	0672 ☐ TSH	SS
0445 ☐ CKMB ISOENZYME	SS	1856 ☐ HIV (ANTIBODY)	SS	2000 ☐ PROSTATE SPECIFIC ANTIGEN (PSA)	SS	0373 ☐ URIC ACID	SS
0161 ☐ CREATININE	SS	0558 ☐ HDL CHOLESTEROL	SS	0310 ☐ PT (PROTHROMBIN TIME)	B	0219 ☐ URINALYSIS	U

CYTOPATHOLOGY

☐ PREGNANT ☐ ABORTION ☐ POST-PARTUM ☐ POST-MENOPAUSE

HISTORY _____

PREV. ABNORMAL CYTOL FINDINGS _____
DATE _____

☐ CONTRACEPTIVES ☐ HORMONES ☐ IUD
☐ HYSTERECTOMY ☐ TOTAL ☐ SUPRA CX
☐ OOPHORECTOMY DATE _____
☐ RADIATION Rx ☐ HORMONES Rx ☐ CHEMO Rx
☐ OTHER _____

LMP: _____
SOURCE ☐ CERVIX DATE COLLECTED: _____
☐ CYTOBRUSH ☐ ENDOCERVIX ☐ VAGINA
☐ OTHER SITE

LAB USE ONLY (DO NOT WRITE BELOW THIS SPACE)

DATE RECEIVED	DATE REPORTED

STATEMENT OF SPECIMEN ADEQUACY

GENERAL CATEGORIZATION

DESCRIPTIVE DIAGNOSIS

HORMONAL EVALUATION   MI

ADDITIONAL COMMENT

CYTOTECHNOLOGIST	PATHOLOGIST

MICROBIOLOGY

THCUL ☐ THROAT	URTHC ☐ URETHRAL	9391 ☐ CHLAMYDIA DNA
EACUL ☐ EAR	VACUL ☐ VAGINAL	9390 ☐ GONORRHEA DNA
EYCUL ☐ EYE	WOCUL ☐ WOUND	9310BR ☐ OCCULT BLOOD
GOCUL ☐ GC	ROCUL ☐ CULTURE (Routine)	0293 ☐ OVA & PARASITE
SPCUL ☐ SPUTUM	URCUL ☐ URINE	WTM ☐ WET MOUNT
STCUL ☐ STOOL	GSP ☐ GRAM STAIN	

SOURCE _____ OTHER _____

DIAGNOSIS OR COMMENTS

BILLING INFORMATION

PRIMARY INSURED	INSURANCE COMPANY

ADDRESS

POLICY NO. & I.D. NO.	ICD9 CODE

LEGEND

SS	Serum Separator	GY	Grey	B	Blue	U	Urine
R	Red	L	Lavender	RB	Royal Blue	G	Green

Form 15

DATE ORDERED _____ AGE _____ **X-RAY REQUEST**   DATE PERFORMED _____

PATIENT _____

X-RAY # _____

CHART# [ ][ ][ ][ ][ ][ ]   DOB _____

13   188

BILL TO: _____

REFERRING
PHYSICIAN: _____

STREET _____

CALL
REPORT EXT: _____

CITY _____

TYPE

✔ NEW ADDRESS [   ]

☐ ASAP   ☐ TODAY

Examination _____

Chief Complaint _____

Clinical Findings _____

✔	SC	Description	CPT	Mod	Fee	✔	SC	Description	CPT	Mod	Fee	✔	SC	Description	CPT	Mod	Fee
		CHEST						**UPPER EXTREMITY**						**HEAD**			
	5085	P.A. & Lat Chest	71020				5158	Shoulder Complete	73030				5042	Facial Bones	70150		
	5083	P.A. Chest	71010				5155	Clavicle	73000				5043	Nose	70160		
	5088	Chest Fluoro	71023				5156	Scapula	73010				5048	Sinuses	70220		
	5098	Ribs Unilateral	71101				5160	A-C Joints	73050				5047	Sinuses, Ltd.	70210		
	5100	Ribs Bilateral	71111				5102	S-C Joints	71130				5051	Skull, Complete	70260		
	5101	Sternum	71120				5161	Humerus	73060				5050	Skull, Ltd.	70250		
	5352	Mammo, Diag	76091				5163	Elbow, Complete	73080				5039	Mastoids	70130		
	5351	Mammo, Unilat	76090				5162	Elbow, 2 views	73070				5046	Orbits	70200		
	5353	Mammo, Screen	76092				5165	Forearm	73090				5037	Mandible	70110		
							5168	Wrist Complete	73110				5056	T.M. Joints	70330		
		ABDOMEN					5167	Wrist, 2 views	73100								
	5204	A.P.	74000				5171	Hand, Complete	73130					**SPINE-PELVIS**			
	5207	Acute Series	74022				5170	Hand, 2 views	73120				5110	C-Spine, Comp	72050		
							5172	Finger(s)	73140				5108	C-Spine, Ltd.	72020		
		GASTROINTESTINAL					5341	Bone Age	76020				5113	T-Spine	72070		
	5212	Swallowing - Eso	74210										5119	L-Spine, Comp	72110		
	5213	Esophagram	74220					**LOWER EXTREMITY**					5118	L-Spine, Ltd.	72100		
	5217	UGI Series	74241				5179	Hip	73510				5140	Pelvis	72170		
	5218	UGI & Sm Bowel	74245				5180	Bilateral Hips	73520				5147	Sacro-Iliac Joints	72202		
	5224	BA Enema	74270				5183	Infant Hips	73540				5148	Sacrum/Coccyx	72220		
	5225	BA Air Contrast	74280				5184	Femur (Thigh)	73550				5112	Scoliosis Study	72069		
	5227	GB Oral	74290				5187	Knee, Complete	73564								
	5228	GB Repeat	74291				5185	Knee, 2 views	73560					**MISCELLANEOUS**			
	5222	Small Bowel	74250				5186	Patella	73562				5337	Fluoroscopy	76000		
	5231	T-Tube Cholangio	74305				5190	Leg (Tibia)	73590				5344	Bone Survey	76062		
	5348	Sinogram	76080				5193	Ankle, Complete	73610				5362	Outside Films	76140		
	5061	Soft Tissue Neck	70360				5192	Ankle, 2 views	73600				5354	Needle Loc	76096		
							5196	Foot, Complete	73630				5356	Specimen Film	76098		
		GENITOURINARY					5195	Foot, 2 views	73620				5159	Shoulder Arthro	73040		
	5242	I.VP.	74400				5197	Os Calcis	73650								
	5258	Salpingogram	74740				5198	Toe(s)	73660					**SUPPLIES**			
	5248	Cystogram	74430				5342	Bone Length Scan	76040								

5-10

Form 16

1. Walter Louis McDougall

2. Marilyn Marvel

3. Ms. Margaret McKinney

4. Roberta Nelson
   6428 Lorraine Rd., Sherman Oaks, XY

5. Rev. Jack Rowe
   462 Twelve Oaks Dr., Encino, XY

6. Renee T. Moore (Mrs. C. H.)

7. Marilyn P. Marvel (Mrs. Paul P.)

8. Roger C. Camp

9. Mrs. John M. White (Jane B.)

10. Anna F. Rolf

11. Mrs. Roger G. Camp (Jane)

12. Raymond E. Stokes Jr.

13. Nancy Jeffers

14. Mrs. Alfred Hall (Martha)

15. Ms. Carla St. John

16. Wm. L. MacPherson

17. Benjamin Thomas

18. L. William McPherson

19. A. Buckley

20. Vincent DeLuca

Form 17

21. John Lee-Barry

22. Alice Buckley

23. Tufo Skroff

24. Mrs. Andrew Hall (Mary Jones)

25. Mrs. Winifred LaSalle (Robert L.)

26. Alice-Ruth Buckely

27. Dr. Jack Rowe
    409 23 St., Encino, XY

28. Robert Nelson III
    321 April Ave., Woodland Hills, XY

29. Professor Carl Starr

30. Margo Hawkins, RN

31. Paul P. Marvel

32. Carl Saintelley

33. Professor Carl Procter

34. Frank Albert

35. Mr. C. H. Moore

36. Larry J. Riley

37. Karen Ruth-Ann Klein

38. Robert Nelson III
    421 April Ave., Woodland Hills, XY

39. Mr. C. Howard Moore

40. Mary Faye Jeffers

Form 18

41. Edward R. Mackey

51. Edward S. Mackey

42. M. Robert DeAriolla

52. Raymond E. Stokes

43. Marvin N. Riley

53. Walter L. McDougall

44. Hannah R. Sentry (Mrs. Randolph E.)

54. Mary MacKay

45. Rock C. Stetson

55. Donald Morris, Mr., II
    26 Avocado Place, Logan, XY

46. Senator Griffith

56. Chas. R. Bennett

47. Mr. Donald Morris, III
    771 So. Main St., Long Beach, XY

57. C. Richard Bennett

48. Dr. John S. Richards

58. Donald Morris
    14 Meridian St., Logan, XY

49. Robert LaVelle

X

50. John C. Richards, MD

X

Form 19

PATIENT RECORD

LAST NAME	FIRST NAME	MIDDLE NAME	BIRTH DATE	SEX	HOME PHONE

ADDRESS	CITY	STATE	ZIP CODE

CELL PHONE	PAGER NO.	FAX NO.	E-MAIL ADDRESS

PATIENT'S SOC. SEC. NO.   **DRIVER'S LICENSE**

PATIENT'S OCCUPATION   **NAME OF COMPANY**

ADDRESS OF EMPLOYER   **PHONE**

SPOUSE OR PARENT   **OCCUPATION**

EMPLOYER   **ADDRESS**   **PHONE**

NAME OF INSURANCE   **INSURED OR SUBSCRIBER**

POLICY/CERTIFICATE NO.   **GROUP NO.**   **REFERRED BY:**

DATE	PROGRESS

Form 20

PATIENT RECORD

LAST NAME	FIRST NAME	MIDDLE NAME	BIRTH DATE	SEX	HOME PHONE

ADDRESS   CITY   STATE   ZIP CODE

CELL PHONE   PAGER NO.   FAX NO.   E-MAIL ADDRESS

PATIENT'S SOC. SEC. NO.   DRIVER'S LICENSE

PATIENT'S OCCUPATION   NAME OF COMPANY

ADDRESS OF EMPLOYER   PHONE

SPOUSE OR PARENT   OCCUPATION

EMPLOYER   ADDRESS   PHONE

NAME OF INSURANCE   INSURED OR SUBSCRIBER

POLICY/CERTIFICATE NO.   GROUP NO.   REFERRED BY:

DATE	PROGRESS

Form 21

MEDICAL RECORD ABSTRACT FORM

Patient's Name: _____

Date(s) of treatment: _____

Patient's physician: _____

Was patient hospitalized? _____ If so, where? _____

_____

Did patient have surgery? _____ If so, what was done? _____

What is the patient's chief complaint? _____

_____

What is the diagnosis? _____

Was any medication prescribed? _____ If, so, what is the name of the

medication and dosage? _____

Does the patient have any drug or food allergies? _____ If so, list them: __

_____

Was any laboratory work performed? _____ If so, list all tests and results:_

_____

What is the prognosis of this case? _____

PATIENT RECORD

LAST NAME	FIRST NAME	MIDDLE NAME	BIRTH DATE	SEX	HOME PHONE

ADDRESS	CITY	STATE	ZIP CODE

CELL PHONE	PAGER NO.	FAX NO.	E-MAIL ADDRESS

PATIENT'S SOC. SEC. NO.   DRIVER'S LICENSE

PATIENT'S OCCUPATION   NAME OF COMPANY

ADDRESS OF EMPLOYER   PHONE

SPOUSE OR PARENT   OCCUPATION

EMPLOYER   ADDRESS   PHONE

NAME OF INSURANCE   INSURED OR SUBSCRIBER

POLICY/CERTIFICATE NO.   GROUP NO.   REFERRED BY:

DATE	PROGRESS

Form 23

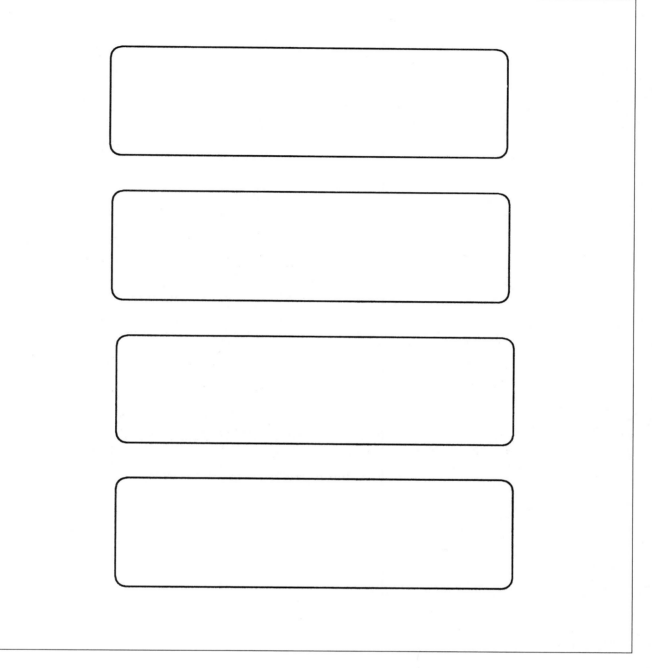

Form 24

PRACTON **M**EDICAL **G**ROUP, **I**NC.

4567 BROAD AVENUE
WOODLAND HILLS, XY 12345-4700

Phone: (555) 486-9002   Fax: (555) 488-7815

NAME _____ DATE _____

ADDRESS _____ CITY _____ STATE _____

Rx

N.E. REP. _____   _____ MD

REP. _____ TIMES   Gerald M. Practon, M.D. C 14021

BNDD NO. H 835190X   Fran T. Practon, M.D.   C 15038

Form 25

PRACTON MEDICAL GROUP, INC.
4567 Broad Avenue
Woodland Hills, XY 12345-4700
Tel. 555/486-9002

Patient's name:

_____

Please bring this card with you
for each appointment.

Your primary physician is:

_____

With so many potent medicines available today, the possibility of undesirable effects of single drugs, or adverse interactions of multiple drugs, is always present. If there is any question of side effects of drugs, or their potential toxicity, feel free to call and discuss this with your physician.

It is vital that you, and all health care professionals involved in your care, know exactly the names and dosages of ALL medicines you are currently taking. Please keep this card with you and show it to your doctor or dentist, during office visits, and to your pharmacist when prescriptions and/or over-the-counter preparations are purchased.

MEDICATION SCHEDULE

Name of Medication	Strength	Times to be Taken					

If you have any questions or problems with medications, please call 486-9002

Form 26

PRACTON MEDICAL GROUP, INC.

4567 BROAD AVENUE • WOODLAND HILLS, XY 12345-4700
OFFICE: (555) 486-9002 • FAX: (555) 488-7815

Fran Practon, M.D.
Gerald Practon, M.D.

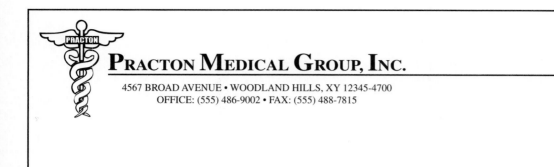

Practon Medical Group, Inc.

4567 BROAD AVENUE • WOODLAND HILLS, XY 12345-4700
OFFICE: (555) 486-9002 • FAX: (555) 488-7815

Fran Practon, M.D.
Gerald Practon, M.D.

Form 28

PRACTON **M**EDICAL **G**ROUP, **I**NC.

4567 BROAD AVENUE • WOODLAND HILLS, XY 12345-4700
OFFICE: (555) 486-9002 • FAX: (555) 488-7815

Fran Practon, M.D.
Gerald Practon, M.D.

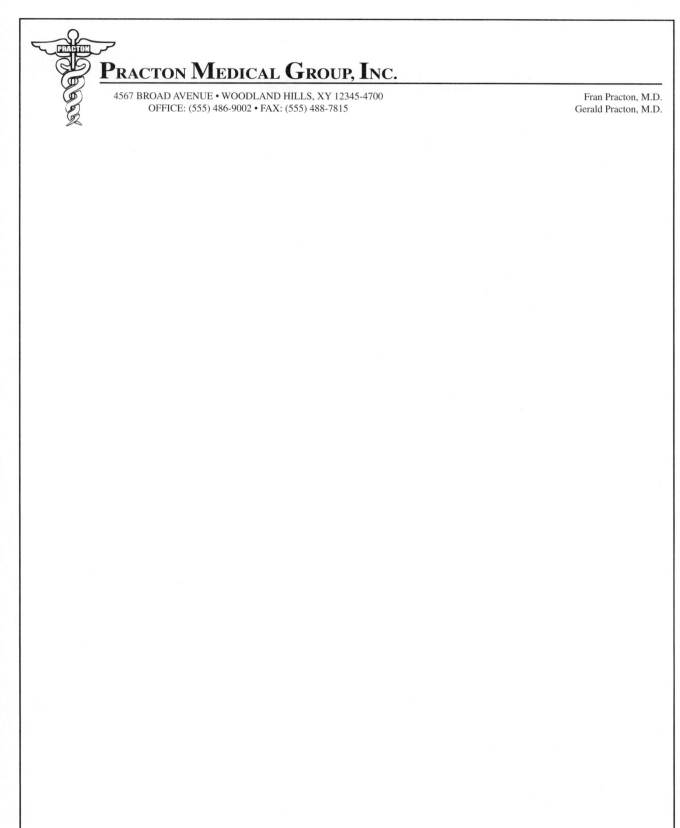

PRACTON MEDICAL GROUP, INC.

4567 BROAD AVENUE • WOODLAND HILLS, XY 12345-4700
OFFICE: (555) 486-9002 • FAX: (555) 488-7815

Fran Practon, M.D.
Gerald Practon, M.D.

Form 30

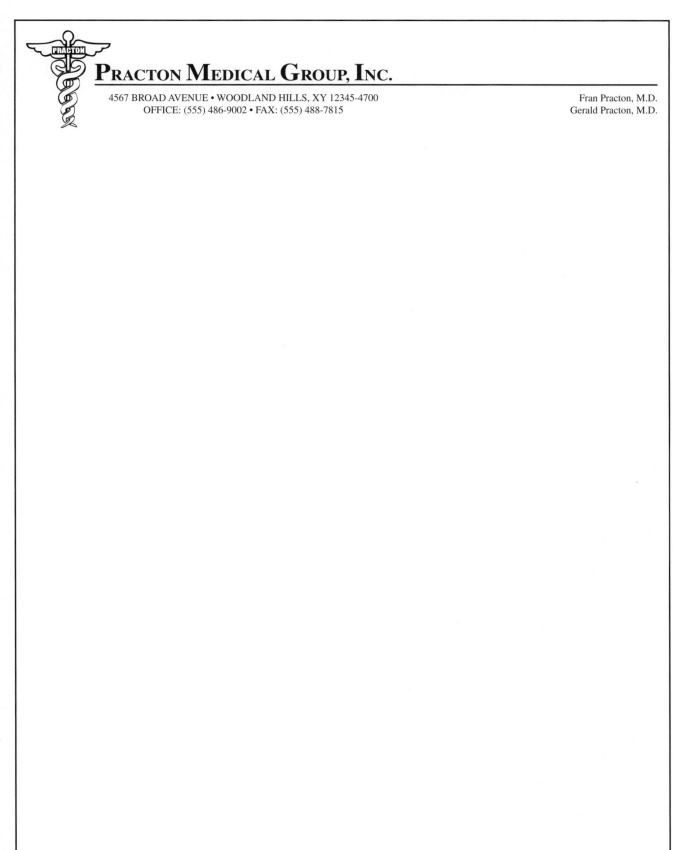

PRACTON MEDICAL GROUP, INC.

4567 BROAD AVENUE • WOODLAND HILLS, XY 12345-4700
OFFICE: (555) 486-9002 • FAX: (555) 488-7815

Fran Practon, M.D.
Gerald Practon, M.D.

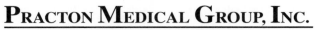

PRACTON MEDICAL GROUP, INC.

4567 BROAD AVENUE
WOODLAND HILLS, XY 12345-4700
TEL: (555) 486-9002
FAX NO. (555) 488-7815

INTEROFFICE MEMO

DATE:

TO:

FROM:

RE:

Form 32

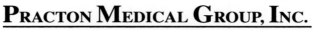

Practon Medical Group, Inc.

4567 BROAD AVENUE
WOODLAND HILLS, XY 12345-4700
TEL: (555) 486-9002
FAX NO. (555) 488-7815

INTEROFFICE MEMO

DATE: TO:

FROM: RE:

Form 33

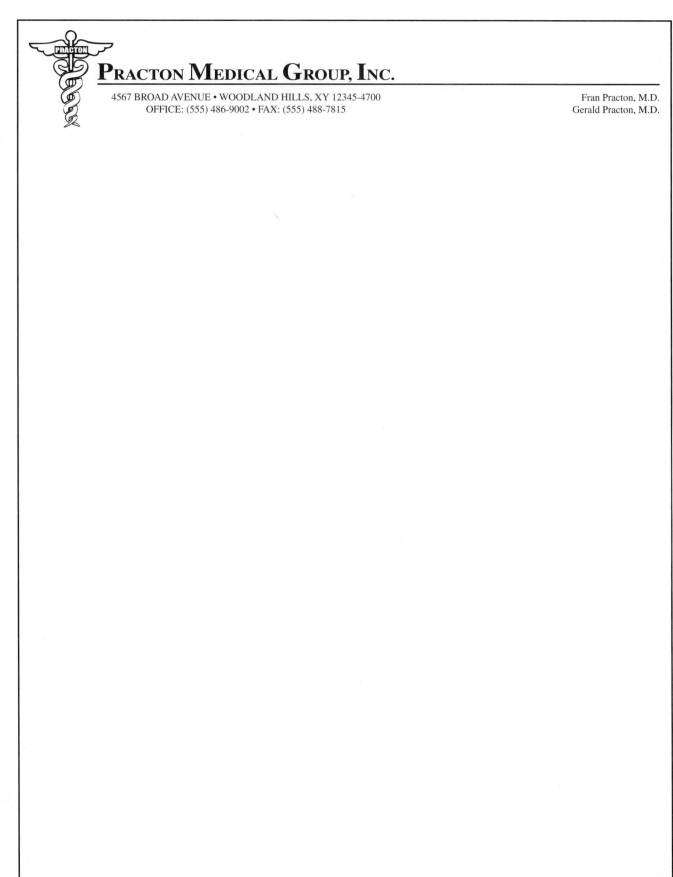

PRACTON MEDICAL GROUP, INC.

4567 BROAD AVENUE • WOODLAND HILLS, XY 12345-4700
OFFICE: (555) 486-9002 • FAX: (555) 488-7815

Fran Practon, M.D.
Gerald Practon, M.D.

Form 34

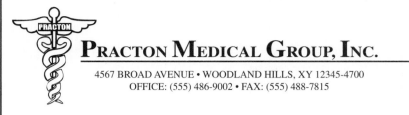

PRACTON MEDICAL GROUP, INC.

4567 BROAD AVENUE • WOODLAND HILLS, XY 12345-4700
OFFICE: (555) 486-9002 • FAX: (555) 488-7815

Fran Practon, M.D.
Gerald Practon, M.D.

Form 35

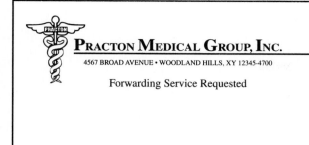

PRACTON MEDICAL GROUP, INC.
4567 BROAD AVENUE • WOODLAND HILLS, XY 12345-4700

Forwarding Service Requested

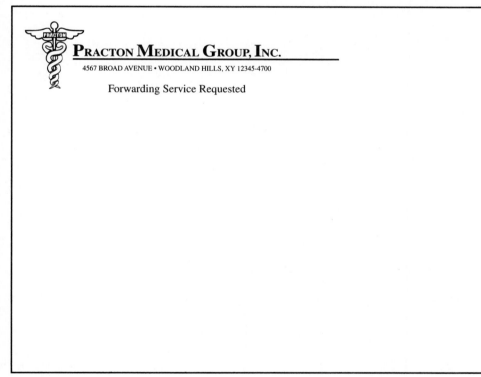

Form 36

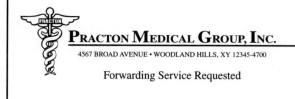

Practon Medical Group, Inc.

4567 BROAD AVENUE • WOODLAND HILLS, XY 12345-4700

Forwarding Service Requested

Form 37

U.S POSTAL SERVICE®
STAMPS BY MAIL® ORDER FORM

Please fill out clearly and completely.

AREA CODE | **DAYTIME PHONE NUMBER**

First Name   Middle Iinitial   Last Name

Company Name (if applicable)

Mailing Address/PO Box   Apt./Suite

City   State   ZIP+4®

ITEM	DESCRIPTION	PRICE	QTY.	COST
1	41c First-Class™ Rate Roll(s) – 100 Stamps per roll – U.S. Flag	$41.00		
2	41c First-Class· Rate Booklet(s) – 20 Stamps per Boooklet – Forever Stamp	$8.20		
3	2c Stamps – 20 Stamps – Navajo Jewelry*	$.40		
4	80c Stamps – 5 Stamps – Mount McKinley**	$4.00		
5	17c Stamps – 10 Stamps – Big Horn Sheep***	$1.70		

*May be combined for the $.41 First-Class Rate
**First ounce for Firdt-Class Rate Flat-Sized Mail
*** Additional ounce for First-Class Rate for Letter and Flat Mail.
  Expected availability - June 2007

Total Cost of Order $ _____

DETACH HERE

PS Form 3227-A – April 2007

Form 38

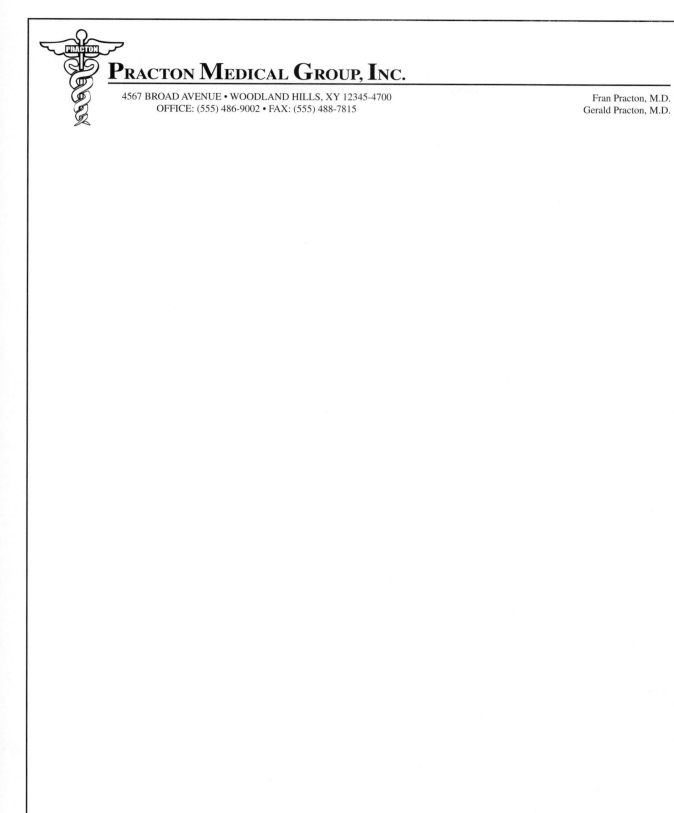

PRACTON MEDICAL GROUP, INC.

4567 BROAD AVENUE • WOODLAND HILLS, XY 12345-4700
OFFICE: (555) 486-9002 • FAX: (555) 488-7815

Fran Practon, M.D.
Gerald Practon, M.D.

Form 39

Form 40

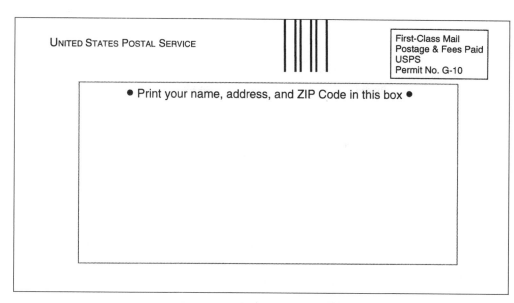

UNITED STATES POSTAL SERVICE

First-Class Mail
Postage & Fees Paid
USPS
Permit No. G-10

● Print your name, address, and ZIP Code in this box ●

SENDER: *COMPLETE THIS SECTION*	*COMPLETE THIS SECTION ON DELIVERY*

- ■ Complete items 1,2, and 3. Also complete item 4 if Restricted Delivery is desired.
- ■ Print your name and address on the reverse so that we can return the card to you.
- ■ Attach this card to the back of the mailpiece, or on the front if space permits.

A. Signature

X

☐ Agent
☐ Addressee

B. Received by *(Printed Name)*   C. Date of Delivery

1. Article Addressed to:

D. Is delivery address different from item 1? ☐ Yes
   If YES, enter delivery address below: ☐ No

3. Service Type
   ☐ Certified Mail   ☐ Express Mail
   ☐ Registered   ☐ Return Receipt for Merchandise
   ☐ Insured Mail   ☐ C.O.D

4. Restricted Delivery? *(Extra Fee)*   ☐ Yes

2. Article Number
   (Transfer from service label)

PS Form 3811, February 2004   Domestic Return Receipt   102595-02-M-1540

PLACE STICKER AT TOP OF ENVELOPE TO THE RIGHT
OF THE RETURN ADDRESS, FOLD AT DOTTED LINE

CERTIFIED MAIL™

7007 0710 0004 3603 0444
7007 0710 0004 3603 0444
7007 0710 0004 3603 0444

U.S. Postal Service™
CERTIFIED MAIL™ **RECEIPT**
(Domestic Mail Only; No Insurance Coverage Provided)

For delivery information visit our website at www.usps.com®

O F F I C I A L   U S E

Postage	$	
Certified Fee		
Return Receipt Fee *(Endorsement Required)*		Postmark Here
Restricted Delivery Fee *(Endorsement Required)*		
Total Postage & Fees	$	

Sent To

Street, Apt. No.;
or PO Box No.

City, State, ZIP+4

PS Form 3800, August 2006   See Reverse for Instructions

Form 41

FAX TRANSMITTAL SHEET

To: _____   Date:_____

Fax Number: _____   Time:_____

Telephone No.:_____

Number of Pages (including this one): _____

From: _____   Telephone No. _____

Note: This transmittal is intended only for the use of the individual or entity to which it is addressed and may contain information that is privileged, confidential, and exempt from disclosure under applicable law. If you are not the intended recipient, any dissemination, distribution, or photocopying of this communication is strictly prohibited. If you have received this communication in error, please notify this office immediately by telephone and return the original fax to us at the address below by U.S. Postal Service. Thank you.

Remarks:_____

_____

_____

If you cannot read this fax or if pages are missing, please contact:

PRACTON MEDICAL GROUP, INC.

4567 BROAD AVENUE • WOODLAND HILLS, XY 12345-4700
OFFICE: (555) 486-9002 • FAX: (555) 488-7815

INSTRUCTIONS TO THE AUTHORIZED RECEIVER: PLEASE COMPLETE THIS STATEMENT OF RECEIPT AND RETURN TO SENDER VIA THE ABOVE FAX NUMBER.

I, _____, verify that I have received _____
(no. of pages including cover sheet)

from _____.
(sending facility's name)

Form 42

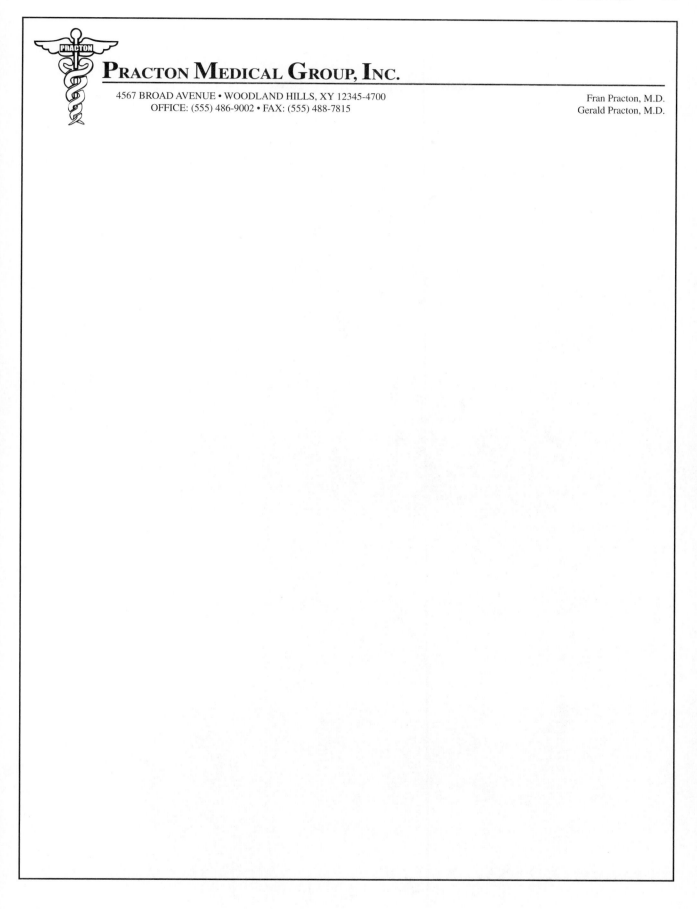

PRACTON MEDICAL GROUP, INC.

4567 BROAD AVENUE • WOODLAND HILLS, XY 12345-4700
OFFICE: (555) 486-9002 • FAX: (555) 488-7815

Fran Practon, M.D.
Gerald Practon, M.D.

Form 43

PRACTON MEDICAL GROUP, INC.

4567 BROAD AVENUE • WOODLAND HILLS, XY 12345-4700

Forwarding Service Requested

Form 44

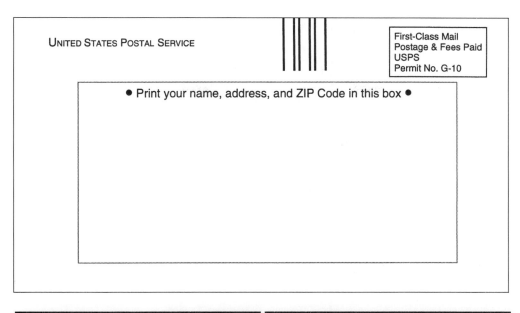

SENDER: *COMPLETE THIS SECTION*

- Complete items 1,2, and 3. Also complete item 4 if Restricted Delivery is desired.
- Print your name and address on the reverse so that we can return the card to you.
- Attach this card to the back of the mailpiece, or on the front if space permits.

1. Article Addressed to:

COMPLETE THIS SECTION ON DELIVERY

A. Signature

X   ☐ Agent   ☐ Addressee

B. Received by *(Printed Name)*   C. Date of Delivery

D. Is delivery address different from item 1? ☐ Yes
   If YES, enter delivery address below: ☐ No

3. Service Type
   ☐ Certified Mail   ☐ Express Mail
   ☐ Registered   ☐ Return Receipt for Merchandise
   ☐ Insured Mail   ☐ C.O.D

4. Restricted Delivery? *(Extra Fee)*   ☐ Yes

2. Article Number
   (Transfer from service label)

PS Form **3811**, February 2004   Domestic Return Receipt   102595-02-M-1540

U.S. Postal Service ™
CERTIFIED MAIL ™ **RECEIPT**
(Domestic Mail Only; No Insurance Coverage Provided)

For delivery information visit our website at www.usps.com®

O F F I C I A L   U S E

Postage $

Certified Fee

Return Receipt Fee
(Endorsement Required)

Restricted Delivery Fee
(Endorsement Required)

Postmark
Here

Total Postage & Fees $

Sent To

Street, Apt. No.;
or PO Box No.

City, State, ZIP+4

PS Form 3800, August 2006   See Reverse for Instructions

7007 0710 0004 3603 0451
7007 0710 0004 3603 0451
7007 0710 0004 3603 0451

PLACE STICKER AT TOP OF ENVELOPE TO THE RIGHT OF THE RETURN ADDRESS, FOLD AT DOTTED LINE

CERTIFIED MAIL ™

Form 45

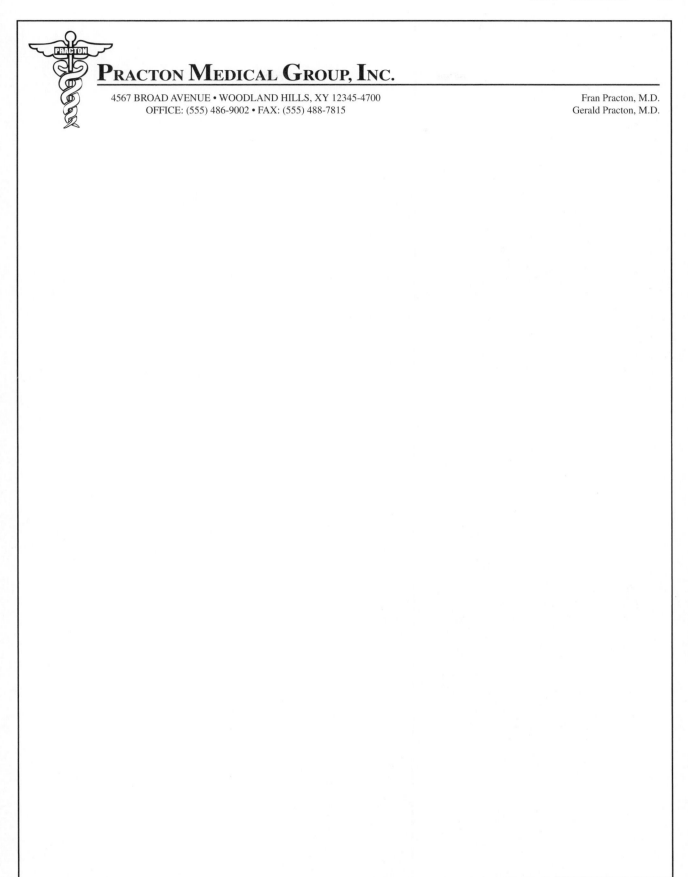

PRACTON MEDICAL GROUP, INC.

4567 BROAD AVENUE • WOODLAND HILLS, XY 12345-4700
OFFICE: (555) 486-9002 • FAX: (555) 488-7815

Fran Practon, M.D.
Gerald Practon, M.D.

Form 46

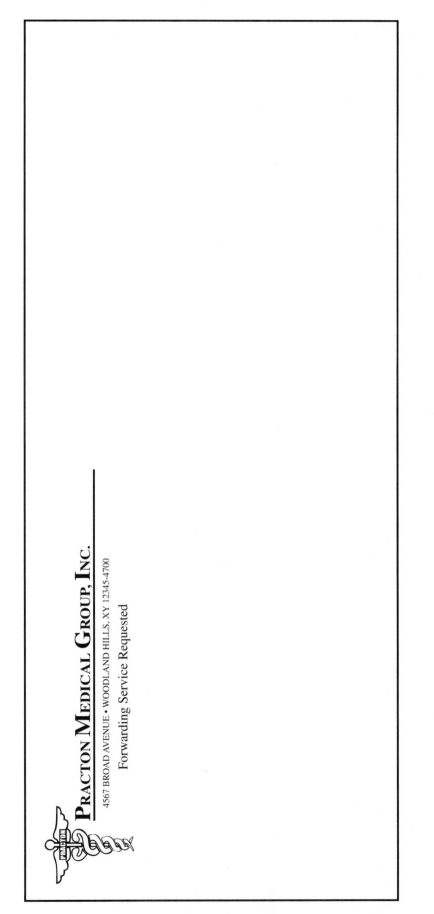

PRACTON MEDICAL GROUP, INC.

4567 BROAD AVENUE • WOODLAND HILLS, XY 12345-4700

Forwarding Service Requested

Form 47

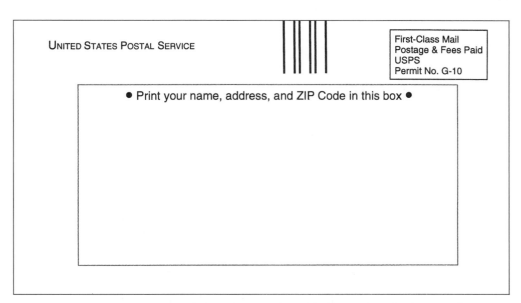

UNITED STATES POSTAL SERVICE

First-Class Mail
Postage & Fees Paid
USPS
Permit No. G-10

● Print your name, address, and ZIP Code in this box ●

SENDER: *COMPLETE THIS SECTION*	COMPLETE THIS SECTION ON DELIVERY

■ Complete items 1,2, and 3. Also complete item 4 if Restricted Delivery is desired.
■ Print your name and address on the reverse so that we can return the card to you.
■ Attach this card to the back of the mailpiece, or on the front if space permits.

A. Signature

X

☐ Agent
☐ Addressee

B. Received by *(Printed Name)*   C. Date of Delivery

1. Article Addressed to:

D. Is delivery address different from item 1? ☐ Yes
   If YES, enter delivery address below: ☐ No

3. Service Type
   ☐ Certified Mail   ☐ Express Mail
   ☐ Registered   ☐ Return Receipt for Merchandise
   ☐ Insured Mail   ☐ C.O.D

4. Restricted Delivery? *(Extra Fee)*   ☐ Yes

2. Article Number
   (Transfer from service label)

PS Form 3811, February 2004   Domestic Return Receipt   102595-02-M-1540

PLACE STICKER AT TOP OF ENVELOPE TO THE RIGHT
OF THE RETURN ADDRESS, FOLD AT DOTTED LINE

CERTIFIED MAIL™

7007 0710 0004 3603 0468
7007 0710 0004 3603 0468
7007 0710 0004 3603 0468

U.S. Postal Service ™
CERTIFIED MAIL ™ **RECEIPT**
(Domestic Mail Only; No Insurance Coverage Provided)

For delivery information visit our website at www.usps.com®

OFFICIAL USE

Postage	$
Certified Fee	
Return Receipt Fee (Endorsement Required)	
Restricted Delivery Fee (Endorsement Required)	
Total Postage & Fees	$

Postmark
Here

Sent To

Street, Apt. No.;
or PO Box No.

City, State, ZIP+4

PS Form 3800, August 2006   See Reverse for Instructions

Form 48

STATEMENT
PRACTON MEDICAL GROUP, INC.
4567 Broad Avenue
Woodland Hills, XY 12345-4700
Tel. 555-486-9002
Fax No. 555-488-7815

Phone No.(H)_____(W)_____ Birthdate_____
Insurance Co._____Policy No._____

	DATE	REFERENCE	DESCRIPTION	CHARGES		CREDITS PYMNTS.		ADJ.		BALANCE	
			BALANCE FORWARD ⟶							25	00
1.	1/25/xx	99213	OV level III	40	20						
2.	1/25/xx	93000	ECG	34	26						
3.	1/25/xx	94010	Spirometry	38	57						
4.	1/25/xx	99000	Handling spec.	5	00						
5.	1/25/xx	81000	Ua Non-auto.& micr.	8	00						
6.	1/26/xx	1/25/xx	Billed Aetna Ins.								
7.	2/12/xx	99212	OV level II	28	55						
8.	2/12/xx	99000	ECG	34	26						
9.	2/12/xx	CK #1692	ROA pt			25	00				
10.	3/2/xx	CK #5093	ROA Aetna ck.			90	74				
11.	3/2/xx	1/25/xx	Aetna adj.					12	60		
12.	3/2/xx	2/12/xx	Billed Aetna								
13.	3/17/xx	CK #1701	ROA pt			22	69				
14.	4/11/xx	CK #7948	ROA Aetna			45	22				
15.	4/11/xx	2/12/xx	Aetna adj.					6	28		

RB40BC-2-96   PLEASE PAY LAST AMOUNT IN BALANCE COLUMN ⟶ ▲

THIS IS A COPY OF YOUR ACCOUNT AS IT APPEARS ON OUR RECORDS

Form 49

STATEMENT

PRACTON MEDICAL GROUP, INC.
4567 Broad Avenue
Woodland Hills, XY 12345-4700
Tel. 555-486-9002
Fax No. 555-488-7815

Phone No.(H)_____(W)_____ Birthdate_____
Insurance Co._____Policy No._____

| DATE | REFERENCE | DESCRIPTION | CHARGES | CREDITS | | BALANCE |
				PYMNTS.	ADJ.	
		BALANCE FORWARD ———————▶				

RB40BC-2-96

PLEASE PAY LAST AMOUNT IN BALANCE COLUMN ———▲

THIS IS A COPY OF YOUR ACCOUNT AS IT APPEARS ON OUR RECORDS

Form 50

DATE	REFERENCE	DESCRIPTION	CHARGES	PYMNTS.	ADJ.	BALANCE	PREVIOUS BALANCE	N A M E
				CREDITS				

This is your RECEIPT for this amount
This is a STATEMENT of your account to date

Please present this slip to receptionist
before leaving office.

PRACTON MEDICAL GROUP, INC.
4567 Broad Avenue
Woodland Hills, XY 12345-4700
Tel. 555-486-9002
Fax. No. 555-488-7815

Thank You!

ROA – Received on Account

OT – Other _____

_____

RB40BC-3-96

NEXT APPOINTMENT _____   **143**

DATE	REFERENCE	DESCRIPTION	CHARGES	PYMNTS.	ADJ.	BALANCE	PREVIOUS BALANCE	N A M E
				CREDITS				

This is your RECEIPT for this amount
This is a STATEMENT of your account to date

Please present this slip to receptionist
before leaving office.

PRACTON MEDICAL GROUP, INC.
4567 Broad Avenue
Woodland Hills, XY 12345-4700
Tel. 555-486-9002
Fax. No. 555-488-7815

Thank You!

ROA – Received on Account

OT – Other _____

_____

RB40BC-3-96

NEXT APPOINTMENT _____   **144**

DATE	REFERENCE	DESCRIPTION	CHARGES	PYMNTS.	ADJ.	BALANCE	PREVIOUS BALANCE	N A M E
				CREDITS				

This is your RECEIPT for this amount
This is a STATEMENT of your account to date

Please present this slip to receptionist
before leaving office.

PRACTON MEDICAL GROUP, INC.
4567 Broad Avenue
Woodland Hills, XY 12345-4700
Tel. 555-486-9002
Fax. No. 555-488-7815

Thank You!

ROA – Received on Account

OT – Other _____

_____

RB40BC-3-96

NEXT APPOINTMENT _____   **145**

DATE	REFERENCE	DESCRIPTION	CHARGES	PYMNTS.	ADJ.	BALANCE	PREVIOUS BALANCE	N A M E
				CREDITS				

This is your RECEIPT for this amount
This is a STATEMENT of your account to date

Please present this slip to receptionist
before leaving office.

PRACTON MEDICAL GROUP, INC.
4567 Broad Avenue
Woodland Hills, XY 12345-4700
Tel. 555-486-9002
Fax. No. 555-488-7815

Thank You!

ROA – Received on Account

OT – Other _____

_____

RB40BC-3-96

NEXT APPOINTMENT _____   **146**

Form 51

PRACTON MEDICAL GROUP, INC.

4567 BROAD AVENUE • WOODLAND HILLS, XY 12345-4700
OFFICE: (555) 486-9002 • FAX: (555) 488-7815

Fran Practon, M.D.
Gerald Practon, M.D.

Form 52

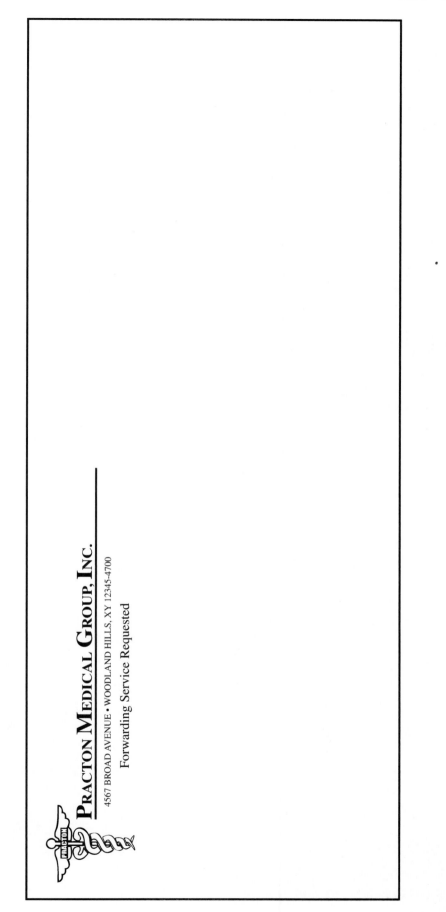

Form 53

STATEMENT
PRACTON MEDICAL GROUP, INC.
4567 Broad Avenue
Woodland Hills, XY 12345-4700
Tel. 555-486-9002
Fax No. 555-488-7815

Phone No.(H)_____(W)_____ Birthdate_____

Insurance Co._____Policy No._____

| DATE | REFERENCE | DESCRIPTION | CHARGES | CREDITS | | BALANCE |
				PYMNTS.	ADJ.	
		BALANCE FORWARD ⟶				

RB40BC-2-96

PLEASE PAY LAST AMOUNT IN BALANCE COLUMN ⟶

THIS IS A COPY OF YOUR ACCOUNT AS IT APPEARS ON OUR RECORDS

Form 54

PRACTON MEDICAL GROUP, INC.

4567 BROAD AVENUE • WOODLAND HILLS, XY 12345-4700
OFFICE: (555) 486-9002 • FAX: (555) 488-7815

Fran Practon, M.D.
Gerald Practon, M.D.

AUTHORIZATION TO CHARGE CREDIT CARD

Patient Name _____

Cardholder Name _____

Credit Card Company_____

Card Number_____ Expiration Date_____

I authorize _____ to charge my credit
card $_____ on the _____ of each month until my
balance of $_____ is paid in full. I understand that if the charge
is not accepted by my credit card company, I will immediately make
the monthly payment to the practice.

I understand that I may cancel this authorization at any time, but by
doing so I acknowledge that the balance owing will be due and
payable in full.

_____   _____
Signature   Date

Form 55

FINANCIAL AGREEMENT

For PROFESSIONAL SERVICES rendered or to be rendered to :

Patient _____

Parent if patient is a minor

Daytime Phone _____

1. Cash price for services .... $ _____
2. Cash down payment .... $ _____
3. Charges covered by insurance service plan ... $ _____
4. Unpaid balance of cash price .... $ _____
5. **Amount financed** (the amount of credit provided to you) .... $ _____
6. **FINANCE CHARGE** (the dollar amount the credit will cost you). ... $ _____
7. **ANNUAL PERCENTAGE RATE** (the cost of credit as a year-ly rate) .... _____ %
8. Total of payments (5 + 6 above- The amount you will have paid when you have made all scheduled payments) .... $ _____
9. Total sales price (1 + 6 above-Sum of cash price, financing charge and any other amounts financed by the creditor, not part of the finance charge) .... $ _____

You have the right at anytime to pay the unpaid balance due under this agreement without penalty.
You have the right at this time to receive an itemization of the amount financed.
☐ I want an itemization   ☐ I do not want an itemization

Total of payments (# 8 above) is payable to Dr. _____
in _____ monthly installments of $ _____
installments of $ _____ each. The first installment being payable on _____ 20 _____ and subsequent installments on the same day of each consecutive month until paid in full.

NOTICE TO PATIENT

Do not sign this agreement if it contains any blank spaces. You are entitled to an exact copy of any agreement you sign. You have the right at any time to pay the unpaid balance due under this agreement.

The patient (parent or guardian) agrees to be and is fully responsible for total payment of services performed in this office including any amounts not covered by any health insurance or prepayment program the responsible party may have. See your contract documents for any additional information about nonpayment, default, any required prepayment in full before the scheduled date and prepayment refunds and penalties.

Signature of patient or one parent if patient is a minor:

X _____ Date: _____

Doctor's Signature _____

Form 1826 • 1982

SCHEDULE OF PAYMENT

No.	Date Due	Amount of Installment	Date Paid	Amount Paid	Balance Owed
D.P.			Total Amount		
1					
2					
3					
4					
5					
6					
7					
8					
9					
10					
11					
12					
13					
14					
15					
16					
17					
18					
19					
20					
21					
22					
23					

Form 56

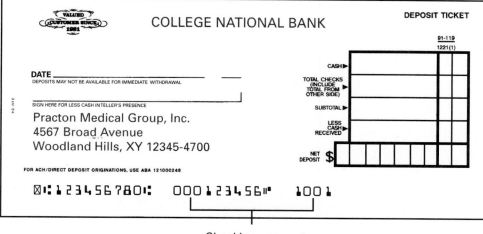

Checking account number

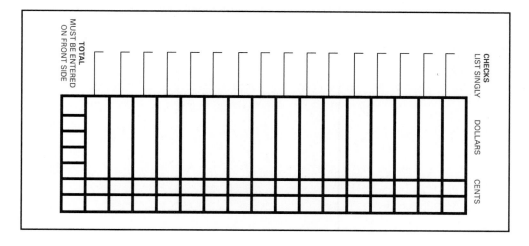

Form 57

Stationer's Corporation
340 West Main Street
Woodland Hills, XY 12345

STATEMENT

5-11-20XX

1 pkg pens	$10.00
1 box 3 x 5 cards	5.50
1 sm file box	8.00
subtotal	23.50
7% tax	1.65

TOTAL BALANCE DUE $25.15

Randolph Electrical Supply
458 State Street
Woodland Hills, XY 12345

STATEMENT

5-11-20XX

Small vacuum	$51.80
subtotal	51.80
7% tax	3.63

TOTAL BALANCE DUE $55.43

PRACTON MEDICAL GROUP, INC.
4567 Broad Avenue
Woodland Hills, XY 12345-4700

FOR INSTRUCTIONAL USE ONLY

DATE	ITEM	AMOUNT

485 $\frac{3-2}{310}$

PAY _____ DOLLARS

PAY TO THE ORDER OF	DATE	GROSS	DISC.	CHECK AMOUNT
				$.

NOT VALID

THE FIRST NATIONAL BANK – Woodland Hills, XY 12345-4700
RB40BC-4-96

⑆123456789⑆   000123456⑈0485

PRACTON MEDICAL GROUP, INC.
4567 Broad Avenue
Woodland Hills, XY 12345-4700

FOR INSTRUCTIONAL USE ONLY

DATE	ITEM	AMOUNT

486 $\frac{3-2}{310}$

PAY _____ DOLLARS

PAY TO THE ORDER OF	DATE	GROSS	DISC.	CHECK AMOUNT
				$.

NOT VALID

THE FIRST NATIONAL BANK – Woodland Hills, XY 12345-4700
RB40BC-4-96

⑆123456789⑆   000123456⑈0486

Form 58

BANK STATEMENT RECONCILIATION

FOUR EASY STEPS TO HELP YOU BALANCE YOUR CHECKBOOK

1. UPDATE YOUR CHECKBOOK

- Compare and check off each transaction recorded in your check register with those listed on this statement. These include checks, direct deposits, direct debits, deposits, ATM transactions, etc.

- Add interest and subtract service charges.

2. DETERMINE OUTSTANDING ITEMS

- Use the charts below to list transactions shown in your check register but not included on this statement.

- Include any from previous months.

OUTSTANDING CHECKS OR OTHER WITHDRAWALS					DEPOSITS NOT CREDITED		
CHECK NO.	AMOUNT		CHECK NO.	AMOUNT	DATE	AMOUNT	
	$			$		$	
				TOTAL	$	TOTAL	$

3. BALANCE YOUR ACCOUNT

- Enter Ending Statement Balance shown on this statement.　　$ _____

- Add deposits listed in your register and not shown on this statement.　　+ _____

- Subtract outstanding checks/withdrawals.　　- _____

- **ADJUSTED TOTAL** (should agree with your checkbook balance)　　$ _____

4. IF THE BALANCE IN YOUR CHECKBOOK DOES NOT AGREE WITH THE ADJUSTED TOTAL, THEN

- Check all addition and subtraction.

- Make sure all outstanding checks, withdrawals, and deposits have been listed in the appropriate chart above.

- Compare the amount of each check, withdrawal, and deposit in your checkbook with the amounts on this statement.

- Review the figures on last month's statement.

IN CASE OF ERRORS OR QUESTIONS ABOUT YOUR ELECTRONIC TRANSFERS, telephone us at the telephone number shown on this statement, or write us at: P.O. Box 30987, City of Industry, CA 91896-7987 as soon as you can if you think your statement or receipt is wrong or if you need more information about a transfer on the statement or receipt. We must hear from you no later than 60 days after we sent you the FIRST statement on which the error or problem appeared. Tell us your name and account number, and describe the error or the transfer you are unsure about. Please explain as clearly as you can why you believe there is an error or why you need more information. You must also tell us the exact dollar amount of the suspected error. If you tell us orally, we require that you send us your complaint or question in writing within 10 business days. If you do not put your complaint or questions in writing or we do not receive it within 10 business days, we may not recredit your account. If we decide that there was no error, we will send you a written explanation within 3 business days after we finish our investigation. You may ask for copies of the documents that we used in our investigation. For purposes of error resolution, our business days are Monday through Friday, 8:30 a.m. to 5:00 p.m., Pacific Time. We are closed Saturdays, Sundays, and federal holidays.

All Non-POS, MasterMoney™ or Foreign Transactions
We will tell you the results of our investigation within 10 business days after we receive your written complaint and will correct any error promptly. If we need more time, however, we may take up to 45 days to investigate your complaint or questions. If we decide we need additional time, we will recredit your account within 10 business days for the amount you think is in error, so that you will have the use of the money during the time it takes us to complete our investigation.

POS, MasterMoney™ and Foreign Transactions
If the transfer results from a point-of-sale transaction, MasterMoney™ transaction, or a transfer initiated outside the United States, we will still correct any error promptly. However, we may take up to 20 business days after we receive your written complaint to tell you the results of our investigation. If we need more time, we may use an additional 90 days. Should we take this additional time, we will recredit your account within 20 business days for the amount you think is in error. This will allow you to have the use of this money while we complete our investigation.

CF 5299F (5/96)

Form 59

STATEMENT
PRACTON MEDICAL GROUP, INC.
4567 Broad Avenue
Woodland Hills, XY 12345-4700
Tel. 555-486-9002
Fax No. 555-488-7815

Phone No.(H)_____ (W)_____ Birthdate_____
Insurance Co._____Policy No._____

DATE	REFERENCE	DESCRIPTION	CHARGES	CREDITS		BALANCE
				Pymnts	Adj	
		BALANCE FORWARD				

STATEMENT
PRACTON MEDICAL GROUP, INC.
4567 Broad Avenue
Woodland Hills, XY 12345-4700
Tel. 555-486-9002
Fax No. 555-488-7815

Phone No.(H)_____ (W)_____ Birthdate_____
Insurance Co._____Policy No._____

DATE	REFERENCE	DESCRIPTION	CHARGES	CREDITS		BALANCE
				Pymnts	Adj	
		BALANCE FORWARD				

Form 60

STATEMENT
PRACTON MEDICAL GROUP, INC.
4567 Broad Avenue
Woodland Hills, XY 12345-4700
Tel. 555-486-9002
Fax No. 555-488-7815

Phone No.(H)_____(W)_____ Birthdate_____
Insurance Co._____Policy No._____

DATE	REFERENCE	DESCRIPTION	CHARGES	CREDITS		BALANCE
				Pymnts	Adj	
		BALANCE FORWARD				

STATEMENT
PRACTON MEDICAL GROUP, INC.
4567 Broad Avenue
Woodland Hills, XY 12345-4700
Tel. 555-486-9002
Fax No. 555-488-7815

Phone No.(H)_____(W)_____ Birthdate_____
Insurance Co._____Policy No._____

DATE	REFERENCE	DESCRIPTION	CHARGES	CREDITS		BALANCE
				Pymnts	Adj	
		BALANCE FORWARD				

Form 61

STATEMENT
PRACTON MEDICAL GROUP, INC.
4567 Broad Avenue
Woodland Hills, XY 12345-4700
Tel. 555-486-9002
Fax No. 555-488-7815

Phone No.(H)_____ (W)_____ Birthdate_____
Insurance Co._____ Policy No._____

DATE	REFERENCE	DESCRIPTION	CHARGES	CREDITS		BALANCE	
				Pymnts	Adj		
		BALANCE FORWARD					

STATEMENT
PRACTON MEDICAL GROUP, INC.
4567 Broad Avenue
Woodland Hills, XY 12345-4700
Tel. 555-486-9002
Fax No. 555-488-7815

Phone No.(H)_____ (W)_____ Birthdate_____
Insurance Co._____ Policy No._____

DATE	REFERENCE	DESCRIPTION	CHARGES	CREDITS		BALANCE	
				Pymnts	Adj		
		BALANCE FORWARD					

Form 62

STATEMENT
PRACTON MEDICAL GROUP, INC.
4567 Broad Avenue
Woodland Hills, XY 12345-4700
Tel. 555 -486-9002
Fax No. 555 -488-7815

Phone No.(H)_____(W)_____ Birthdate_____
Insurance Co._____Policy No._____

DATE	REFERENCE	DESCRIPTION	CHARGES	CREDITS		BALANCE	
				Pymnts	Adj		
		BALANCE FORWARD					

STATEMENT
PRACTON MEDICAL GROUP, INC.
4567 Broad Avenue
Woodland Hills, XY 12345-4700
Tel. 555 -486-9002
Fax No. 555 -488-7815

Phone No.(H)_____(W)_____ Birthdate_____
Insurance Co._____Policy No._____

DATE	REFERENCE	DESCRIPTION	CHARGES	CREDITS		BALANCE	
				Pymnts	Adj		
		BALANCE FORWARD					

Form 63

STATEMENT
PRACTON MEDICAL GROUP, INC.
4567 Broad Avenue
Woodland Hills, XY 12345-4700
Tel. 555-486-9002
Fax No. 555-488-7815

Phone No.(H)_____ (W)_____ Birthdate_____
Insurance Co._____Policy No._____

DATE	REFERENCE	DESCRIPTION	CHARGES	CREDITS		BALANCE	
				Pymnts	Adj		
		BALANCE FORWARD					

STATEMENT
PRACTON MEDICAL GROUP, INC.
4567 Broad Avenue
Woodland Hills, XY 12345-4700
Tel. 555-486-9002
Fax No. 555-488-7815

Phone No.(H)_____ (W)_____ Birthdate_____
Insurance Co._____Policy No._____

DATE	REFERENCE	DESCRIPTION	CHARGES	CREDITS		BALANCE	
				Pymnts	Adj		
		BALANCE FORWARD					

Form 64

STATEMENT
PRACTON MEDICAL GROUP, INC.
4567 Broad Avenue
Woodland Hills, XY 12345-4700
Tel. 555-486-9002
Fax No. 555-488-7815

Phone No.(H)_____ (W)_____ Birthdate_____
Insurance Co._____Policy No._____

DATE	REFERENCE	DESCRIPTION	CHARGES	CREDITS		BALANCE	
				Pymnts	Adj		
		BALANCE FORWARD					

STATEMENT
PRACTON MEDICAL GROUP, INC.
4567 Broad Avenue
Woodland Hills, XY 12345-4700
Tel. 555-486-9002
Fax No. 555-488-7815

Phone No.(H)_____ (W)_____ Birthdate_____
Insurance Co._____Policy No._____

DATE	REFERENCE	DESCRIPTION	CHARGES	CREDITS		BALANCE	
				Pymnts	Adj		
		BALANCE FORWARD					

Form 65

STATEMENT
PRACTON MEDICAL GROUP, INC.
4567 Broad Avenue
Woodland Hills, XY 12345-4700
Tel. 555-486-9002
Fax No. 555-488-7815

Phone No.(H)_____(W)_____ Birthdate_____
Insurance Co._____Policy No._____

DATE	REFERENCE	DESCRIPTION	CHARGES	CREDITS		BALANCE	
				Pymnts	Adj		
		BALANCE FORWARD					

STATEMENT
PRACTON MEDICAL GROUP, INC.
4567 Broad Avenue
Woodland Hills, XY 12345-4700
Tel. 555-486-9002
Fax No. 555-488-7815

Phone No.(H)_____(W)_____ Birthdate_____
Insurance Co._____Policy No._____

DATE	REFERENCE	DESCRIPTION	CHARGES	CREDITS		BALANCE	
				Pymnts	Adj		
		BALANCE FORWARD					

Form 66

STATEMENT
PRACTON MEDICAL GROUP, INC.
4567 Broad Avenue
Woodland Hills, XY 12345-4700
Tel. 555-486-9002
Fax No. 555-488-7815

Phone No.(H)_____ (W)_____ Birthdate_____
Insurance Co._____Policy No._____

DATE	REFERENCE	DESCRIPTION	CHARGES	CREDITS		BALANCE	
				Pymnts	Adj		
		BALANCE FORWARD					

STATEMENT
PRACTON MEDICAL GROUP, INC.
4567 Broad Avenue
Woodland Hills, XY 12345-4700
Tel. 555-486-9002
Fax No. 555-488-7815

Phone No.(H)_____ (W)_____ Birthdate_____
Insurance Co._____Policy No._____

DATE	REFERENCE	DESCRIPTION	CHARGES	CREDITS		BALANCE	
				Pymnts	Adj		
		BALANCE FORWARD					

Form 67

STATEMENT
PRACTON MEDICAL GROUP, INC.
4567 Broad Avenue
Woodland Hills, XY 12345-4700
Tel. 555 -486-9002
Fax No. 555 -488-7815

Phone No.(H)_____(W)_____ Birthdate_____
Insurance Co._____Policy No._____

DATE	REFERENCE	DESCRIPTION	CHARGES	CREDITS		BALANCE
				Pymnts	Adj	
		BALANCE FORWARD				

STATEMENT
PRACTON MEDICAL GROUP, INC.
4567 Broad Avenue
Woodland Hills, XY 12345-4700
Tel. 555 -486-9002
Fax No. 555 -488-7815

Phone No.(H)_____(W)_____ Birthdate_____
Insurance Co._____Policy No._____

DATE	REFERENCE	DESCRIPTION	CHARGES	CREDITS		BALANCE
				Pymnts	Adj	
		BALANCE FORWARD				

Form 68

STATEMENT
PRACTON MEDICAL GROUP, INC.
4567 Broad Avenue
Woodland Hills, XY 12345-4700
Tel. 555 -486-9002
Fax No. 555 -488-7815

Phone No.(H)_____(W)_____ Birthdate_____
Insurance Co._____Policy No._____

DATE	REFERENCE	DESCRIPTION	CHARGES	CREDITS		BALANCE
				Pymnts	Adj	
		BALANCE FORWARD				

STATEMENT
PRACTON MEDICAL GROUP, INC.
4567 Broad Avenue
Woodland Hills, XY 12345-4700
Tel. 555 -486-9002
Fax No. 555 -488-7815

Phone No.(H)_____(W)_____ Birthdate_____
Insurance Co._____Policy No._____

DATE	REFERENCE	DESCRIPTION	CHARGES	CREDITS		BALANCE
				Pymnts	Adj	
		BALANCE FORWARD				

Form 69

STATEMENT
PRACTON MEDICAL GROUP, INC.
4567 Broad Avenue
Woodland Hills, XY 12345-4700
Tel. 555-486-9002
Fax No. 555-488-7815

Phone No.(H)_____(W)_____ Birthdate_____
Insurance Co._____Policy No._____

DATE	REFERENCE	DESCRIPTION	CHARGES	CREDITS		BALANCE
				Pymnts	Adj	
		BALANCE FORWARD				

STATEMENT
PRACTON MEDICAL GROUP, INC.
4567 Broad Avenue
Woodland Hills, XY 12345-4700
Tel. 555-486-9002
Fax No. 555-488-7815

Phone No.(H)_____(W)_____ Birthdate_____
Insurance Co._____Policy No._____

DATE	REFERENCE	DESCRIPTION	CHARGES	CREDITS		BALANCE
				Pymnts	Adj	
		BALANCE FORWARD				

Form 70

STATEMENT
PRACTON MEDICAL GROUP, INC.
4567 Broad Avenue
Woodland Hills, XY 12345-4700
Tel. 555-486-9002
Fax No. 555-488-7815

Phone No.(H)_____(W)_____ Birthdate_____
Insurance Co._____Policy No._____

DATE	REFERENCE	DESCRIPTION	CHARGES	CREDITS		BALANCE
				Pymnts	Adj	
		BALANCE FORWARD				

STATEMENT
PRACTON MEDICAL GROUP, INC.
4567 Broad Avenue
Woodland Hills, XY 12345-4700
Tel. 555-486-9002
Fax No. 555-488-7815

Phone No.(H)_____(W)_____ Birthdate_____
Insurance Co._____Policy No._____

DATE	REFERENCE	DESCRIPTION	CHARGES	CREDITS		BALANCE
				Pymnts	Adj	
		BALANCE FORWARD				

Form 71

STATEMENT
PRACTON MEDICAL GROUP, INC.
4567 Broad Avenue
Woodland Hills, XY 12345-4700
Tel. 555-486-9002
Fax No. 555-488-7815

Phone No.(H)_____(W)_____ Birthdate_____
Insurance Co._____ Policy No._____

DATE	REFERENCE	DESCRIPTION	CHARGES	CREDITS		BALANCE	
				Pymnts	Adj		
		BALANCE FORWARD					

STATEMENT
PRACTON MEDICAL GROUP, INC.
4567 Broad Avenue
Woodland Hills, XY 12345-4700
Tel. 555-486-9002
Fax No. 555-488-7815

Phone No.(H)_____(W)_____ Birthdate_____
Insurance Co._____ Policy No._____

DATE	REFERENCE	DESCRIPTION	CHARGES	CREDITS		BALANCE	
				Pymnts	Adj		
		BALANCE FORWARD					

Form 72

STATEMENT
PRACTON MEDICAL GROUP, INC.
4567 Broad Avenue
Woodland Hills, XY 12345-4700
Tel. 555-486-9002
Fax No. 555-488-7815

Phone No.(H)_____ (W)_____ Birthdate_____
Insurance Co._____ Policy No._____

DATE	REFERENCE	DESCRIPTION	CHARGES	CREDITS		BALANCE
				Pymnts	Adj	
		BALANCE FORWARD				

STATEMENT
PRACTON MEDICAL GROUP, INC.
4567 Broad Avenue
Woodland Hills, XY 12345-4700
Tel. 555-486-9002
Fax No. 555-488-7815

Phone No.(H)_____ (W)_____ Birthdate_____
Insurance Co._____ Policy No._____

DATE	REFERENCE	DESCRIPTION	CHARGES	CREDITS		BALANCE
				Pymnts	Adj	
		BALANCE FORWARD				

Form 73

FAMILY HEALTH MAGAZINE
3490 Broadway Street
New York, NY 10010

0136

June 26, 20XX

16-66/1220

PAY TO THE ORDER OF *Gerald Practon, M.D.* $50.00

Fifty and No/100 ————————————— DOLLARS

BANK OF AMERICA NT&SA

VOID

⑈122000661⑈0136⑈ 10386⑈60402⑈

COLONY BOYS SCHOOL
659 Manchester Avenue
Woodland Hills, XY 12345

785

June 26,   20XX   16-36/208
                    ‾‾‾‾‾‾
                    1220

Pay to the
Order of Fran Practon, M. D. ——————— $ 75.00

Seventy-five and no/100——————— ———————————— Dollars

⬥ BARCLAYS BANK

VOID

memo lecture

⑈122000360⑈0785 208913379⑈

Adrienne Cane
6502 North J Street
Woodland Hills, XY 12345
Tel. 555/498-2110

0425

June 26, 20XX

16-4
‾‾‾‾
1220

PAY TO THE
ORDER OF *Practon Medical Group, Inc.* $50.00

Fifty and no/100 ————————— DOLLARS

SECURITY PACIFIC NATIONAL BANK ◼

VOID

Adrienne Cane

⑈122000043⑈0425⑈ 229⑈048596⑈

Betty K. Lawson
6400 Best Way
Woodland Hills, XY 12345
Tel:555/459-9533

192

June 28, 20XX $\frac{90\text{-}1692}{1222}$

PAY TO THE
ORDER OF *Practon Medical Group Inc.* $15.00

Fifteen and No/100 ———— V O I D ———————————— DOLLARS

UCB · UNITED   BANK

MEMO _____   *Betty K. Lawson*

⑊ ⑈1222⑈ 1692⑈: 20441361⑈ 0192 11

DELUXE CHECK PRINTERS - LH

Jody F. Swinney
4300 Saunders Road
Woodland Hills, XY 12345
Tel: 555/908-6605

No. 150

June 28, 20XX   16-8/1220

Pay to
the order of *Practon Medical Group, Inc.* $15.00

Fifteen and No/100 ———— V O I D ———————— DOLLARS

◈ CROCKER NATIONAL BANK

Memo _____   *Jody. F. Swinney*

⑈122000085⑈:0150 14005060⑈ 0150

Form 75

DATE	REFERENCE	DESCRIPTION	CHARGES	PYMNTS.	ADJ.	BALANCE	PREVIOUS BALANCE	N A M E
				CREDITS				

This is your RECEIPT for this amount
This is a STATEMENT of your account to date

Please present this slip to receptionist
before leaving office.

PRACTON MEDICAL GROUP, INC.
4567 Broad Avenue
Woodland Hills, XY 12345-4700
Tel. 555-486-9002
Fax. No. 555-488-7815

Thank You!

ROA – Received on Account

OT – Other _____

NEXT APPOINTMENT _____

RB40BC-3-96

147

DATE	REFERENCE	DESCRIPTION	CHARGES	PYMNTS.	ADJ.	BALANCE	PREVIOUS BALANCE	N A M E
				CREDITS				

This is your RECEIPT for this amount
This is a STATEMENT of your account to date

Please present this slip to receptionist
before leaving office.

PRACTON MEDICAL GROUP, INC.
4567 Broad Avenue
Woodland Hills, XY 12345-4700
Tel. 555-486-9002
Fax. No. 555-488-7815

Thank You!

ROA – Received on Account

OT – Other _____

NEXT APPOINTMENT _____

RB40BC-3-96

148

DATE	REFERENCE	DESCRIPTION	CHARGES	PYMNTS.	ADJ.	BALANCE	PREVIOUS BALANCE	N A M E
				CREDITS				

This is your RECEIPT for this amount
This is a STATEMENT of your account to date

Please present this slip to receptionist
before leaving office.

PRACTON MEDICAL GROUP, INC.
4567 Broad Avenue
Woodland Hills, XY 12345-4700
Tel. 555-486-9002
Fax. No. 555-488-7815

Thank You!

ROA – Received on Account

OT – Other _____

NEXT APPOINTMENT _____

RB40BC-3-96

149

DATE	REFERENCE	DESCRIPTION	CHARGES	PYMNTS.	ADJ.	BALANCE	PREVIOUS BALANCE	N A M E
				CREDITS				

This is your RECEIPT for this amount
This is a STATEMENT of your account to date

Please present this slip to receptionist
before leaving office.

PRACTON MEDICAL GROUP, INC.
4567 Broad Avenue
Woodland Hills, XY 12345-4700
Tel. 555-486-9002
Fax. No. 555-488-7815

Thank You!

ROA – Received on Account

OT – Other _____

NEXT APPOINTMENT _____

RB40BC-3-96

150

Form 76

DAYSHEET (RECORD OF CHARGES AND RECEIPTS)

PAGE NO _____ OF _____ DATE _____

RECORD OF DEPOSITS

BUSINESS ANALYSIS SUMMARIES
(OPTIONAL)

DATE	REFERENCE	DESCRIPTION	CHARGES	CREDITS		BALANCE	√	PREVIOUS BALANCE	N A M E
				PYMNTS.	ADJ.				

CHARGES — Col. A
CREDITS — PYMNTS. Col. B-1 — ADJ. Col. B-2
BALANCE — Col. C
PREVIOUS BALANCE — Col. D

	RECEIPT NUMBER
1	
2	
3	
4	
5	
6	
7	
8	
9	
10	
11	
12	
13	
14	
15	
16	
17	
18	
19	
20	
21	
22	
23	
24	
25	
26	
27	
28	

DATE: _____

	CASH	CHECKS
TOTAL CASH		
TOTAL CHECKS		
TOTAL DEPOSIT		

TOTALS THIS PAGE
PREVIOUS PAGE
MONTH-TO-DATE

PREPARED BY

PROOF OF POSTING

COL. D TOTAL	$
PLUS COL. A TOTAL	$
SUB TOTAL	$
LESS COLS. B-1 & B-2	$
MUST EQUAL COL. C	$

ACCOUNTS RECEIVABLE CONTROL

PREVIOUS DAY'S TOTAL	$
PLUS COL. A	$
SUB TOTAL	$
LESS COLS. B-1 & B-2	$
TOTAL ACCTS. REC.	$

ACCOUNTS RECEIVABLE PROOF

ACCTS. REC. 1ST OF MONTH	$
PLUS COL. A - MONTH TO DATE	$
SUB TOTAL	$
LESS B-1 & B-2 MO. TO DATE	$
TOTAL ACCTS. REC.	$

CASH PAID OUT

	$
	$

CASH CONTROL

Beginning Cash On Hand	$
Receipts Today (Col. B-1)	$
Total	$
Less Paid Outs	$
Less Bank Deposit	$
Closing Cash On Hand	$

RB40BC-6-96

Form 77

DAYSHEET (RECORD OF CHARGES AND RECEIPTS)

PAGE NO _____ OF _____ DATE _____

RECORD OF DEPOSITS

BUSINESS ANALYSIS SUMMARIES (OPTIONAL)

DATE	REFERENCE	DESCRIPTION	CHARGES	CREDITS		BALANCE		PREVIOUS BALANCE	√	N A M E	RECEIPT NUMBER	DATE:		
				PYMNTS.	ADJ.								CASH	CHECKS

Col. A Col. B-1 Col. B-2 Col. C Col. D

TOTALS THIS PAGE
PREVIOUS PAGE
MONTH-TO-DATE

PREPARED BY

TOTAL CASH
TOTAL CHECKS
TOTAL DEPOSIT

PROOF OF POSTING

COL. D TOTAL	$
PLUS COL. A TOTAL	$
SUB TOTAL	$
LESS COLS. B-1 & B-2	$
MUST EQUAL COL. C	$

ACCOUNTS RECEIVABLE CONTROL

PREVIOUS DAY'S TOTAL	$
PLUS COL. A	$
SUB TOTAL	$
LESS COLS. B-1 & B-2	$
TOTAL ACCTS. REC.	$

ACCOUNTS RECEIVABLE PROOF

ACCTS. REC. 1ST OF MONTH	$
PLUS COL. A - MONTH TO DATE	$
SUB TOTAL	$
LESS B-1 & B-2 MO. TO DATE	$
TOTAL ACCTS. REC.	$

CASH PAID OUT

	$
	$
	$

CASH CONTROL

Beginning Cash On Hand	$
Receipts Today (Col. B-1)	$
Total	$
Less Paid Outs	$
Less Bank Deposit	$
Closing Cash On Hand	$

RB40BC-6-96

Form 78

Roger T. Simpson
792 Baker Street
Woodland Hills, XY 12345
555/549-0879

3000

June 29, 20XX   16-1493/343
                  1220

PAY TO THE
ORDER OF *Practon Medical Group, Inc.* $ *15.00*

Fifteen and NO/100   VOID   DOLLARS

Channel Islands Office
UNION BANK

MEMO *Copay*   *Roger T. Simpson*

⑆ 1220 1493 2 951 7800 0 17 3000

Bank of A. Levy

№ 553

June 29, 20XX   90-372/1222

Pay to the Order of Practon Medical Group, Inc. $

Two and no/100   VOID   *Dollars*

Jack J. Johnson
5490 Olive Mill Road
Woodland Hills, XY 12345

Memo Copay   *Signed Jack J. Johnson*

⑆ 122203727 0553 2145 878

Prudential Insurance Company
4680 Cowper Street
Woodland Hills, XY 12345

189

June 27, 20XX   90-3219
                1222

PAY TO THE
ORDER OF   Practon Medical Group, Inc.----- ---------- $ 15.00

Fifteen and No/100-------------- -------   VOID   ---------------- DOLLARS

OJAI VALLEY STATE BANK

FOR completion life ins form

122232196 0189 260 10074 2

Form 79

RECORD OF DEPOSITS

DAYSHEET (RECORD OF CHARGES AND RECEIPTS)

PAGE NO. _____ OF _____ DATE _____

BUSINESS ANALYSIS SUMMARIES
(OPTIONAL)

DATE	REFERENCE	DESCRIPTION	CHARGES	CREDITS		BALANCE	√	PREVIOUS BALANCE	N A M E	RECEIPT NUMBER	RECORD OF DEPOSITS	
				PYMNTS	ADJ.						CASH	CHECKS

CREDITS

DATE:

	CASH	CHECKS
TOTAL CASH		
TOTAL CHECKS		
TOTAL DEPOSIT		

CASH PAID OUT

		$
		$
		$

PREPARED BY

TOTALS THIS PAGE
PREVIOUS PAGE
MONTH-TO-DATE

Col. A Col. B-1 Col. B-2 Col. C Col. D

PROOF OF POSTING

COL. D TOTAL	$	
PLUS COL. A TOTAL	$	
SUB TOTAL	$	
LESS COLS. B-1 & B-2	$	
MUST EQUAL COL. C	$	

ACCOUNTS RECEIVABLE CONTROL

PREVIOUS DAY'S TOTAL	$	
PLUS COL. A	$	
SUB TOTAL	$	
LESS COLS. B-1 & B-2	$	
TOTAL ACCTS. REC.	$	

ACCOUNTS RECEIVABLE PROOF

ACCTS. REC. 1ST OF MONTH	$	
PLUS COL. A - MONTH TO DATE	$	
SUB TOTAL	$	
LESS B-1 & B-2 MO. TO DATE	$	
TOTAL ACCTS. REC.	$	

CASH CONTROL

Beginning Cash On Hand	$	
Receipts Today (Col. B-1)	$	
Total	$	
Less Paid Outs	$	
Less Bank Deposit	$	
Closing Cash On Hand	$	

RB40BC-6-96

Form 80

Rachel T. O'Brien
5598 East 17 Street
Woodland Hills, XY 12345
555/566-2119

16-21/204
1220

4800

June 30, 20XX

pay to the order of *Practon Medical Group, Inc.* $ *10.00*

Ten and NO/100 _____ dollars

V O I D

UB CB **UNITED BANK**

Rachel T. O'Brien

⑆122000218⑆20450 2843⑈ 4800 11

Recycled and Recyclable

Joseph C. Smith
P.O. Box 4301
Woodland Hills, XY 12345
555/549-1124

217

90-2055
1222

June 30, 20XX

PAY TO THE ORDER OF *Practon Medical Group, Inc.* $ *75.00*

Seventy five and no/100 _____ *V O I D* _____ **DOLLARS**

SECURITY PACIFIC NATIONAL BANK **S**

SAMPLE VOID

For PE + lab test

Joseph C. Smith

⑈000217⑈ ⑆1222⑈20550⑈437⑈ 23456⑈

Form 81

DAYSHEET (RECORD OF CHARGES AND RECEIPTS)

PAGE NO _____ OF _____ DATE _____

R8408C-6-98

	Col. A	Col. B-1	Col. B-2	Col. C	Col. D
TOTALS THIS PAGE					
PREVIOUS PAGE					
MONTH-TO-DATE					

PREPARED BY _____

PROOF OF POSTING	
COL. D TOTAL	$
PLUS COL. A TOTAL	$
SUB TOTAL	$
LESS COLS. B-1 & B-2	$
MUST EQUAL COL. C	$

ACCOUNTS RECEIVABLE CONTROL	
PREVIOUS DAY'S TOTAL	$
PLUS COL. A	$
SUB TOTAL	$
LESS COLS. B-1 & B-2	$
TOTAL ACCTS. REC.	$

ACCOUNTS RECEIVABLE PROOF	
ACCTS. REC. 1ST OF MONTH	$
PLUS COL. A-MONTH TO DATE	$
SUB TOTAL	$
LESS B-1 & B-2 MO. TO DATE	$
TOTAL ACCTS. REC.	$

Form 82

MANAGED CARE PLAN
TREATMENT AUTHORIZATION REQUEST

**TO BE COMPLETED BY PRIMARY CARE PHYSICIAN
OR OUTSIDE PROVIDER**

Health Net	☐	Met Life	☐
Pacificare	☐	Travelers	☐
Secure Horizons	☐	Pru Care	☐

Patient Name_____Date_____

M____ F____ Birthdate_____ Home telephone number_____

Address_____

Primary Care Physician_____Member ID#_____

Referring Physician_____Member ID#_____

Referred to_____ Address_____

_____ Office telephone no._____

Diagnosis Code_____ Diagnosis_____

Diagnosis Code_____ Diagnosis_____

Treatment Plan_____

Authorization requested for procedures/tests/visits:

Procedure Code_____ Description_____

Procedure Code_____ Description_____

Facility to be used_____Estimated length of stay_____

Office ☐   Outpatient ☐   Inpatient ☐   Other ☐

List of potential consultants (e.g., anesthetists, assistants, or medical/surgical):

_____

Physician's signature_____

TO BE COMPLETED BY PRIMARY CARE PHYSICIAN

PCP Recommendations_____PCP Initials_____

Eligibility checked_____Effective date_____

TO BE COMPLETED BY UTILIZATION MANAGEMENT

Authorized_____ Not authorized_____

Deferred_____ Modified_____

Authorization Request #_____

Comments_____

Form 83

1500

HEALTH INSURANCE CLAIM FORM

APPROVED BY NATIONAL UNIFORM CLAIM COMMITTEE 08/05

| | PICA | | | | | | | | PICA | | |

1. MEDICARE □ (Medicare #) MEDICAID □ (Medicaid #) TRICARE CHAMPUS □ (Sponsor's SSN) CHAMPVA □ (Member ID#) GROUP HEALTH PLAN □ (SSN or ID) FECA BLK LUNG □ (SSN) OTHER □ (ID)

1a. INSURED'S I.D. NUMBER   (For Program in Item 1)

2. PATIENT'S NAME (Last Name, First Name, Middle Initial)

3. PATIENT'S BIRTH DATE   MM | DD | YY   SEX   M □   F □

4. INSURED'S NAME (Last Name, First Name, Middle Initial)

5. PATIENT'S ADDRESS (No., Street)

6. PATIENT RELATIONSHIP TO INSURED   Self □   Spouse □   Child □   Other □

7. INSURED'S ADDRESS (No., Street)

CITY   STATE

8. PATIENT STATUS   Single □   Married □   Other □
Employed □   Full-Time Student □   Part-Time Student □

CITY   STATE

ZIP CODE   TELEPHONE (Include Area Code) (   )

ZIP CODE   TELEPHONE (Include Area Code) (   )

9. OTHER INSURED'S NAME (Last Name, First Name, Middle Initial)

10. IS PATIENT'S CONDITION RELATED TO:

11. INSURED'S POLICY GROUP OR FECA NUMBER

a. OTHER INSURED'S POLICY OR GROUP NUMBER

a. EMPLOYMENT? (Current or Previous)   YES □   NO □

a. INSURED'S DATE OF BIRTH   MM | DD | YY   SEX   M □   F □

b. OTHER INSURED'S DATE OF BIRTH   MM | DD | YY   SEX   M □   F □

b. AUTO ACCIDENT?   PLACE (State)   YES □   NO □

b. EMPLOYER'S NAME OR SCHOOL NAME

c. EMPLOYER'S NAME OR SCHOOL NAME

c. OTHER ACCIDENT?   YES □   NO □

c. INSURANCE PLAN NAME OR PROGRAM NAME

d. INSURANCE PLAN NAME OR PROGRAM NAME

10d. RESERVED FOR LOCAL USE

d. IS THERE ANOTHER HEALTH BENEFIT PLAN?   YES □   NO □   *If yes,* return to and complete item 9 a-d.

READ BACK OF FORM BEFORE COMPLETING & SIGNING THIS FORM.

12. PATIENT'S OR AUTHORIZED PERSON'S SIGNATURE I authorize the release of any medical or other information necessary to process this claim. I also request payment of government benefits either to myself or to the party who accepts assignment below.

SIGNED _____   DATE _____

13. INSURED'S OR AUTHORIZED PERSON'S SIGNATURE I authorize payment of medical benefits to the undersigned physician or supplier for services described below.

SIGNED _____

14. DATE OF CURRENT: MM | DD | YY   ILLNESS (First symptom) OR INJURY (Accident) OR PREGNANCY(LMP)

15. IF PATIENT HAS HAD SAME OR SIMILAR ILLNESS. GIVE FIRST DATE   MM | DD | YY

16. DATES PATIENT UNABLE TO WORK IN CURRENT OCCUPATION   FROM MM | DD | YY   TO MM | DD | YY

17. NAME OF REFERRING PROVIDER OR OTHER SOURCE

17a.
17b. NPI

18. HOSPITALIZATION DATES RELATED TO CURRENT SERVICES   FROM MM | DD | YY   TO MM | DD | YY

19. RESERVED FOR LOCAL USE

20. OUTSIDE LAB?   YES □   NO □ $ CHARGES

21. DIAGNOSIS OR NATURE OF ILLNESS OR INJURY (Relate Items 1, 2, 3 or 4 to Item 24E by Line)
1. |___.___   3. |___.___
2. |___.___   4. |___.___

22. MEDICAID RESUBMISSION CODE   ORIGINAL REF. NO.

23. PRIOR AUTHORIZATION NUMBER

24. A. DATE(S) OF SERVICE						B. PLACE OF SERVICE	C. EMG	D. PROCEDURES, SERVICES, OR SUPPLIES (Explain Unusual Circumstances)		E. DIAGNOSIS POINTER	F. $ CHARGES	G. DAYS OR UNITS	H. EPSDT Family Plan	I. ID. QUAL.	J. RENDERING PROVIDER ID. #
From			To					CPT/HCPCS	MODIFIER						
MM	DD	YY	MM	DD	YY										
1														NPI	
2														NPI	
3														NPI	
4														NPI	
5														NPI	
6														NPI	

25. FEDERAL TAX I.D. NUMBER   SSN □ EIN □

26. PATIENT'S ACCOUNT NO.

27. ACCEPT ASSIGNMENT? (For govt. claims, see back)   YES □   NO □

28. TOTAL CHARGE $

29. AMOUNT PAID $

30. BALANCE DUE $

31. SIGNATURE OF PHYSICIAN OR SUPPLIER INCLUDING DEGREES OR CREDENTIALS (I certify that the statements on the reverse apply to this bill and are made a part thereof.)

SIGNED _____   DATE _____

32. SERVICE FACILITY LOCATION INFORMATION

a. NPI   b.

33. BILLING PROVIDER INFO & PH # (   )

a. NPI   b.

NUCC Instruction Manual available at: www.nucc.org

APPROVED OMB-0938-0999 FORM CMS-1500 (08-05)

Form 84

1500

HEALTH INSURANCE CLAIM FORM

APPROVED BY NATIONAL UNIFORM CLAIM COMMITTEE 08/05

CARRIER

☐☐☐ PICA   PICA ☐☐☐

| 1. MEDICARE ☐ (Medicare #)   MEDICAID ☐ (Medicaid #)   TRICARE CHAMPUS ☐ (Sponsor's SSN)   CHAMPVA ☐ (Member ID#)   GROUP HEALTH PLAN ☐ (SSN or ID)   FECA BLK LUNG ☐ (SSN)   OTHER ☐ (ID) | 1a. INSURED'S I.D. NUMBER   (For Program in Item 1) |

2. PATIENT'S NAME (Last Name, First Name, Middle Initial)

3. PATIENT'S BIRTH DATE   MM | DD | YY   SEX   M ☐   F ☐

4. INSURED'S NAME (Last Name, First Name, Middle Initial)

5. PATIENT'S ADDRESS (No., Street)

6. PATIENT RELATIONSHIP TO INSURED   Self ☐   Spouse ☐   Child ☐   Other ☐

7. INSURED'S ADDRESS (No., Street)

CITY   STATE

8. PATIENT STATUS   Single ☐   Married ☐   Other ☐
Employed ☐   Full-Time Student ☐   Part-Time Student ☐

CITY   STATE

ZIP CODE   TELEPHONE (Include Area Code)   (   )

ZIP CODE   TELEPHONE (Include Area Code)   (   )

9. OTHER INSURED'S NAME (Last Name, First Name, Middle Initial)

10. IS PATIENT'S CONDITION RELATED TO:

11. INSURED'S POLICY GROUP OR FECA NUMBER

a. OTHER INSURED'S POLICY OR GROUP NUMBER

a. EMPLOYMENT? (Current or Previous)   YES ☐   NO ☐

a. INSURED'S DATE OF BIRTH   MM | DD | YY   SEX   M ☐   F ☐

b. OTHER INSURED'S DATE OF BIRTH   MM | DD | YY   SEX   M ☐   F ☐

b. AUTO ACCIDENT?   PLACE (State)   YES ☐   NO ☐

b. EMPLOYER'S NAME OR SCHOOL NAME

c. EMPLOYER'S NAME OR SCHOOL NAME

c. OTHER ACCIDENT?   YES ☐   NO ☐

c. INSURANCE PLAN NAME OR PROGRAM NAME

d. INSURANCE PLAN NAME OR PROGRAM NAME

10d. RESERVED FOR LOCAL USE

d. IS THERE ANOTHER HEALTH BENEFIT PLAN?   YES ☐   NO ☐   *If yes*, return to and complete item 9 a-d.

READ BACK OF FORM BEFORE COMPLETING & SIGNING THIS FORM.

12. PATIENT'S OR AUTHORIZED PERSON'S SIGNATURE I authorize the release of any medical or other information necessary to process this claim. I also request payment of government benefits either to myself or to the party who accepts assignment below.

SIGNED _____   DATE _____

13. INSURED'S OR AUTHORIZED PERSON'S SIGNATURE I authorize payment of medical benefits to the undersigned physician or supplier for services described below.

SIGNED _____

PATIENT AND INSURED INFORMATION

14. DATE OF CURRENT: MM | DD | YY   ◄ ILLNESS (First symptom) OR INJURY (Accident) OR PREGNANCY(LMP)

15. IF PATIENT HAS HAD SAME OR SIMILAR ILLNESS. GIVE FIRST DATE   MM | DD | YY

16. DATES PATIENT UNABLE TO WORK IN CURRENT OCCUPATION   MM | DD | YY   FROM   TO   MM | DD | YY

17. NAME OF REFERRING PROVIDER OR OTHER SOURCE

17a.
17b. NPI

18. HOSPITALIZATION DATES RELATED TO CURRENT SERVICES   MM | DD | YY   FROM   TO   MM | DD | YY

19. RESERVED FOR LOCAL USE

20. OUTSIDE LAB?   YES ☐   NO ☐ $ CHARGES

21. DIAGNOSIS OR NATURE OF ILLNESS OR INJURY (Relate Items 1, 2, 3 or 4 to Item 24E by Line)

1. |____.____   3. |____.____

2. |____.____   4. |____.____

22. MEDICAID RESUBMISSION CODE   ORIGINAL REF. NO.

23. PRIOR AUTHORIZATION NUMBER

24. A. DATE(S) OF SERVICE						B. PLACE OF SERVICE	C. EMG	D. PROCEDURES, SERVICES, OR SUPPLIES (Explain Unusual Circumstances) CPT/HCPCS	MODIFIER	E. DIAGNOSIS POINTER	F. $ CHARGES	G. DAYS OR UNITS	H. EPSDT Family Plan	I. ID. QUAL.	J. RENDERING PROVIDER ID. #
From MM DD YY			To MM DD YY												
1														NPI	
2														NPI	
3														NPI	
4														NPI	
5														NPI	
6														NPI	

25. FEDERAL TAX I.D. NUMBER   SSN ☐ EIN ☐

26. PATIENT'S ACCOUNT NO.

27. ACCEPT ASSIGNMENT? (For govt. claims, see back)   YES ☐   NO ☐

28. TOTAL CHARGE $

29. AMOUNT PAID $

30. BALANCE DUE $

31. SIGNATURE OF PHYSICIAN OR SUPPLIER INCLUDING DEGREES OR CREDENTIALS (I certify that the statements on the reverse apply to this bill and are made a part thereof.)

SIGNED _____   DATE _____

32. SERVICE FACILITY LOCATION INFORMATION

a. NPI   b.

33. BILLING PROVIDER INFO & PH #   (   )

a. NPI   b.

PHYSICIAN OR SUPPLIER INFORMATION

NUCC Instruction Manual available at: www.nucc.org

APPROVED OMB-0938-0999 FORM CMS-1500 (08-05)

Form 85

1500

HEALTH INSURANCE CLAIM FORM

APPROVED BY NATIONAL UNIFORM CLAIM COMMITTEE 08/05

☐☐ PICA

PICA ☐☐

1. MEDICARE ☐ (Medicare #) MEDICAID ☐ (Medicaid #) TRICARE CHAMPUS ☐ (Sponsor's SSN) CHAMPVA ☐ (Member ID#) GROUP HEALTH PLAN ☐ (SSN or ID) FECA BLK LUNG ☐ (SSN) OTHER ☐ (ID)

1a. INSURED'S I.D. NUMBER   (For Program in Item 1)

2. PATIENT'S NAME (Last Name, First Name, Middle Initial)

3. PATIENT'S BIRTH DATE   SEX
MM | DD | YY   M ☐   F ☐

4. INSURED'S NAME (Last Name, First Name, Middle Initial)

5. PATIENT'S ADDRESS (No., Street)

6. PATIENT RELATIONSHIP TO INSURED
Self ☐   Spouse ☐   Child ☐   Other ☐

7. INSURED'S ADDRESS (No., Street)

CITY   STATE

8. PATIENT STATUS
Single ☐   Married ☐   Other ☐
Employed ☐   Full-Time Student ☐   Part-Time Student ☐

CITY   STATE

ZIP CODE   TELEPHONE (Include Area Code)
( )

ZIP CODE   TELEPHONE (Include Area Code
( )

9. OTHER INSURED'S NAME (Last Name, First Name, Middle Initial)

10. IS PATIENT'S CONDITION RELATED TO:

11. INSURED'S POLICY GROUP OR FECA NUMBER

a. OTHER INSURED'S POLICY OR GROUP NUMBER

a. EMPLOYMENT? (Current or Previous)
☐ YES   ☐ NO

a. INSURED'S DATE OF BIRTH
MM | DD | YY   SEX   M ☐   F ☐

b. OTHER INSURED'S DATE OF BIRTH
MM | DD | YY   SEX   M ☐   F ☐

b. AUTO ACCIDENT?   PLACE (State)
☐ YES   ☐ NO

b. EMPLOYER'S NAME OR SCHOOL NAME

c. EMPLOYER'S NAME OR SCHOOL NAME

c. OTHER ACCIDENT?
☐ YES   ☐ NO

c. INSURANCE PLAN NAME OR PROGRAM NAME

d. INSURANCE PLAN NAME OR PROGRAM NAME

10d. RESERVED FOR LOCAL USE

d. IS THERE ANOTHER HEALTH BENEFIT PLAN?
☐ YES   ☐ NO   *If yes*, return to and complete item 9 a-d.

READ BACK OF FORM BEFORE COMPLETING & SIGNING THIS FORM.
12. PATIENT'S OR AUTHORIZED PERSON'S SIGNATURE I authorize the release of any medical or other information necessary to process this claim. I also request payment of government benefits either to myself or to the party who accepts assignment below.

SIGNED _____   DATE _____

13. INSURED'S OR AUTHORIZED PERSON'S SIGNATURE I authorize payment of medical benefits to the undersigned physician or supplier for services described below.

SIGNED _____

14. DATE OF CURRENT:
MM | DD | YY   ILLNESS (First symptom) OR INJURY (Accident) OR PREGNANCY(LMP)

15. IF PATIENT HAS HAD SAME OR SIMILAR ILLNESS.
GIVE FIRST DATE   MM | DD | YY

16. DATES PATIENT UNABLE TO WORK IN CURRENT OCCUPATION
MM | DD | YY   MM | DD | YY
FROM   TO

17. NAME OF REFERRING PROVIDER OR OTHER SOURCE

17a.
17b. NPI

18. HOSPITALIZATION DATES RELATED TO CURRENT SERVICES
MM | DD | YY   MM | DD | YY
FROM   TO

19. RESERVED FOR LOCAL USE

20. OUTSIDE LAB? $ CHARGES
☐ YES   ☐ NO

21. DIAGNOSIS OR NATURE OF ILLNESS OR INJURY (Relate Items 1, 2, 3 or 4 to Item 24E by Line)

1. |___.___   3. |___.___

2. |___.___   4. |___.___

22. MEDICAID RESUBMISSION CODE   ORIGINAL REF. NO.

23. PRIOR AUTHORIZATION NUMBER

24. A. DATE(S) OF SERVICE			B. PLACE OF SERVICE	C. EMG	D. PROCEDURES, SERVICES, OR SUPPLIES (Explain Unusual Circumstances)		E. DIAGNOSIS POINTER	F. $ CHARGES	G. DAYS OR UNITS	H. EPSDT Family Plan	I. ID. QUAL.	J. RENDERING PROVIDER ID. #
From MM DD YY	To MM DD YY				CPT/HCPCS	MODIFIER						
1											NPI	
2											NPI	
3											NPI	
4											NPI	
5											NPI	
6											NPI	

25. FEDERAL TAX I.D. NUMBER   SSN ☐ EIN ☐

26. PATIENT'S ACCOUNT NO.

27. ACCEPT ASSIGNMENT? (For govt. claims, see back)
☐ YES   ☐ NO

28. TOTAL CHARGE $

29. AMOUNT PAID $

30. BALANCE DUE $

31. SIGNATURE OF PHYSICIAN OR SUPPLIER INCLUDING DEGREES OR CREDENTIALS
(I certify that the statements on the reverse apply to this bill and are made a part thereof.)

SIGNED _____   DATE _____

32. SERVICE FACILITY LOCATION INFORMATION

a. NPI   b.

33. BILLING PROVIDER INFO & PH # ( )

a. NPI   b.

NUCC Instruction Manual available at: www.nucc.org

APPROVED OMB-0938-0999 FORM CMS-1500 (08-05)

CARRIER / PATIENT AND INSURED INFORMATION / PHYSICIAN OR SUPPLIER INFORMATION

Form 86

medical arts press®

ORDER FORM
67000_B

SOURCE CODE	CUSTOMER NUMBER

1-A BILL TO: Party responsible for payment. If name and address are not correct, please make changes below. We cannot ship to a P.O. Box. If P.O. Box is shown, please fill in street address in "Ship To" area at right.

Name(s) _____
(include Dergee/Title) _____

Address _____
_____

City/State/ZIP _____

Office Phone (____) _____ **FAX Phone** (____) _____

E-Mail Address: _____

For question...
Call _____

To serve you bettter...
Practice Specialty _____

Phone (____) _____ No. of Doctors _____

1-B SHIP TO: (Fill in only if different from "BILL TO".) For delivery, We must have a street address. We cannot ship to a P.O. Box.

Name(s) _____
_____

Address _____
_____
_____

City _____

State/Zip _____

2 PLEASE SEND ME: Fill in only those areas that apply to you order.

Please Fill In As Applicable

QUANTITY	CATALOG NUMBER	DESCRIPTION	MESSAGE	INK COLOR(S)	TYPE STYLE	LAYOUT NO.	LOGO NO.	PRODUCT COLOR	SIZE	YEAR	START NO.	TOTAL AMOUNT

COUPON CODE(S) If you have any coupon or discount codes, please enter them here:

*For Rush Delivery specify: ☐ **UPS Next Day** ☐ **UPS 2nd Day** Check the box at left if desired. You will be billed for rush shipping and handling charges.

☐ **RX BLANKS** (Complete the following information 85 it pertains to your state requirements)

DEA No. _____

License No. _____

☐ **MEDICAL INSURANCE CLAM FORMS** (Only complete the following if tou want it printed on your forms.)

Box 25:
SSN No. _____
or
Group No. _____

Box 33:
PIN No. _____
or
EIN No. _____

MERCHANDISE TOTAL	
Handling Fee	FREE
Sales Tax: Medical Arts Press collects tax in all states that have a sales/use tax. Please add tax at applicable rate.	
*Rush Delivery	
TOTAL	

Form 87

ORDER FORM

photocopy this form for ordering convenience

24 HOUR FAX LINE: 555.638.0116

TOLL FREE DIRECT ORDER LINE

1.555.800.4930

MSI, Incorporated
20 Main Street, Third Floor
Irvine, California 92714

**PLEASE FILL IN YOUR CUSTOMER NUMBER IF
YOU HAVE PURCHASED FROM US BEFORE:**

NAME _____

ADDRESS _____

CITY/STATE/ZIP _____

SPECIALTY _____

TELEPHONE _____

SHIP TO(IF DIFFERENT FROM ABOVE)_____

If you are a new customer, or have recently moved, help us expedite your order by providing us with your state registration number.

State License # _____

Expiration Date _____

PRODUCT PART NUMBER	PAGE #	PRODUCT DESCRIPTION	PKG SIZE	UNITS	QTY	EXTN

TOTAL OF MERCHANDISE	
STATE TAX (CA, IN, KY, OH, WA, WV)	
SHIPPING & HANDLING	
TOTAL	

IF YOU WISH TO PAY FOR YOUR ORDER BY CREDIT CARD, PLEASE COMPLETE THE FOLLOWING INFORMATION:

☐ VISA   ☐ MASTERCARD   ☐ DISCOVER   ☐ PREFERRED CUSTOMER CARD

YOUR CARD # : ☐☐☐☐☐☐☐☐☐☐☐☐☐☐☐☐☐☐☐

SIGNATURE _____ CARD EXP. DATE _____

THANK YOU FOR YOUR ORDER!

Form 88

medical arts press® — ORDER FORM
67000_B

SOURCE CODE   **CUSTOMER NUMBER**

1-A BILL TO: Party responsible for payment. If name and address are not correct, please make changes below. We cannot ship to a P.O. Box. If P.O. Box is shown, please fill in street address in "Ship To" area at right.

Name(s) _____
(include Dergee/Title)

Address _____
_____

City/State/ZIP _____

Office Phone (_____) _____ FAX Phone (_____) _____

E-Mail Address: _____

For question...
Call _____
Phone (_____) _____

To serve you bettter...
Practice Specialty _____
_____ No. of Doctors _____

1-B SHIP TO: (Fill in only if different from "BILL TO".) For delivery, We must have a street address. We cannot ship to a P.O. Box.

Name(s) _____
_____

Address _____
_____

City _____

State/Zip _____

2 PLEASE SEND ME: Fill in only those areas that apply to you order.

Please Fill In As Applicable

QUANTITY	CATALOG NUMBER	DESCRIPTION	MESSAGE	INK COLOR(S)	TYPE STYLE	LAYOUT NO.	LOGO NO.	PRODUCT COLOR	SIZE	YEAR	START NO.	TOTAL AMOUNT

COUPON CODE(S) If you have any coupon or discount codes, please enter them here:

*For Rush Delivery specify: ☐ **UPS Next Day** ☐ **UPS 2nd Day**   Check the box at left if desired. You will be billed for rush shipping and handling charges.

☐ **RX BLANKS** (Complete the following information 85 it pertains to your state requirements)

DEA No. _____

License No. _____

☐ **MEDICAL INSURANCE CLAM FORMS** (Only complete the following if tou want it printed on your forms.)

Box 25: _____
SSN No. _____
or
Group No. _____

Box 33: _____
PIN No. _____
or
EIN No. _____

MERCHANDISE TOTAL	
Handling Fee	FREE
Sales Tax: Medical Arts Press collects tax in all states that have a sales/use tax. Please add tax at applicable rate.	
*Rush Delivery	
TOTAL	

Form 89

medical arts press®

ORDER FORM
67000_B

1-A BILL TO: Party responsible for payment. If name and address are not correct, please make changes below. We cannot ship to a P.O. Box. If P.O. Box is shown, please fill in street address in "Ship To" area at right.

SOURCE CODE	CUSTOMER NUMBER

Name(s) _____
(include Dergee/Title)
_____

Address _____
_____

City/State/ZIP _____

Office Phone ( ) _____ FAX Phone ( ) _____

E-Mail Address: _____

1-B SHIP TO: (Fill in only if different from "BILL TO".) For delivery, We must have a street address. We cannot ship to a P.O. Box.

Name(s) _____
_____

Address _____
_____
_____

City _____

State/Zip _____

For question...
Call _____
Phone ( ) _____

To serve you bettter...
Practice Specialty _____
_____ No. of Doctors _____

2 PLEASE SEND ME: Fill in only those areas that apply to you order.

Please Fill In As Applicable

QUANTITY	CATALOG NUMBER	DESCRIPTION	MESSAGE	INK COLOR(S)	TYPE STYLE	LAYOUT NO.	LOGO NO.	PRODUCT COLOR	SIZE	YEAR	START NO.	TOTAL AMOUNT

COUPON CODE(S) If you have any coupon or discount codes, please enter them here:

MERCHANDISE TOTAL	
Handling Fee	FREE
Sales Tax: Medical Arts Press collects tax in all states that have a sales/use tax. Please add tax at applicable rate.	
*Rush Delivery	
TOTAL	

*For Rush Delivery specify: ☐ **UPS Next Day** ☐ **UPS 2nd Day**
Check the box at left if desired.
You will be billed for rush shipping and handling charges.

☐ **RX BLANKS** (Complete the following information 85 it pertains to your state requirements)

DEA No. _____

License No. _____

☐ **MEDICAL INSURANCE CLAM FORMS** (Only complete the following if tou want it printed on your forms.)

Box 25:
SSN No. _____
or
Group No. _____

Box 33:
PIN No. _____
or
EIN No. _____

Form 90

TRAVEL EXPENSE REPORT

TRIP BEGINNING _____   TRIP ENDING _____

DATE	SAT		SUN		MON		TUES		WED		THURS		FRI		SAT		TOTALS
LODGING																	
BREAKFAST																	
LUNCH																	
DINNER																	
LOCAL FARES																	
AUTO EXPENSES																	
PARKING FEES																	
PHONE/E-MAIL																	
ENTERTAINMENT																	
TIPS																	
TOLLS																	
OTHER/MISC.																	
TOTALS																	

Description of Business Purpose/Locations

Form 91

RECORD OF CHECKS DRAWN ON_____   CHECK REGISTER

MONTH OF_____   _____PAGE NO._____

	Paid to	Date	Gross Amount	Discount		Amount of check	Check Number
						Balance Forward ⟶	
1							
2							
3							
4							
5							
6							
7							
8							
9							
10							
11							
12							
13							
14							
15							
16							
17							
18							
19							
20							
21							
22							
23							
24							
25							
26							
27							
28							
29							
30							
			Ⓐ	Ⓑ		Ⓒ	

PROOF FORMULAS:

　　　　DISBURSEMENTS – COL'S Ⓑ + Ⓒ = Ⓐ

　　　　　　COL Ⓐ TOTAL = TOTAL OF COLUMNS USED FOR EXPENSE DISTRIBUTION

Form 92

MONTH OF _____ 20XX

(MEMO) BANK BALANCE			(MEMO) BANK DEPOSIT		1 Medical Supplies	2 OFC Upkeep	3 Salaries	4 Rent Upkeep	5 Utilities	6 Office Supplies	7 Taxes	8 Books Journals	9 Auto Upkeep	10 Laundry Cleaning	11 Promo & Entertain.
			DATE	AMOUNT											
		1													
		2													
		3													
		4													
		5													
		6													
		7													
		8													
		9													
		10													
		11													
		12													
		13													
		14													
		15													
		16													
		17													
		18													
		19													
		20													
		21													
		22													
		23													
		24													
		25													
		26													
		27													
		28													
		29													
		30													

Form 93

MONTH OF _____ 20_____

	Business Travel	Collections	NSF Checks	Equip. & Maintenance	Prof. Meetings	Bus. Insurance	Contribu- tions	Parking	Telephone	Life. Insurance			MISCELLANEOUS DESCRIPTION	AMOUNT
1														
2														
3														
4														
5														
6														
7														
8														
9														
10														
11														
12														
13														
14														
15														
16														
17														
18														
19														
20														
21														
22														
23														
24														
25														
26														
27														
28														
29														
30														

Form 94

PRACTON MEDICAL GROUP, INC.
4567 Broad Avenue
Woodland Hills, XY 12345-4700

FOR INSTRUCTIONAL USE ONLY

DATE	ITEM	AMOUNT

479

3-2
310

PAY _____ **DOLLARS**

PAY TO THE ORDER OF	DATE	GROSS	DISC.	CHECK AMOUNT
				$.

NOT VALID

THE FIRST NATIONAL BANK – Woodland Hills, XY 12345-4700
RB40BC-4-96

⑈123450⑈ 000123456⑈ 0479

PRACTON MEDICAL GROUP, INC.
4567 Broad Avenue
Woodland Hills, XY 12345-4700

FOR INSTRUCTIONAL USE ONLY

DATE	ITEM	AMOUNT

480

3-2
310

PAY _____ **DOLLARS**

PAY TO THE ORDER OF	DATE	GROSS	DISC.	CHECK AMOUNT
				$.

NOT VALID

THE FIRST NATIONAL BANK – Woodland Hills, XY 12345-4700
RB40BC-4-96

⑈123450⑈ 000123456⑈ 0480

PRACTON MEDICAL GROUP, INC.
4567 Broad Avenue
Woodland Hills, XY 12345-4700

FOR INSTRUCTIONAL USE ONLY

DATE	ITEM	AMOUNT

481

3-2
310

PAY _____ **DOLLARS**

PAY TO THE ORDER OF	DATE	GROSS	DISC.	CHECK AMOUNT
				$.

NOT VALID

THE FIRST NATIONAL BANK – Woodland Hills, XY 12345-4700
RB40BC-4-96

⑈123450⑈ 000123456⑈ 0481

Form 95

PRACTON MEDICAL GROUP, INC.
4567 Broad Avenue
Woodland Hills, XY 12345-4700

FOR INSTRUCTIONAL USE ONLY

DATE	ITEM	AMOUNT

482

3-2
310

PAY _____ **DOLLARS**

PAY TO THE ORDER OF	DATE	GROSS	DISC.	CHECK AMOUNT
				$

NOT VALID

_____

_____

THE FIRST NATIONAL BANK – Woodland Hills, XY 12345-4700
RB40BC-4-96

⑆123456780⑆ 000123456⑈   0482

PRACTON MEDICAL GROUP, INC.
4567 Broad Avenue
Woodland Hills, XY 12345-4700

FOR INSTRUCTIONAL USE ONLY

DATE	ITEM	AMOUNT

483

3-2
310

PAY _____ **DOLLARS**

PAY TO THE ORDER OF	DATE	GROSS	DISC.	CHECK AMOUNT
				$

NOT VALID

_____

_____

THE FIRST NATIONAL BANK – Woodland Hills, XY 12345-4700
RB40BC-4-96

⑆123456780⑆ 000123456⑈   0483

PRACTON MEDICAL GROUP, INC.
4567 Broad Avenue
Woodland Hills, XY 12345-4700

FOR INSTRUCTIONAL USE ONLY

DATE	ITEM	AMOUNT

484

3-2
310

PAY _____ **DOLLARS**

PAY TO THE ORDER OF	DATE	GROSS	DISC.	CHECK AMOUNT
				$

NOT VALID

_____

_____

THE FIRST NATIONAL BANK – Woodland Hills, XY 12345-4700
RB40BC-4-96

⑆123456780⑆ 000123456⑈   0484

Form 96

PRACTON MEDICAL GROUP, INC.
4567 Broad Avenue
Woodland Hills, XY 12345-4700

FOR INSTRUCTIONAL USE ONLY

DATE	ITEM	AMOUNT

485

3-2
310

PAY _____ **DOLLARS**

PAY TO THE ORDER OF	DATE	GROSS	DISC.

CHECK AMOUNT

$ _____ . _____

NOT VALID

THE FIRST NATIONAL BANK – Woodland Hills, XY 12345-4700
RB40BC-4-96

⑆123456780⑆ 000123456⑈   0485

PRACTON MEDICAL GROUP, INC.
4567 Broad Avenue
Woodland Hills, XY 12345-4700

FOR INSTRUCTIONAL USE ONLY

DATE	ITEM	AMOUNT

486

3-2
310

PAY _____ **DOLLARS**

PAY TO THE ORDER OF	DATE	GROSS	DISC.

CHECK AMOUNT

$ _____ . _____

NOT VALID

THE FIRST NATIONAL BANK – Woodland Hills, XY 12345-4700
RB40BC-4-96

⑆123456780⑆ 000123456⑈   0486

PRACTON MEDICAL GROUP, INC.
4567 Broad Avenue
Woodland Hills, XY 12345-4700

FOR INSTRUCTIONAL USE ONLY

DATE	ITEM	AMOUNT

487

3-2
310

PAY _____ **DOLLARS**

PAY TO THE ORDER OF	DATE	GROSS	DISC.

CHECK AMOUNT

$ _____ . _____

NOT VALID

THE FIRST NATIONAL BANK – Woodland Hills, XY 12345-4700
RB40BC-4-96

⑆123456780⑆ 000123456⑈   0487

Form 97

PRACTON MEDICAL GROUP, INC.
4567 Broad Avenue
Woodland Hills, XY 12345-4700

FOR INSTRUCTIONAL USE ONLY

DATE	ITEM	AMOUNT

488

3-2
310

PAY _____ **DOLLARS**

PAY TO THE ORDER OF	DATE	GROSS		DISC.	

CHECK AMOUNT

$ [.   ]

NOT VALID

THE FIRST NATIONAL BANK – Woodland Hills, XY 12345-4700
RB40BC-4-96

⑆123456780⑆ 000123456⑈   0488

PRACTON MEDICAL GROUP, INC.
4567 Broad Avenue
Woodland Hills, XY 12345-4700

FOR INSTRUCTIONAL USE ONLY

DATE	ITEM	AMOUNT

489

3-2
310

PAY _____ **DOLLARS**

PAY TO THE ORDER OF	DATE	GROSS		DISC.	

CHECK AMOUNT

$ [.   ]

NOT VALID

THE FIRST NATIONAL BANK – Woodland Hills, XY 12345-4700
RB40BC-4-96

⑆123456780⑆ 000123456⑈   0489

PRACTON MEDICAL GROUP, INC.
4567 Broad Avenue
Woodland Hills, XY 12345-4700

FOR INSTRUCTIONAL USE ONLY

DATE	ITEM	AMOUNT

490

3-2
310

PAY _____ **DOLLARS**

PAY TO THE ORDER OF	DATE	GROSS		DISC.	

CHECK AMOUNT

$ [.   ]

NOT VALID

THE FIRST NATIONAL BANK – Woodland Hills, XY 12345-4700
RB40BC-4-96

⑆123456780⑆ 000123456⑈   0490

Form 98

PRACTON MEDICAL GROUP, INC.
4567 Broad Avenue
Woodland Hills, XY 12345-4700

FOR INSTRUCTIONAL USE ONLY

DATE	ITEM	AMOUNT

491 3-2 / 310

PAY _____ DOLLARS

PAY TO THE ORDER OF	DATE	GROSS		DISC.	

CHECK AMOUNT

$ _____ . ____

NOT VALID

THE FIRST NATIONAL BANK – Woodland Hills, XY 12345-4700
RB40BC-4-96

⑈123456780⑈ 000123456⑈   0491

PRACTON MEDICAL GROUP, INC.
4567 Broad Avenue
Woodland Hills, XY 12345-4700

FOR INSTRUCTIONAL USE ONLY

DATE	ITEM	AMOUNT

492 3-2 / 310

PAY _____ DOLLARS

PAY TO THE ORDER OF	DATE	GROSS		DISC.	

CHECK AMOUNT

$ _____ . ____

NOT VALID

THE FIRST NATIONAL BANK – Woodland Hills, XY 12345-4700
RB40BC-4-96

⑈123456780⑈ 000123456⑈   0492

PRACTON MEDICAL GROUP, INC.
4567 Broad Avenue
Woodland Hills, XY 12345-4700

FOR INSTRUCTIONAL USE ONLY

DATE	ITEM	AMOUNT

493 3-2 / 310

PAY _____ DOLLARS

PAY TO THE ORDER OF	DATE	GROSS		DISC.	

CHECK AMOUNT

$ _____ . ____

NOT VALID

THE FIRST NATIONAL BANK – Woodland Hills, XY 12345-4700
RB40BC-4-96

⑈123456780⑈ 000123456⑈   0493

Form 99

PRACTON MEDICAL GROUP, INC.
4567 Broad Avenue
Woodland Hills, XY 12345-4700

FOR INSTRUCTIONAL USE ONLY

DATE	ITEM	AMOUNT

494

$\frac{3\text{-}2}{310}$

PAY _____ **DOLLARS**

PAY TO THE ORDER OF	DATE	GROSS	DISC.		CHECK AMOUNT
				$	

NOT VALID

THE FIRST NATIONAL BANK – Woodland Hills, XY 12345-4700
RB40BC-4-96

⑈123456780⑆ 000123456⑈ 0494

PRACTON MEDICAL GROUP, INC.
4567 Broad Avenue
Woodland Hills, XY 12345-4700

FOR INSTRUCTIONAL USE ONLY

DATE	ITEM	AMOUNT

495

$\frac{3\text{-}2}{310}$

PAY _____ **DOLLARS**

PAY TO THE ORDER OF	DATE	GROSS	DISC.		CHECK AMOUNT
				$	

NOT VALID

THE FIRST NATIONAL BANK – Woodland Hills, XY 12345-4700
RB40BC-4-96

⑈123456780⑆ 000123456⑈ 0495

Form 100

PETTY CASH RECEIPT ENVELOPE

From _____ 20XX To _____ 20XX   **Paid by Check No.** _____

Entered		Audited		Approved		Paid	

Date	No.	Paid to:	Item	Account	Amount

Office Fund Amount $ _____   **Receipts Paid** $ _____

Total Receipts and Cash $ _____   **Cash on Hand** $ _____

(Over or Short) $ _____   **TOTAL** $ _____

DISTRIBUTION OF PETTY CASH

										Totals

Form 101

BANK STATEMENT RECONCILIATION

FOUR EASY STEPS TO HELP YOU BALANCE YOUR CHECKBOOK

1. UPDATE YOUR CHECKBOOK

- Compare and check off each transaction recorded in your check register with those listed on this statement. These include checks, direct deposits, direct debits, deposits, ATM transactions, etc.

- Add interest and subtract service charges.

2. DETERMINE OUTSTANDING ITEMS

- Use the charts below to list transactions shown in your check register but not included on this statement.

- Include any from previous months.

OUTSTANDING CHECKS OR OTHER WITHDRAWALS					DEPOSITS NOT CREDITED		
CHECK NO.	AMOUNT		CHECK NO.	AMOUNT	DATE	AMOUNT	
	$			$		$	
			TOTAL	$	TOTAL	$	

3. BALANCE YOUR ACCOUNT

- Enter Ending Statement Balance shown on this statement. $ _____

- Add deposits listed in your register and not shown on this statement.   + _____

- Subtract outstanding checks/withdrawals.   - _____

- **ADJUSTED TOTAL** (should agree with your checkbook balance) $ _____

4. IF THE BALANCE IN YOUR CHECKBOOK DOES NOT AGREE WITH THE ADJUSTED TOTAL, THEN

- Check all addition and subtraction.

- Make sure all outstanding checks, withdrawals, and deposits have been listed in the appropriate chart above.

- Compare the amount of each check, withdrawal, and deposit in your checkbook with the amounts on this statement.

- Review the figures on last month's statement.

IN CASE OF ERRORS OR QUESTIONS ABOUT YOUR ELECTRONIC TRANSFERS, telephone us at the telephone number shown on this statement, or write us at: P.O. Box 30987, City of Industry, CA 91896-7987 as soon as you can if you think your statement or receipt is wrong or if you need more information about a transfer on the statement or receipt. We must hear from you no later than 60 days after we sent you the FIRST statement on which the error or problem appeared. Tell us your name and account number, and describe the error or the transfer you are unsure about. Please explain as clearly as you can why you believe there is an error or why you need more information. You must also tell us the exact dollar amount of the suspected error. If you tell us orally, we require that you send us your complaint or question in writing within 10 business days. If you do not put your complaint or questions in writing or we do not receive it within 10 business days, we may not recredit your account. If we decide that there was no error, we will send you a written explanation within 3 business days after we finish our investigation. You may ask for copies of the documents that we used in our investigation. For purposes of error resolution, our business days are Monday through Friday, 8:30 a.m. to 5:00 p.m., Pacific Time. We are closed Saturdays, Sundays, and federal holidays.

All Non-POS, MasterMoney™ or Foreign Transactions
We will tell you the results of our investigation within 10 business days after we receive your written complaint and will correct any error promptly. If we need more time, however, we may take up to 45 days to investigate your complaint or questions. If we decide we need additional time, we will recredit your account within 10 business days for the amount you think is in error, so that you will have the use of the money during the time it takes us to complete our investigation.

POS, MasterMoney™ and Foreign Transactions
If the transfer results from a point-of-sale transaction, MasterMoney™ transaction, or a transfer initiated outside the United States, we will still correct any error promptly. However, we may take up to 20 business days after we receive your written complaint to tell you the results of our investigation. If we need more time, we may use an additional 90 days. Should we take this additional time, we will recredit your account within 20 business days for the amount you think is in error. This will allow you to have the use of this money while we complete our investigation.

CF 5299F (5/96)

Form 102

PAYROLL REGISTER FOR PERIOD ENDING: _____

EMPLOYEE NAME	EARNINGS						DEDUCTIONS							
	No. of Exempts	Hours Worked	Hourly Rate	Reg. Pay	Over-time	Gross Pay	FICA	Fed. Inc. Tax	State Inc. Tax	SDI	Medicare	Other	TOTAL DEDUC.	Check No.	NET PAY

Form 103

EMPLOYEE EARNING RECORD

Name_____

Address_____

_____

Telephone_____

Social Security Number_____

Date of Hire_____

Date of Birth_____

Position_____PT/FT

No. of Exemptions_____S/M

Rate of Pay_____ hr/wk/mo

Period Ended	Hours Worked	EARNINGS			DEDUCTIONS							NET PAY	Year to Date
		Reg. Pay	Over-time	Gross Pay	FICA	Fed. Inc. Tax	State Inc. Tax	SDI	Medicare	Other	TOTAL DEDUC.		

Form 104

Form W-4 (2006)

Purpose. Complete Form W-4 so that your employer can withhold the correct federal income tax from your pay. Because your tax situation may change, you may want to refigure your withholding each year.

Exemption from withholding. If you are exempt, complete only lines 1, 2, 3, 4, and 7 and sign the form to validate it. Your exemption for 2006 expires February 16, 2007. See Pub. 505, Tax Withholding and Estimated Tax.

Note. You cannot claim exemption from withholding if (a) your income exceeds $850 and includes more than $300 of unearned income (for example, interest and dividends) and (b) another person can claim you as a dependent on their tax return.

Basic instructions. If you are not exempt, complete the **Personal Allowances Worksheet** below. The worksheets on page 2 adjust your withholding allowances based on itemized deductions, certain credits, adjustments to income, or two-

earner/two-job situations. Complete all worksheets that apply. However, you may claim fewer (or zero) allowances.

Head of household. Generally, you may claim head of household filing status on your tax return only if you are unmarried and pay more than 50% of the costs of keeping up a home for yourself and your dependent(s) or other qualifying individuals. See line **E** below.

Tax credits. You can take projected tax credits into account in figuring your allowable number of withholding allowances. Credits for child or dependent care expenses and the child tax credit may be claimed using the **Personal Allowances Worksheet** below. See Pub. 919, How Do I Adjust My Tax Withholding, for information on converting your other credits into withholding allowances.

Nonwage income. If you have a large amount of nonwage income, such as interest or dividends, consider making estimated tax payments using Form 1040-ES, Estimated Tax for Individuals. Otherwise, you may owe additional tax.

Two earners/two jobs. If you have a working spouse or more than one job, figure the total number of allowances you are entitled to claim on all jobs using worksheets from only one Form W-4. Your withholding usually will be most accurate when all allowances are claimed on the Form W-4 for the highest paying job and zero allowances are claimed on the others.

Nonresident alien. If you are a nonresident alien, see the Instructions for Form 8233 before completing this Form W-4.

Check your withholding. After your Form W-4 takes effect, use Pub. 919 to see how the dollar amount you are having withheld compares to your projected total tax for 2006. See Pub. 919, especially if your earnings exceed $130,000 (Single) or $180,000 (Married).

Recent name change? If your name on line 1 differs from that shown on your social security card, call 1-800-772-1213 to initiate a name change and obtain a social security card showing your correct name.

Personal Allowances Worksheet (Keep for your records.)

A Enter "1" for **yourself** if no one else can claim you as a dependent . . . . **A** _____

B Enter "1" if:
- You are single and have only one job; or
- You are married, have only one job, and your spouse does not work; or
- Your wages from a second job or your spouse's wages (or the total of both) are $1,000 or less.

B _____

C Enter "1" for your **spouse.** But, you may choose to enter "-0-" if you are married and have either a working spouse or more than one job. (Entering "-0-" may help you avoid having too little tax withheld.) . . . . **C** _____

D Enter number of **dependents** (other than your spouse or yourself) you will claim on your tax return . . . . . **D** _____

E Enter "1" if you will file as **head of household** on your tax return (see conditions under **Head of household** above) . **E** _____

F Enter "1" if you have at least $1,500 of **child or dependent care expenses** for which you plan to claim a credit . . **F** _____

(**Note.** Do **not** include child support payments. See **Pub. 503,** Child and Dependent Care Expenses, for details.)

G **Child Tax Credit** (including additional child tax credit):
- If your total income will be less than $55,000 ($82,000 if married), enter "2" for each eligible child.
- If your total income will be between $55,000 and $84,000 ($82,000 and $119,000 if married), enter "1" for each eligible child plus "1" **additional** if you have four or more eligible children. **G** _____

H Add lines A through G and enter total here. (**Note.** This may be different from the number of exemptions you claim on your tax return.) ▶ **H** _____

For accuracy, complete all worksheets that apply.
- If you plan to **itemize or claim adjustments to income** and want to reduce your withholding, see the **Deductions and Adjustments Worksheet** on page 2.
- If you have **more than one job** or are **married and you and your spouse both work** and the combined earnings from all jobs exceed $35,000 ($25,000 if married) see the **Two-Earner/Two-Job Worksheet** on page 2 to avoid having too little tax withheld.
- If **neither** of the above situations applies, **stop here** and enter the number from line H on line 5 of Form W-4 below.

- - - - - - - - - - - - - - - - - - Cut here and give Form W-4 to your employer. Keep the top part for your records. - - - - - - - - - - - - - - - - -

Form **W-4**	**Employee's Withholding Allowance Certificate**	OMB No. 1545-0074
Department of the Treasury Internal Revenue Service	▶ Whether you are entitled to claim a certain number of allowances or exemption from withholding is subject to review by the IRS. Your employer may be required to send a copy of this form to the IRS.	2006

1 Type or print your first name and middle initial.	Last name	**2** Your social security number

Home address (number and street or rural route)	**3** ☐ Single ☐ Married ☐ Married, but withhold at higher Single rate.
	Note. If married, but legally separated, or spouse is a nonresident alien, check the "Single" box.
City or town, state, and ZIP code	**4** If your last name differs from that shown on your social security card, check here. You must call 1-800-772-1213 for a new card. ▶ ☐

5 Total number of allowances you are claiming (from line **H** above **or** from the applicable worksheet on page 2) **5** _____

6 Additional amount, if any, you want withheld from each paycheck - - - - - - - - - - - **6** $ _____

7 I claim exemption from withholding for 2006, and I certify that I meet **both** of the following conditions for exemption.
- Last year I had a right to a refund of **all** federal income tax withheld because I had **no** tax liability **and**
- This year I expect a refund of **all** federal income tax withheld because I expect to have **no** tax liability.

If you meet both conditions, write "Exempt" here - - - - - - - - - - - - ▶ **7** _____

Under penalties of perjury, I declare that I have examined this certificate and to the best of my knowledge and belief, it is true, correct, and complete.

Employee's signature
(Form is not valid unless you sign it.) ▶ _____ **Date** ▶ _____

8 Employer's name and address (Employer: Complete lines 8 and 10 only if sending to the IRS.)	**9** Office code (optional)	**10** Employer identification number (EIN)

For Privacy Act and Paperwork Reduction Act Notice, see page 2. Cat. No. 10220Q Form **W-4** (2006)

Form 105

EMPLOYEE BENEFITS

Benefit	Employer Pays	Employee Pays
Medical Insurance	$_____	$_____
Life Insurance	$_____	$_____
Accident Insurance	$_____	$_____
Disability Insurance	$_____	$_____
Worker's Compensation	$_____	$_____
Holiday # _____	$_____	$_____
Vacation # _____	$_____	$_____
Sick Leave # _____	$_____	$_____
Personal Leave	$_____	$_____
Education	$_____	$_____
Incentive Bonus	$_____	$_____
Retirement	$_____	$_____
Uniforms	$_____	$_____
Other	$_____	$_____
Total benefits	$_____	$_____

Wage of employee $_____

Gross wage for 20____ $_____

Total employment package $_____

Employee Name:_____   Date:_____

Form 106

EMPLOYMENT APPLICATION FORM

Directions: Answer all questions using black ink (print).

PERSONAL INFORMATION

(LAST NAME)	(FIRST NAME)	(MI)	
ADDRESS – STREET	CITY	STATE	ZIP

PHONE NUMBER: SOCIAL SECURITY NUMBER:

POSITION DESIRED:

EXPECTED SALARY OR HOURLY WAGE:

EDUCATION

NAME OF SCHOOL	ADDRESS	DATE(S)	DEGREE/CERTIFICATE
HIGH SCHOOL			
VOCATIONAL/TECHNICAL			
COLLEGE			
OTHER			

WORK EXPERIENCE – Give present position (or last position held) first.

JOB TITLE	EMPLOYER	ADDRESS	DATES

DUTIES PERFORMED:

JOB TITLE	EMPLOYER	ADDRESS	DATES

DUTIES PERFORMED:

JOB TITLE	EMPLOYER	ADDRESS	DATES

DUTIES PERFORMED:

REFERENCES – List three persons (other than relatives) who have known you for at least 2 years.

NAME/TITLE	ADDRESS	TELEPHONE NUMBER

APPLICANT'S SIGNATURE _____ DATE_____

Form 107

PREEMPLOYMENT WORKSHEET

Employment objective: _____

Driver's license number: _____

Date of birth: _____   U.S. citizen? Yes _____ No ___

Physical disabilities that need to be taken into consideration for job modifications: _____

_____

Volunteer activities: _____

Memberships in professional organizations: _____

_____

Personal interests: _____

_____

SKILLS: _____

    Typing/Keying rate: _____WPM   _____

    Other:_____   _____

    _____   _____

    _____   _____

    _____   _____

    _____   _____

    _____   _____

    _____   _____

    _____   _____

    _____   _____

Form 108

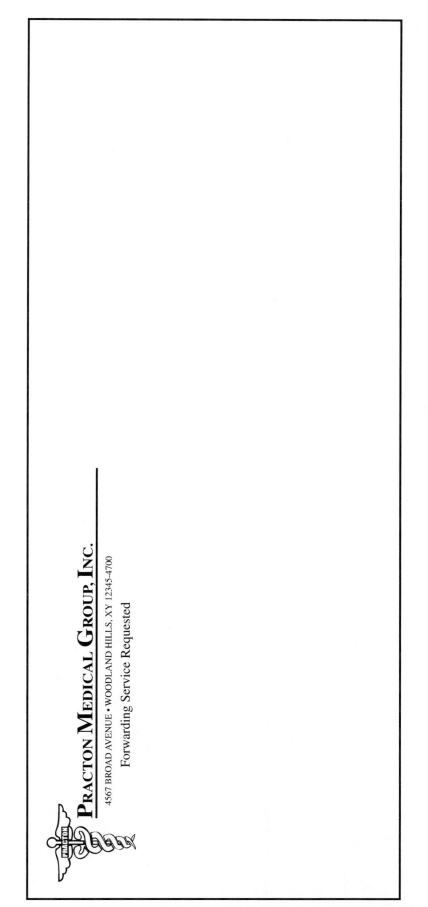

Form 109

Practon Medical Group, Inc.
4567 BROAD AVENUE • WOODLAND HILLS, XY 12345-4700
Forwarding Service Requested

Form 110

PART III

Competency Grids

- CAAHEP Curriculum Competencies
- ABHES Curriculum Competencies
- CMA Certification Examination Content
- RMA Certification Examination Competencies
- CMAS Examination Specifications
- AAMA Role Delineation Study

CAAHEP CURRICULUM COMPETENCIES

The Commission on Accreditation and Allied Health Education Programs (CAAHEP) have established standards and guidelines for medical assisting educational programs. The 2003 minimum curriculum standards have been adopted by the American Association of Medical Assistants (AAMA) and used in the accreditation process for programs who train individuals to enter the medical assisting profession. Following are entry-level competencies for medical assistants.* These are cross-referenced in a chapter-by-chapter grid (see Table III-1) to help locate them in the *Administrative Medical Assisting* textbook and *Workbook*.

III.C.3.a. ADMINISTRATIVE COMPETENCIES
(1) Perform Clerical Functions
- (1)(a) Schedule and manage appointments
- (1)(b) Schedule inpatient and outpatient admissions and procedures
- (1)(c) Organize a patient's medical records
- (1)(d) File medical records

(2) Perform Bookkeeping Procedures
- (2)(a) Prepare a bank deposit
- (2)(b) Post entries on a daysheet
- (2)(c) Perform accounts receivable procedures
- (2)(d) Perform billing and collection procedures
- (2)(e) Post adjustments
- (2)(f) Process credit balance
- (2)(g) Process refunds
- (2)(h) Post NSF checks
- (2)(i) Post collection agency payments

(3) Process Insurance Claims
- (3)(a) Apply managed care policies and procedures
- (3)(b) Apply third party guidelines
- (3)(c) Perform procedural coding
- (3)(d) Perform diagnostic coding
- (3)(e) Complete insurance claim forms

III.C.3.b. CLINICAL COMPETENCIES†
(1) Fundamental Procedures
- (1)(d) Dispose of biohazardous materials

(4) Patient Care

- (4)(c) Obtain and record patient history
- (4)(h) Maintain medication and immunization records

III.C.3.c GENERAL COMPETENCIES
(1) Professional Communications
- (1)(a) Respond to and initiate written communications
- (1)(b) Recognize and respond to verbal communications
- (1)(c) Recognize and respond to nonverbal communications
- (1)(d) Demonstrate telephone techniques

(2) Legal Concepts
- (2)(a) Identify and respond to issues of confidentiality
- (2)(b) Perform within legal and ethical boundaries
- (2)(c) Establish and maintain the medical record
- (2)(e) Document appropriately
- (2)(f) Demonstrate knowledge of federal and state health care legislation and regulations

(3) Patient Instruction
- (3)(a) Explain general office policies
- (3)(b) Instruct individuals according to their needs
- (3)(c) Provide instruction for health maintenance and disease prevention
- (3)(d) Identify community resources

(4) Operational Functions
- (4)(a) Perform an inventory of supplies and equipment
- (4)(b) Perform routine maintenance of administrative and clinical equipment
- (4)(c) Utilize computer software to maintain office systems
- (4)(d) Use methods of quality control

*The competencies are reprinted with permission from the Commission on Accreation for Allied Health Programs.
†Only those clinical competencies that apply to this text are listed.

TABLE III-1

Commission on Accreditation of Allied Health Education Programs (CAAHEP) Standards and Guidelines
for Medical Assisting Educational Programs, 2003

		III.C.3.a. ADMINISTRATIVE COMPETENCIES			III.C.3.b. CLINICAL COMPETENCIES	III.C.3.c. GENERAL COMPETENCIES			
Administrative Medical Assisting, 6ed.									
Ch	Title	1. Perform Clerical Functions	2. Perform Bookkeeping Procedures	3. Process Insurance Claims	Clinical	1. Professional Communi- cation	2. Legal Concepts	3. Patient Instruction	4. Opera- tional Functions
1	A Career As an Administrative Medical Assistant	a, b, c, d	e	b			a	a, b, c, d	c
2	The Health Care Environment: Past, Present, and Future	a, b, c, d					d	b	
3	Medicolegal and Ethical Responsibilities	✓					a, b, d, e		c
4	The Art of Communication					b, c	a	b	
5	The Receptionist	a, d					a, d	a, b, c, d	
6	Telephone Procedures	c, d, e				b, d, e			
7	Appointments	a, b				a, b, d	d	a	
8	Filing Procedures	c, d	a, c						
9	Medical Records	c, d	c, e				b, c, d		
10	Drug and Prescription Records				(1)e, (4)c, h		d	b	
11	Written Correspondence					a			
12	Processing Mail and Telecommunications	✓				a			c
13	Fees, Credit, and Collection	✓	c, d, e, f, g, h, i			a, b			
14	Banking	✓	a, e–i						
15	Bookkeeping	✓	b, c, e–i						
16	Health Insurance Systems			a, b, c, d, e					
17	Office Managerial Responsibilities	✓		a		a	e		a, b, d
18	Financial Management of the Medical Practice	✓	a, b				e		
19	Seeking a Position As an Administrative Medical Assistant	✓				a, b, c	b		

ABHES CURRICULUM COMPETENCIES

The Accrediting Bureau of Health Education Schools (ABHES) is a nationally recognized, independent, non-profit accrediting agency of institutions and educational programs that predominantly provide allied health education. Policies, procedures and standards have been developed for the accreditation of medical assisting programs and the 2006 entry-level competencies required for successful completion are outlined as follows.* These are cross-referenced in a chapter-by-chapter grid (see Table III-2) to help locate them in the *Administrative Medical Assisting* textbook and *Workbook*.

VI.B.1.a.1.   PROFESSIONALISM

1(a)   Project a positive attitude
1(b)   Maintain confidentiality at all times
1(c)   Be a "team player"
1(d)   Be cognizant of ethical boundaries
1(e)   Exhibit initiative
1(f)   Adapt to change
1(g)   Evidence a responsible attitude
1(h)   Be courteous and diplomatic
1(i)   Conduct work within scope of education, training, and ability

VI.B.1.a.2.   COMMUNICATION

2(a)   Be attentive, listen, and learn
2(b)   Be impartial and show empathy when dealing with patients
2(c)   Adapt what is said to the recipient's level of comprehension
2(d)   Serve as liaison between physician and others
2(e)   Use proper telephone techniques
2(f)   Interview effectively
2(g)   Use appropriate medical terminology
2(h)   Receive, organize, prioritize, and transmit information expediently
2(i)   Recognize and respond to verbal and non-verbal communication
2(j)   Use correct grammar, spelling and formatting techniques in written works
2(k)   Use principles of verbal and nonverbal communication
2(l)   (duplicate i)
2(m) Adapt to individualized needs
2(n)   Apply electronic technology

2(o)   Use fundamental writing skills
2(p)   Exhibit professional components
2(q)   Understand allied health professions and credentialing

VI.B.1.a.3.   ADMINISTRATIVE DUTIES

3(a)   Perform basic secretarial skills
3(b)   Prepare and maintain medical records
3(c)   Schedule and monitor appointments
3(d)   Apply computer concepts for office procedures
3(e)   Perform medical transcription
3(f)   Locate resources and information for patients and employers
3(g)   Manage physicians' professional schedule and travel
3(h)   Schedule inpatient and outpatient admissions
3(i)   File medical records
3(j)   Prepare a bank statement and deposit record
3(k)   Reconcile a bank statement
3(l)   Post entries on a day sheet
3(m) Perform billing and collection procedures
3(n)   Prepare a check
3(o)   Establish and maintain a petty cash fund
3(p)   Post adjustments
3(q)   Process credit balance
3(r)   Process refunds
3(s)   Post NSF checks
3(t)   Post collection agency payments
3(u)   Apply managed care policies and procedures
3(v)   Obtain managed care referrals and pre-certification
3(w) Perform diagnostic coding
3(x)   Complete insurance claim forms
3(y)   Use physician fee schedule

VI.B.1.a.4.   CLINICAL DUTIES†

4(a)   Interview and record patient history
4(e)   Recognize emergencies
4(l)   Screen and follow up patient test results
4(n)   Maintain medication and immunization records
4(q)   Dispose of biohazardous materials
4(r)   Practice standard precautions

---

*The competencies are reprinted with permission from the Accrediting Bureau of Health Education Schools.
†Only those clinical competencies that apply to this text are listed.

VI.B.1.a.5. LEGAL CONCEPTS

5(a) Determine needs for documentation and reporting

5(b) Document accurately

5(c) Use appropriate guidelines when releasing records or information

5(d) Follow established policy in initiating or terminating medical treatment

5(e) Dispose of controlled substances in compliance with government regulations

5(f) Maintain licenses and accreditation

5(g) Monitor legislation related to current healthcare issues and practices

5(h) Perform risk management procedures

VI.B.1.a.6. OFFICE MANAGEMENT

6(a) Maintain physical plant

6(b) Operate and maintain facilities and perform routine maintenance of administrative and clinical equipment safely

6(c) Inventory equipment and supplies

6(d) Evaluate and recommend equipment and supplies for practice

6(e) Maintain liability coverage

6(f) Exercise efficient time management

VI.B.1.a.7. INSTRUCTION

7(a) Orient patients to office policies and procedures

7(b) Instruct patients with special needs

7(c) Teach patients methods of health promotion and disease prevention

7(d) Orient and train personnel

VI.B.1.a.8. FINANCIAL MANAGEMENT

8(a) Use manual and computerized bookkeeping systems

8(b) Implement current procedural terminology and *ICD-9* coding

8(c) Analyze and use current third-party guidelines for reimbursement

8(d) Manage accounts payable and receivable

8(e) Maintain records for accounting and banking purposes

8(f) Process employee payroll

TABLE III-2
Accrediting Bureau of Health Education Schools (ABHES) Competencies
for Medical Assisting Programs, 2006

Administrative Medical Assisting, 6ed. Ch / Title	VI.B.1.a.1. Professional-ism	VI.B.1.a.2. Commun-ication	VI.B.1.a.3. Administra-tive Duties	VI.B.1.a.4. Clinical Duties	VI.B.1.a.5. Legal Concepts	VI.B.1.a.6. Office Management	VI.B.1.a.7. Instruction	VI.B.1.a 8. Financial Management
1 A Career As an Administrative Medical Assistant	a, b, d, e, f, g, h, i	b, d, g, h, j, m, n, o, p, q	a, d, f		f		a, b, c	
2 The Health Care Environment: Past, Present, and Future	c	a, c, d, g	e, u	a	g		b	
3 Medicolegal and Ethical Responsibilities	a, d	j, n		a, d	b, c, d, g, h			
4 The Art of Communication	a, b, h	a, b, c, d, f, g, h, i, k, l, m, p				a, b		
5 The Receptionist	a, b, c, h	e, f, g, m	a, f	e	g	a, b, c		
6 Telephone Procedures	b, h	a, e, h, j, k	a	e	b			
7 Appointments	h	a, d, g, h, j, n	a, c, d, g, h	e	a		a	
8 Filing Procedures		h	b, i		c			
9 Medical Records		g, i, j, n, o	b, e, i	a	a, b, c			
10 Drug and Prescription Records		g, j	b, f, j	n, q	b, e, f	c	c	
11 Written Correspondence		g, j, n, o	a, d, e					
12 Processing Mail and Telecommunications		g, h, j, o	a					
13 Fees, Credit, and Collection		a, b, d, g, i, j, k, o	a, m, p, q, r, s, t, y				a	
14 Banking			a, j, k, n, p, q, r, s, t					d, e
15 Bookkeeping		n	a, j, l, o–t, y					a, d, e
16 Health Insurance Systems			u, v, w, x, y					b, c
17 Office Managerial Responsibilities		o	g	q, r	g, h	a–f	a, d	
18 Financial Management of the Medical Practice	h		d, j, k, o, n, u		g	✓		d, e, f
19 Seeking a Position As an Administrative Medical Assistant	a, c, d, e, g, h	a, c, i, j, k, o, p	a					

CMA CERTIFICATION EXAMINATION CONTENT

The American Association of Medical Assistants (AAMA) has developed a content outline for the Certified Medical Assistant (CMA) certification examination as follows.* These are cross-referenced in a chapter-by-chapter grid (see Table III-3) to help locate them in the *Administrative Medical Assisting* textbook and *Workbook*.

I. GENERAL

A. Medical Terminology
  1. Word building and definitions
     a. Basic structure
        (1) roots or stems
        (2) prefixes
        (3) suffixes
        (4) plurals
        (5) abbreviations
        (6) symbols
     b. Surgical procedures
     c. Diagnostic procedures
     d. Medial specialties
     e. Common diseases and pathology
  2. Uses of technology
     a. Spelling and pronunciation
     b. Selection and use
     c. Reference sources
B. Anatomy and Physiology†
  1. Body as a whole, including multiple systems
  2. Systems, including structure, function, related conditions and diseases
C. Psychology
  1. Basic principles
     a. Meaning of individual self-worth
     b. Understanding human behavior—Maslow's hierarchy of needs
     c. Social needs of people
     d. Understanding emotional behavior
  2. Developmental stages of the life cycle
     a. Developmental theories used to explain behavior and development
     b. Human growth and development
  3. Hereditary, cultural, and environmental influences on behavior
     a. Helping patients adjust to illness
     b. Cultural influences on behavior
     c. Importance of recognizing cultural differences and attitudes toward the health care system
     d. Recognizing social and environmental influences on behavior

  4. Defense mechanisms
     a. Recognition
     b. Management
D. Professionalism
  1. Displaying professional attitude
     a. Supporting professional organization
     b. Accepting responsibility for own actions
  2. Job readiness and seeking employment
     a. Resumé and cover letter
     b. Methods of job searching
     c. Interviewing as a job candidate
     d. Professional presentation
  3. Performing within ethical boundaries
     a. Ethical standards
        (1) AAMA Code of Ethics
        (2) AMA Code of Ethics
     b. Patient rights
     c. Current issues in medical bioethics
  4. Maintaining confidentiality
     a. Agent of physician
        (1) patient rights
        (2) releasing patient information
     b. Intentional tort
        (1) invasion of privacy
        (2) slander and libel
  5. Working as a team member to achieve goals
     a. Member responsibility
     b. Promoting competent patient care
     c. Utilizing principles of group dynamics
E. Communication
  1. Adapting communication to an individual's ability to understand
     a. Blind
     b. Deaf
     c. Elderly
     d. Children
     e. Seriously ill
     f. Mentally impaired
     g. Illiterate
     h. Non-English-speaking
     i. Anxious
     j. Angry/Distraught
     k. Motor impaired
  2. Recognizing and responding to verbal and nonverbal communication
     a. Positive body language
     b. Listening skills
     c. Eye contact
     d. Barriers to effective communication
     e. Identifying needs of others
  3. Patient instructions
     a. Explaining general office policies

*The competencies are reprinted with permission from the American Association of Medical Assistants.
†Only those anatomy and physiology competencies that apply to this text are listed.

b.   Instructing individuals according to their needs

c.   Instruction and demonstrating the use and care of patient equipment

d.   Providing instruction for health maintenance and disease prevention

e.   Identifying community resources

4.   Professional communication and behavior

a.   Professional situations

(1)   tact

(2)   diplomacy

(3)   courtesy

(4)   responsibility

b.   Therapeutic relationships

(1)   impartial behavior

(2)   effective responses to cultural differences

(3)   empathy

5.   Evaluating and understanding communication

a.   Observation

b.   Active listening

c.   Feedback

6.   Interviewing techniques

a.   Guiding, controlling and ending interviews

b.   Using questions

c.   Specific interviews

(1)   interviewee

(2)   setting

d.   Legal restrictions

7.   Receiving, organizing, prioritizing and transmitting information

a.   Modalities for incoming and outgoing data

b.   Prioritizing incoming and outgoing data

8.   Telephone techniques

a.   Incoming calls management criteria

(1)   screening

(2)   effective conversation

(3)   maintaining confidentiality

(4)   gathering data

(5)   multiple-line competency

(6)   transferring appropriate calls

(7)   screening and referral

(8)   identifying caller, office, and self

(9)   taking messages

(10)   ending calls

b.   Monitoring special calls

(1)   problem calls

(2)   emergency calls

9.   Fundamental writing skills

a.   Sentence structure

b.   Gammar

c.   Punctuation

d.   Spelling

F.   Medicolegal Guidelines and Requirements

1.   Licenses and accreditation

a.   Medical practice acts

b.   Renewal of license

c.   Revocation/suspension of license

(1)   criminal/unprofessional conduct

(2)   professional/personal incapacity

d.   Facility accreditation

(1)   state requirements (certificate of need/laboratory registration)

(2)   federal requirements (ambulatory surgical center/physician office laboratory)

2.   Legislation

a.   State compliance

(1)   personnel standards, hiring and termination

(2)   Medicare/Medicaid reimbursement policies

(3)   acts (living wills/anatomical gifts)

(4)   reportable incidences (public health statutes/criminal acts)

b.   Federal compliance

(1)   OSHA

(2)   right to privacy

(3)   controlled substances

(4)   Medicare/Medicaid regulations

(5)   Clinical Laboratory Improvement Act

(6)   Americans with Disabilities Act

(7)   Health Insurance Portability and Accountability Act

3.   Documentation/reporting

a.   Sources of information

b.   Drug Enforcement Administration

c.   Internal Revenue Service

d.   Employment laws

e.   Personal injury occurrences

f.   Workers' compensation

g.   Medical records

(1)   patient activity

(2)   patient care

(3)   patient confidentiality

(4)   ownership

h.   Personnel records

(1)   evaluation

(2)   privacy

4.   Releasing medical information

a.   Consent

(1)   patient written authorization

(2) state and federal codes
b. Rescinding authorization for release
5. Physician-patient relationship
  a. Contract
    (1) legal obligations
    (2) consequences for noncompliance
  b. Responsibility and rights
    (1) patient
    (2) physician
    (3) medical assistant
  c. Guidelines for third-party agreements
  d. Professional liability
    (1) current standard of care
    (2) current legal standards
    (3) informed consent
  e. Arbitration agreements
  f. Affirmative defenses
    (1) statute of limitations
    (2) comparative/contributory negligence
    (3) assumption of risk
  g. Termination of medical care
    (1) establishing policy
    (2) elements for withdrawal
    (3) patient notification and documentation

II. ADMINISTRATIVE

G. Data Entry
1. Keyboard fundamentals and functions
  a. Alpha, numeric and symbol keys
  b. Spacing and margins
  c. Horizontal and vertical centering
  d. Tabulation
2. Formats
  a. Letters
  b. Memos
  c. Reports
  d. Manuscripts
  e. Envelopes
  f. Chart notes
  g. Templates
3. Proofreading
  a. Proofreader's marks
  b. Making corrections from rough draft
H. Equipment
1. Equipment operation
  a. Calculator
  b. Photocopier
  c. Computer/Word processor
  d. Fax machine
  e. Telephone services and use
    (1) multi-button telephone

(2) types of calls
(3) features
f. Scanners
2. Maintenance and repairs
  a. Contents of instruction material
  b. Routine maintenance
    (1) agreements
    (2) warranty
    (3) repair service
I. Computer Concepts
1. Computer components
  a. Terminology
  b. Central processing unit, monitor, keyboard
  c. Scanner
  d. Printers
  e. Disk drive
  f. Storage devices
  g. Operating systems
  h. Basic commands*
2. Care and maintenance of computer
  a. Main unit and components
  b. Protection/safety
  c. Maintenance agreements
  d. Support
  e. Leasing
3. Computer applications
  a. Word processing
  b. Database
  c. Spreadsheets, graphics
  d. Electronic mail
  e. Networks
  f. Multi-user/Multi-task system
  g. Security/Password
  h. Training programs
  i. Medical management software
    (1) file maintenance
    (2) new patient entry
    (3) diagnostic and procedural code entry
    (4) payment/entry transaction
    (5) electronic claims
    (6) routine billing (superbill/itemized statements to third parties/monthly statements)
    (7) report generation (monthly revenue/accounts receivable)
    (8) utilities
4. Internet services
J. Records Management
1. Needs, purposes and terminology of filing systems
  a. Basic filing systems
    (1) alphabetic
    (2) numeric
    (3) geographic
    (4) subject

*Only those computer basic command competencies that apply to this text are listed.

b. Special filing systems
   (1) color-code
   (2) tickler file
   (3) electronic data processing files
   (4) cross-reference/master file
2. Process for filing documents
3. Organization of patient's medical record
4. Filing guidelines
   a. Storing
   b. Protecting/safekeeping
   c. Transferring
   d. Retaining
   e. Purging
   f. Destroying
5. Medical records
   a. Types
      (1) problem oriented
      (2) source oriented
   b. Collecting information
   c. Making corrections
   d. Retaining and purging
      (1) statute of limitations
      (2) deceased patients
K. Screening and Processing Mail
   1. US Postal Service
      a. Regulations
      b. Classifications
      c. Types of mail services
      d. Tracing mail
      e. Recalling mail
   2. Private services
      a. Alternate delivery
      b. Fax services
   3. Postal machine/meter
   4. Processing incoming mail
   5. Preparing outgoing mail
      a. Labels
      b. Optical Character Reader guidelines
L. Scheduling and Monitoring Appointments
   1. Utilizing appointment schedules/types
      a. Stream
      b. Wave
      c. Modified wave
      d. Open booking
      e. Categorization
   2. Appointment guidelines
      a. Legal aspects
      b. New/Established patient
      c. Patient needs/preference
      d. Physician preference/habits
      e. Facilities/equipment requirements
   3. Appointment protocol
      a. Follow-up visits
         (1) routine
         (2) urgent
      b. Emergency/Acutely ill

c. Physician referrals
d. Cancellations/No-shows
e. Physician delay/unavailability
f. Outside services
g. Reminders/Recalls
   (1) appointment cards
   (2) tickler file
M. Resource Information and Community Services
   1. Services available
   2. Appropriate referrals
   3. Follow-up
   4. Patient advocate
N. Managing Physician's Professional Schedule and Travel
   1. Arranging meetings
   2. Scheduling travel
   3. Integrating meetings and travel with office schedule
      a. Matrix appointment schedule
      b. Arranging professional coverage
      c. Return schedule requirements
O. Managing the Office
   1. Maintaining the physical plant
      a. Office environment
      b. Personnel
         (1) recruiting
         (2) interviewing
         (3) hiring
         (4) evaluating performance
         (5) disciplining
         (6) terminating
         (7) documenting
      c. Facilities and equipment
         (1) maintenance and repair
         (2) safety regulations (OSHA/CDC/ADA/fire/security)
   2. Equipment and supply inventory
      a. Inventory control
      b. Storage and security
      c. Purchasing
   3. Maintaining liability coverage
      a. Types of coverage
      b. Recordkeeping
   4. Time management
      a. Establishing priorities
      b. Managing routine duties
P. Office Policies and Procedures
   1. Patient information booklet
   2. Patient education
   3. Instructions for patients with special needs
   4. Personnel manual
   5. Policy and procedures manuals/protocols
   6. Compliance plan
Q. Managing Practice Finances
   1. Bookkeeping systems

a. Demographic data
b. Day sheets, charge slips, receipts, ledgers, etc.
   (1) charges, payments and adjustments
   (2) transactions
   (3) identifying and correcting errors
c. Petty cash

2. Coding systems
   a. Types
      (1) *Current Procedure Terminology (CPT)*
      (2) *International Classification of Diseases, Clinical Modification (ICD-CM)*
      (3) *Healthcare Financing Common Procedural Coding Systems (HCPCS Level II)*
   b. Relationship between procedures and diagnostic codes

3. Third-party billing
   a. Types
      (1) capitated plans
      (2) commercial carriers
      (3) government plans (Medicare/Medicaid/TRICARE/CAMPVA)
      (4) prepaid HMO, PPO, POS
      (5) workers' compensation
   b. Processing claims
      (1) manual and electronic preparation of claims
      (2) tracing claims
      (3) sequence of filing
      (4) reconciling payments/rejections
      (5) inquiry and appeal process
   c. Applying managed care policies and procedures
      (1) referrals
      (2) precertification
      (3) contracts and fees
   d. Fee schedules
      (1) methods for establishing fees (RVS/RBRVS/DRG)
      (2) updating fee schedules

4. Accounting and banking procedures
   a. Accounts receivable
      (1) collecting/updating demographic data
      (2) billing procedures (itemization/billing cycles)
      (3) aging/controlling accounts receivable
      (4) collection procedures (analysis/office efforts/agencies/consumer protection acts)

b. Accounts payable
   (1) ordering goods and services
   (2) monitoring invoices
   (3) tracking merchandise
   (4) paying accounts
   (5) writing checks
c. Banking procedures
   (1) processing accounts receivable
   (2) preparing bank deposits
   (3) electronic banking
   (4) reconciling bank statement
   (5) maintaining financial records

5. Employee payroll
   a. Maintaining payroll records
   b. Calculating wages and taxes
   c. Preparing payroll checks and earning statements
   d. Depositing taxes
   e. Filing and mailing tax reports

III.   CLINICAL*

R. Principles of Infection Control
   3. Disposal of biohazardous material
S. Treatment Area
   3. Restocking supplies
U. Patient History Interview
   1. Components of patient history
      a. Personal data
      b. Chief complaint
      c. Past, present, family and social history
      d. Review of systems
   2. Documentation guidelines
W. Preparing and Administering Medications
   1. Pharmacology
      a. Classes of drugs
      b. Drug forms
      c. Drug action/uses
      d. Side effects/adverse reactions
      e. Emergency use
      f. Substance abuse
      g. Calculation of dosage
      h. Immunizations
   3. Prescriptions
      a. Prescription parts
      b. Safekeeping
      c. Recordkeeping
      d. Reordering
      e. Controlled substances
   4. Maintaining medication and immunization records
   5. Medication disposal
X. Emergencies
   1. Preplanned action
      a. Policies and procedures

*Only those clinical competencies that apply to this text are listed.

TABLE III-3

American Association of Medical Assistants (AAMA) Certified Medical Assistant (CMA) Examination Content Outline

		I. General					
Administrative Medical Assisting, 6ed.							
Ch	Title	A. Medical Terminology	B. A & P	C. Psychology	D. Professionalism	E. Communication	F. Medicolegal Guidelines & Requirements
1	A Career As an Administrative Medical Assistant	1a5, 2a	1, 2	1a, 1d, 2, 3a	1, 2d	2e, 3, 4a, 4b3	1b
2	The Health Care Environment: Past, Present, and Future	1a5, 1d, 2			5		
3	Medicolegal and Ethical Responsibilities	1a5, 2			3, 4		1a; 2b-2/7; 4, 5
4	The Art of Communication	1a5, 2a, b		1, 2b, 3, 4	1b	1, 2, 3a, b, 4, 5, 6b	
5	The Receptionist	1a5, 2a		3d	1, 4, 5b	3a, b, d, e, 4a, 6c1, 7a, b	3g3
6	Telephone Procedures	1a5			1, 4a2	3a, b, 4, 6a, b, c2, 7a, 8a1-10, b1-2	3g1-3, 4
7	Appointments	1a5, 7, 1e, 2b				2, 3a, 7a, 8	
8	Filing Procedures	1a5			4a2	7b	4
9	Medical Records	1a5	2a-j		4a2		2a3a, 3g
10	Drug and Prescription Records	1a5					1d, 2b3, 3b
11	Written Correspondence	1a5, 2a					
12	Processing Mail and Telecommunications	1a5				7a, b	
13	Fees, Credit, and Collection	1a5				8	
14	Banking	1a5					
15	Bookkeeping	1a5					
16	Health Insurance Systems	1a5					2a2, 2b4, 7, 3e, f
17	Office Managerial Responsibilities	1a5			1a, 5c	3a, 4a1-4, 4b1-3, 6a, c, d	2a1, 2b1, 6, 7, 3d
18	Financial Management of the Medical Practice	1a5			1, 5		3c, d
19	Seeking a Position As an Administrative Medical Assistant				1b, 2a-d, 5	1, 2, 4a1-4, 6d, 9a-d	

TABLE III-3 (*continued*)
American Association of Medical Assistants (AAMA) Certified Medical Assistant (CMA) Examination Content Outline

											III. Clinical
G. Data Entry	H. Equipment	I. Computer Concepts	J. Records Management	K. Screening and Processing Mail	L. Scheduling and Monitoring Appointments	M. Resource Information & Community Services	N. Managing Physicians' Professional Schedule and Travel	O. Managing the Office	P. Office Policies and Procedures	Q. Managing Practice Finances	R—Z Clinical
2c	1c	3a, 4						2, 3			
						2				3a-4	
									6		
	1b, c, d, e	3e, i2, i6a	1a1		3b, e	1, 5			2, 5	1b,	
	1e1-3								1, 2, 4		
	1c, e	3i-2			1, 2, 3		3a		2		
		3i1	1a, b, 2, 3, 4a-f, 5d1-2								
2f, g	1f		3, 5a, c								U1, 2
		3b									R3, S3, W1a, b, c, d, f, 3, 4, 5
1a-d, 2a, b, e		1d, f, 3a, b									
2e	1b, d	3d, g		1a-d, 2a-b, 3, 4, 5a-b							
										1b1-2, 4a1, 2, 3, 4	
	1a									4c1-5	
	1a									1a, b1-3, 4a, b5	
										2a1-3, 2b, 3a1-3, 3a4, 5, 3b1-5, 3c1-3, 3d1a-c, 2d2	
	2a, b1-3	2a-d, 3, 7					1-3	1a-c, 1c2d, e, 2a-c, 3a-b, 4a-b	1, 4, 5, 6	4b1-4	W-4, X-1
								4a3, 5a-e			
1, 2, 3	3a										

RMA CERTIFICATION EXAMINATION COMPETENCIES

The American Medical Technologists (AMT) have established (2005) competencies and construction parameters for the Registered Medical Assistant (RMA) certification examination as follows.* These are cross-referenced in a chapter-by-chapter grid (see Table III-4) to help locate them in the *Administrative Medical Assisting* textbook and *Workbook*.

I. GENERAL MEDICAL ASSISTING KNOWLEDGE

  A. Anatomy and Physiology†
   1. Body systems
    a. Skeletal
    b. Muscular
    c. Endocrine
    d. Urinary
    e. Reproductive
    f. Gastrointestinal
    g. Nervous
    h. Respiratory
    i. Cardiovascular
    j. Integumentary
    k. Special senses
  B. Medical Terminology
   1. Word parts
    a. Identify word parts: root, prefixes, and suffixes
   2. Definitions
    a. Define medical terms
   3. Common abbreviations and symbols
    a. Identify and understand utilization of medical abbreviations and symbols
   4. Spelling
    a. Spell medical terms accurately
  C. Medical Law
   1. Medical law
    a. Types of consent used in medical practice
    b. Disclosure laws and regulations
    c. Laws, regulations, and acts pertaining to the practice of medicine
    d. Scope of practice acts regarding medical assisting
    e. Patient Bill of Rights legislation
   2. Licensure, certification, and registration
    a. Identify credentialing requirements of medical professional
    b. Understand the application of the Clinical Laboratory Improvement Amendments of 1988

   3. Terminology
    a. Define terminology associated with medical law
  D. Medical Ethics
   1. Principles of medical ethics and ethical conduct
    a. Identify and employ proper ethics in practice as a medical assistant
    b. Identify the principles of ethics established by the American Medical Association
    c. Identify and understand the application of the AMA Patient Bill of Rights
    d. Recognize unethical practices and identify the proper response
    e. Recognize the importance of professional development through continuing education
  E. Human Relations
   1. Patient relations
    a. Identify age-group specific responses and support
    b. Identify and employ professional conduct in all aspects of patient care
    c. Understand and properly apply communication methods
   2. Interpersonal relations
    a. Employ appropriate interpersonal skills with:
     (1) employer/administration
     (2) co-workers
     (3) vendors
     (4) business associates
    b. Observe and respect cultural diversity in the workplace
  F. Patient Education
   1. Patient instruction
    a. Health and wellness
    b. Nutrition
    c. Hygiene
    d. Treatment and medications
    e. Pre- and post-operative care
    f. Body mechanics
    g. Personal and physical safety
   2. Patient resource materials
    a. Develop, assemble, and maintain appropriate patient brochures and informational material
   3. Documentation
    a. Understand and utilize proper documentation of patient encounters and instruction

*The competencies are reprinted with permission from the American Medical Technologists.
†Only those anatomy and physiology competencies that apply to this text are listed.

II. ADMINISTRATIVE MEDICAL ASSISTING

A. Insurance
1. Terminology
   a. Identify and define terminology associated with various insurance types in the medical office
2. Plans
   a. Identify and understand the application of medical, disability, and accident insurance plans
   b. Identify and appropriately apply plan policies and regulations for programs including
      (1) HMO, PPO, EPO, indemnity, open, etc.
      (2) short-term and long-term disability
      (3) Family Medical Leave Act (FMLA)
      (4) workers' compensation (first report/follow-up reports)
      (5) Medicare (including Advance Beneficiary Notice [ABN])
      (6) Medicaid
      (7) CHAMPUS/TRICARE
3. Claims
   a. Complete and file insurance claims
      (1) file claims for paper and Electronic Data Interchange
      (2) understand and adhere to HIPAA Security and Uniformity Regulations
   b. Evaluate claims response
      (1) understand and evaluate explanation of benefits
      (2) evaluate claims rejection and utilize proper follow-up procedures
4. Coding
   a. Identify HIPAA-mandated coding systems
      (1) *ICD-9-CM*
      (2) *CPT*
      (3) *HCPCS*
   b. Properly apply diagnosis and procedure codes to insurance claims
5. Insurance finance applications
   a. Identify and comply with contractual requirements of insurance plans
   b. Process insurance payments and contractual write-off amounts
   c. Track unpaid claims
   d. Generate aging reports
B. Financial Bookkeeping
1. Terminology
   a. Understand terminology associated with medical financial bookkeeping
2. Patient billing
   a. Maintain and explain physician's fee schedules
   b. Collect and post payments
   c. Manage patient ledgers and accounts
   d. Understand and prepare Truth in Lending Statements
   e. Prepare and mail itemized statements
   f. Understand and employ available billing methods
   g. Understand and employ billing cycles
3. Collections
   a. Prepare aging reports and identify delinquent accounts
   b. Perform skip tracing
   c. Understand application of the Fair Debt Collection Practices Act
   d. Identify and understand bankruptcy and small claims procedures
   e. Understand and perform appropriate collection procedures
4. Fundamental medical office accounting procedures
   a. Employ appropriate accounting procedures
      (1) pegboard/double entry bookkeeping
      (2) computerized
   b. Perform daily balancing procedures
   c. Prepare monthly trial balance
   d. Apply accounts receivable and payable principles
5. Banking procedures
   a. Understand and manage petty cash account
   b. Prepare and make bank deposits
   c. Maintain checking accounts
   d. Reconcile bank statements
   e. Understand check processing procedures and requirements
      (1) non-sufficient funds
      (2) endorsements
   f. Process payables and practice obligations
   g. Understand and maintain disbursement accounts
6. Employee payroll
   a. Prepare employee payroll
      (1) understand hourly and salary payroll procedures
      (2) understand and apply payroll withholding and deductions

b. Understand and maintain payroll records
    (1) prepare and maintain payroll tax deduction records
    (2) prepare employee tax forms
    (3) prepare quarterly tax forms and deposits
c. Understand terminology pertaining to payroll and payroll tax

7. Financial mathematics
   a. Understand and perform appropriate calculations related to patient and practice accounts

C. Medical Receptionist/Secretarial/Clerical
   1. Terminology
      a. Understand and correctly apply terminology associated with medical receptionist and secretarial duties
   2. Reception
      a. Employ appropriate communication skills when receiving and greeting patients
      b. Understand basic emergency triage in coordinating patient arrivals
      c. Screen visitors and sales persons arriving at the office
      d. Obtain patient demographics and information
      e. Understand and maintain patient confidentiality during check-in procedures
      f. Prepare patient record
      g. Assist patients into examination rooms
   3. Scheduling
      a. Employ appointment scheduling system
          (1) identify and employ various scheduling styles
      b. Employ proper procedures for cancellations and missed appointments
      c. Understand referral and authorization process
      d. Understand and manage patient recall system
      e. Schedule non-office appointments
   4. Oral and written communication
      a. Employ appropriate telephone etiquette
      b. Perform appropriate telephone procedures
      c. Instruct patients via telephone
      d. Inform patients of test results per physician instruction
      e. Receive, process, and document results received from outside provider
      f. Compose correspondence employing acceptable business format
      g. Employ effective written communication skills adhering to ethics and laws of confidentiality
      h. Employ active listening skills

   5. Records and chart management
      a. Manage patient medical record system
      b. Record diagnostic test results in patient chart
      c. File patient and physician communication in chart
      d. File materials according to proper system
          (1) chronological
          (2) alphabetical
          (3) problem-oriented medical records
          (4) subject
      e. Protect, store, and retain medical records according to proper conventions and HIPAA privacy regulations
      f. Prepare and release private health information as required, adhering to state and Federal guidelines
      g. Chart information
   6. Transcription and dictation
      a. Transcribe notes from dictation system
      b. Transcribe letter or notes from direct dictation
   7. Supplies and equipment management
      a. Maintain inventory of medical office supplies and equipment
      b. Coordinate maintenance and repair of office equipment
      c. Maintain equipment maintenance logs according to OSHA regulations
   8. Computer applications
      a. Identify and understand hardware components
      b. Identify and understand application of basic software and operating systems
      c. Recognize software application for patient record maintenance, bookkeeping, patient accounting system
      d. Employ procedures for integrity of information and compliance with HIPAA Security and Privacy regulations
          (1) encryption
          (2) firewall software and hardware
          (3) personnel passwords

(4)   access restrictions
(5)   activity logs
9.   Office safety
   a.   Maintain office sanitation and comfort
   b.   Develop and maintain office safety manual*
   c.   Develop emergency procedures and policies
   d.   Employ procedures in compliance with Occupational Safety and Health Administration guidelines and regulations
      (1)   hazard communication
      (2)   engineering and work practice controls
      (3)   employee training program
      (4)   standard precautions
   e.   Maintain records of biohazardous waste and chemical disposal

III.   CLINICAL MEDICAL ASSISTING†

E.   Physical Examinations
   1.   Medical history
      a.   Obtain patient history employing appropriate terminology and abbreviations
      b.   Differentiate between subjective and objective information
      c.   Understand and employ SOAP charting system for recording information
   3.   Methods of examination
      a.   Define methods of examination
         (1)   auscultation

(2)   palpation
(3)   mensuration
(4)   percussion
   b.   Understand use of each examination method
F.   Clinical Pharmacology
   3.   Prescriptions
      a.   Identify and define drug schedules and legal prescription requirements for each
      b.   Understand procedures for completing prescriptions and authorization of medical refills
      c.   Identify and perform proper documentation of medication transactions
   4.   Drugs
      a.   Identify Drug Enforcement Agency regulations for ordering, dispensing, prescribing, storing, and documenting regulated drugs
      b.   Identify and define drug categories
      c.   Identify commonly used drugs
      d.   Identify and describe routes of medication administration
         (1)   parenteral
         (2)   rectal
         (3)   topical
         (4)   vaginal
         (5)   sublingual
         (6)   oral
         (7)   inhalation
         (8)   installation
      e.   Demonstrate ability to use drug references (*Physician's Desk Reference*)

*Denotes advanced skills.
†Only those clinical competencies that apply to this text are listed.

TABLE III-4

American Medical Technologists (AMT) Competencies and Construction Parameters
for the Registered Medical Assistant (RMA) Examination

Ch	Title	I. GENERAL MEDICAL ASSISTING KNOWLEDGE						II. ADMINISTRATIVE MEDICAL ASSISTING			III. CLINICAL MEDICAL ASSISTING
	Administrative Medical Assisting, 6ed.	A. A & P	B. Medical Terminology	C. Medical Law	D. Medical Ethics	E. Human Relations	F. Patient Education	A. Insurance	B. Financial Bookkeeping	C. Medical Receptionist, Secretarial, Clerical	A.–K.
1	A Career As an Administrative Medical Assistant	1	1, 2, 3, 4	1d, 2a	1a, 1e	1b, 2a	1a-g				
2	The Health Care Environment: Past, Present, and Future		1, 2, 3, 4				1, 3	2b(1)			
3	Medicolegal and Ethical Responsibilities		1, 2, 3, 4	1a, b, c, e, 3a	1a, b, c, d		1			2e, 4g, 5f	
4	The Art of Communication		1, 2, 3, 4			1, 2				2a, 4h	
5	The Receptionist		1, 2, 3, 4			1b, c	2a, 3a			1a, 2a, b, c, d, e, f, g	
6	Telephone Procedures		1, 2, 3, 4	1b		1c	1, 3a			1a, 4a, b, c, g, h, 5g	
7	Appointments		3a			2a(3), (4)	1, 3a			1a, 3a(1), 4a, b, c	
8	Filing Procedures		1							5a-g	
9	Medical Records	1a-k	1, 3				3a			2d, 4h, 5a, c, d(1-4), e, f, g, 6a, 8d(1), (3)	E1, 3
10	Drug and Prescription Records		1, 2, 3, 4				1, 3a			5g, 6a	F3a, b, c, 4a, b, d, e
11	Written Correspondence		1, 2, 3, 4							4f, g, 6a, b, 8b	
12	Processing Mail and Telecommunications		2, 3							4f, 8d(1-3)	
13	Fees, Credit, and Collection		2, 3					5b, d	2a-g, 3a-e		
14	Banking		2, 3						2b, c, 5b-f		
15	Bookkeeping		2, 3						2a, b, 4a(1-2), b, c, d, 5a, b, 7a		
16	Health Insurance Systems		2, 3					1a, 2a, b(1-7), 3a(1-2), 3b(1-2), 4a(1-3), 4b, 5a, c		3c	
17	Office Managerial Responsibilities		2, 3	1b, c	e	2a(1-4)	2a	2b(3)	7a	7a, c, 8, 9a-e	A2, I1c
18	Financial Management of the Medical Practice		2, 3						1a, 4a, d, 5g, 6a(1-2), b(1-3), c, 7a		
19	Seeking a Position As an Administrative Medical Assistant		2			2a(1)				4f, h	

CMAS EXAMINATION SPECIFICATIONS

The American Medical Technologists (AMT) have developed (2003) competencies and examination specifications for the Certified Medical Administrative Specialist (CMAS) as follows.* These are cross referenced in a chapter-by-chapter grid (see Table III-5) to help locate them in the *Administrative Medical Assisting* textbook and *Workbook*.

I. MEDICAL ASSISTING FOUNDATIONS
A. Medical Terminology
1. Use and spell basic medical terms appropriately
2. Identify root words, prefixes, and suffixes
3. Define basic medical terms
B. Anatomy and Physiology
1. Know basic structures and functions of body systems
2. Know various disorders of the body
C. Legal and Ethical Considerations
1. Apply principles of medical law and ethics to the health care setting
2. Recognize legal responsibilities of, and know scope of practice for the medical administrative specialist
3. Know basic laws pertaining to medical practice
4. Know and observe disclosure laws
5. Know the principles of medical ethics established by the AMA
6. Recognize unethical practices and identify ethical responses for situations in the medical office
D. Professionalism
1. Employ human relations skills appropriate to the health care setting
2. Display behaviors of a professional medical administrative specialist
3. Participate in appropriate continuing education

II. BASIC CLINICAL MEDICAL OFFICE ASSISTING
A. Basic Health History Interview
1. Obtain preliminary health histories from patients
B. Basic Charting
1. Chart patient information
C. Vital Signs and Measurements
1. Measure vital signs
2. Obtain other vital measurements (weight, height)
D. Asepsis in the medical office
1. Understand concepts of asepsis, sanitization, disinfection, and sterilization
2. Understand prevention of disease transmission
3. Observe standard precautions
E. Examination Preparation
1. Prepare patients for clinical examinations
F. Medical Office Emergencies
1. Recognize and respond to medical emergencies
2. Employ first aid and CPR appropriately
3. Report emergencies as required by law
G. Pharmacology
1. Understand basic pharmacological concepts and terminology

III. MEDICAL OFFICE CLERICAL ASSISTING
A. Appointment Management and Scheduling
1. Schedule and monitor patient and visitor appointments
2. Address cancellations and missed appointments
3. Prepare information for referrals and preauthorizations
4. Arrange hospital admissions and surgery, and schedule patients for out-patient diagnostic tests
5. Manage recall system and file
B. Reception
1. Receive and process patients and visitors
2. Screen visitors and vendors requesting to see physician
3. Coordinate patient flow into examining rooms
C. Communication
1. Employ effective written and oral communication
2. Address and process incoming telephone calls from outside providers, pharmacies, and vendors
3. Employ appropriate telephone etiquette when screening patient calls and addressing office business
4. Recognize and employ proper protocols for telephone emergencies
5. Format business documents and correspondence appropriately

*The competencies are reprinted with permission from the American Medical Technologists.

6. Process incoming and outgoing mail

D. Patient Information and Community Resources
   1. Order and organize patient informational materials
   2. Maintain list of community referral resources

IV. MEDICAL RECORDS MANAGEMENT

A. Systems
   1. Demonstrate knowledge of and manage patient medical records systems
   2. Manage documents and patient charts using paper methods
   3. Manage documents and patient charts using computerized methods

B. Procedures
   1. File records alphabetically, numerically, by subject, and by color
   2. Employ rules of indexing
   3. Arrange contents of patient charts in appropriate order
   4. Document and file laboratory results and patient communication in charts
   5. Perform corrections and additions to records
   6. Store, protect, retain, and destroy records appropriately
   7. Transfer files
   8. Perform daily chart management
   9. Prepare charts for external review and audits

C. Confidentiality
   1. Observe and maintain confidentiality of records, charts, and test results
   2. Observe special regulations regarding the confidentiality of protected information

V. HEALTH CARE INSURANCE PROCESSING, CODING, AND BILLING

A. Insurance Processing
   1. Understand private/commercial health care insurance plans (PPO, HMO, traditional indemnity)
   2. Understand government health care insurance plans (Medicare, Medicaid, Veteran's Administration, CHAMPUS, TRICARE, use of Advance Beneficiary Notices)
   3. Process patient claims using appropriate forms and time frames
   4. Process workers' compensation/disability reports and forms
   5. Submit claims for third-party reimbursements including the use of electronic transmission methods

B. Coding
   1. Understand procedure and diagnosis coding
   2. Employ *Current Procedural Terminology* (*CPT*) and Evaluation and Management codes appropriately
   3. Employ *International Classification of Diagnostic* (*ICD-9-CM*) codes appropriately
   4. Employ *Health Care Financing Administration Common Procedure Coding System* (*HCPCS*) codes appropriately

C. Insurance Billing and Finances
   1. Understand health care insurance terminology
   2. Understand billing requirements for health care insurance plans
   3. Process insurance payments
   4. Track unpaid claims and file and track appeals
   5. Understand fraud and abuse regulations

VI. MEDICAL OFFICE FINANCIAL MANAGEMENT

A. Fundamental Financial Management
   1. Understand basic principles of accounting
   2. Perform bookkeeping procedures including balancing accounts
   3. Perform financial computations
   4. Manage accounts payable
   5. Manage accounts receivable
   6. Prepare monthly trial balance reports
   7. Understand basic audit controls
   8. Understand professional fee structures
   9. Understand physician/practice owner compensation provisions
   10. Understand credit arrangements
   11. Manage other financial aspects of office management

B. Patient Accounts
   1. Manage patient accounts/ledgers
   2. Manage patient billing
   3. Manage collections in compliance with state and federal regulations

C. Banking
   1. Understand banking services and procedures
   2. Manage petty cash

D. Payroll
1. Prepare employee payroll and reports
2. Maintain payroll tax deduction procedures and records

VII. MEDICAL OFFICE INFORMATION PROCESSING
A. Fundamentals of Computing
1. Possess fundamental knowledge of computing in the medical office including keyboarding, data entry, and retrieval
2. Possess fundamental knowledge of PC-based environment
3. Possess fundamental knowledge of word processing, spreadsheet, database, and presentation graphics applications
4. Employ procedures for ensuring the integrity and confidence of computer-stored information
B. Medical Office Computer Applications
1. Employ medical office software applications
2. Use computer for billing and financial transactions
3. Employ e-mail applications

VIII. MEDICAL OFFICE MANAGEMENT
A. Office Communications*
1. Facilitate staff meetings and in-service, and ensure communication of essential information to staff
B. Business Organization Management*
1. Manage medical office business functions
2. Manage office mailing and shipping services

3. Manage outside vendors and supplies
4. Manage contracts and relationships with associated health care providers
5. Comply with licensure and accreditation requirements
C. Human Resources*
1. Manage/supervise medical office staff
2. Conduct performance reviews and disciplinary action
3. Maintain office policy manual
4. Manage staff payroll and scheduling
5. Manage staff recruiting in compliance with state and federal laws
6. Orient and train new staff
7. Manage employee benefits
D. Safety
1. Maintain office safety, maintain office safety manual, and post emergency instructions
2. Observe emergency safety requirements
3. Maintain records of biohazardous waste, hazardous chemicals, and safety conditions
4. Comply with Occupational Safety and Health Act guidelines and regulations
E. Supplies and Equipment
1. Manage medical and office supply inventories and order supplies
2. Maintain office equipment and arrange for equipment maintenance and repair
F. Physical Office Plant
1. Maintain office facilities and environment
G. Risk Management and Quality Assurance
1. Understand and employ risk management and quality assurance concepts

---

*Job functions may or may not be entry-level; however, the competent specialist should have sound knowledge of these management functions at certification level.

TABLE III-5
American Medical Technologists (AMT) Competencies and Examination Specifications
for the Certified Medical Administrative Specialist (CMAS) Examination

*Administrative Medical
Assisting, 6ed.*

Ch	Title	I. Medical Assisting Foundation	II. Basic Clinical Medical Office Assisting	III. Medical Office Clerical Assisting	IV. Medical Records Management	V. Health Care Insurance Processing, Coding, and Billing	VI. Medical Office Financial Management	VII. Medical Office Information Processing	VIII. Medical Office Management
1	A Career As an Administrative Medical Assistant	A, B1, D1, 2, 3	B-1	D2				A1, A2	B-5
2	The Health Care Environment: Past, Present, and Future	A1, 3	C-2	A3		A1			
3	Medicolegal and Ethical Responsibilities	A1, 3, C1, 3, 4, 5, 6			C-2				G-1
4	The Art of Communication	A1, 3, D1, 4		C1					
5	The Receptionist	A1, 3, C4, D1, 2	A1, F1	B, D	B8, C			A4, B3	D2, 3, F1
6	Telephone Procedures	A1, D1	B, F1	C1, 3, 4	A2, C1				
7	Appointments	A1, D1	B1, F1	A1, 2, 3, 4, 5, B2-3, C3	A2			B1	
8	Filing Procedures				A1-3, B1-4, 6-8, C1-2				
9	Medical Records	A1, B1-2	A1, B1		A1-3. B3, 5, 9, C1			A4	
10	Drug and Prescription Records	A1	B1, G1		A2, 3, B8				
11	Written Correspondence	A1	C1, 5					A1, 2, 3, B1	
12	Processing Mail and Telecommunications	A1		C1, 6	C2			A4, B1, 3	B2
13	Fees, Credit, and Collection	A1					A5, 8, 10, B1-3		
14	Banking	A1					A3-5, B1, C1		
15	Bookkeeping	A1					A1-7, B1, C2	B1, 2	
16	Health Insurance Systems	A1				A1-5, B1-4, C1-4			
17	Office Managerial Responsibilities	A1, D3	D2, F	D1					A1, B1-3, C1-3, 6, 7, D1-7, E1-2, F1
18	Financial Management of the Medical Practice	A1					A1, 3, 4, C1, D1, 2		
19	Seeking a Position As an Administrative Medical Assistant	A1, D2		C1, 5				A2	C2

AAMA ROLE DELINEATION STUDY

Competencies required to practice medical assisting were first described in the American Association of Medical Assistants' 1979 DACUM (**D**eveloping **A** Cur-ricul**UM**). In 1996 and 1997 the AAMA began to do a major occupational analysis of the practice of medical assisting, titled the Role Delineation Study (2003). Content of the information from the study was categorized into the following areas of competency for entry-level medical assistants. These are cross-referenced in a chapter-by-chapter grid (see Table III-6) to help locate them in the *Administrative Medical Assisting* text-book and *Workbook*.

In addition, the books meet the requirements and standards set forth by the National Health Care Skill Standards Project for multiskilling and multitasking for the Information Services Cluster for the occupation of medical assisting.

I. ADMINISTRATIVE

A. Administrative Procedures
1. Perform basic administrative medical assisting functions
2. Schedule, coordinate and monitor appointments
3. Schedule inpatient/outpatient admissions and procedures
4. Understand and apply third-party guidelines
5. Obtain reimbursement through accurate claims submission
6. Monitor third-party reimbursement
7. Understand and adhere to managed care policies and procedures
8. Negotiate managed care contracts*

B. Practice Finances
1. Perform procedural and diagnostic coding
2. Apply bookkeeping principles
3. Manage accounts receivable
4. Manage accounts payable*
5. Process payroll*
6. Document and maintain accounting and banking records*
7. Develop and maintain fee schedules*
8. Manage renewals of business and professional insurance policies*
9. Manage personnel benefits and maintain records*
10. Perform marketing, financial, and strategic planning*

III. CLINICAL†

C. Patient Care
7. Maintain medication and immunization records
8. Recognize and respond to emergencies
9. Coordinate patient care information with other health care providers

III. GENERAL

A. Professionalism
1. Display a professional manner and image
2. Demonstrate initiative and responsibility
3. Work as a member of the health care team
4. Prioritize and perform multiple tasks
5. Adapt to change
6. Promote the CMA credential
7. Enhance skills through continuing education
8. Treat all patients with compassion and empathy
9. Promote and practice through positive public relations

B. Communication Skills
1. Recognize and respect cultural diversity
2. Adapt communications to individual's ability to understand
3. Use a professional telephone technique
4. Recognize and respond effectively to verbal, nonverbal, and written communications
5. Use medical terminology appropriately
6. Utilize electronic technology to receive, organize, prioritize and transmit information
7. Serve as liaison

C. Legal Concepts
1. Perform within legal and ethical boundaries
2. Prepare and maintain medical records
3. Document accurately
4. Follow employer's established policies dealing with the health care contract
5. Implement and maintain federal and state health care legislation and regulations
6. Comply with established risk management and safety procedures
7. Recognize professional credentialing criteria
8. Develop and maintain personnel, policy and procedure manuals

*Denotes advanced skills.
†Only those clinical competencies that apply to this text are listed.

D. Instruction
1. Instruct individuals according to their needs
2. Explain office policies and procedures
3. Teach methods of health promotion and disease prevention
4. Locate community resources and disseminate information
5. Develop educational materials*
6. Conduct continuing education activities*

E. Operational Functions

1. Perform inventory of supplies and equipment
2. Perform routine maintenance of administrative and clinical equipment
3. Apply computer techniques to support office operations
4. Perform personnel management functions*
5. Negotiate leases and prices for equipment and supply contracts*

*Denotes advanced skills.

TABLE III-6
American Association of Medical Assistants (AAMA) Role Delineation Study
Developed to provide a current analysis of the profession in the workplace (updated 2002)

Administrative Medical Assisting, 6ed.		I. Administrative		II. Clinical	III. General				
Ch	Title	A. Administrative Procedures	B. Practice Finances	A. B. C. Clinical	A. Professionalism	B. Communication Skills	C. Legal Concepts	D. Instruction	E. Operational Functions
1	A Career As an Administrative Medical Assistant	1		C1-9	1, 2, 4, 5, 6, 7, 8, 9	2, 5, 7	1, 7	1, 2, 3, 4	
2	The Health Care Environment: Past, Present, and Future	1, 7			3	5	3	1	
3	Medicolegal and Ethical Responsibilities	1				5	1, 5, 6	1	
4	The Art of Communication	1			4, 8, 9	1, 2, 4, 5, 7	4	4	
5	The Receptionist	1, 7		C8	1, 3, 4, 5, 8, 9	5, 6, 7	2, 4, 5, 6	2, 3, 4	
6	Telephone Procedures	1		C8	4, 8, 9	2, 3, 4, 5, 6	2, 3	1, 2	
7	Appointments	1, 2, 3		C8, 9		3, 5, 6, 7	2, 3	1, 2	
8	Filing Procedures	1				5, 6	2, 3		
9	Medical Records	1		C2, 7		5, 6	2, 3		3
10	Drug and Prescription Records	1		C7		5, 6	1, 2, 3, 6, 7	1, 2	1
11	Written Correspondence	1				4, 5			
12	Processing Mail and Telecommunications	1				4, 5, 6			3
13	Fees, Credit, and Collection	1	2, 3, 7			5			3
14	Banking	1	2, 3, 4, 6						
15	Bookkeeping	1	2, 3, 4, 7						3
16	Health Insurance Systems	1, 4, 5, 6, 7	1			6			
17	Office Managerial Responsibilities	1	8, 9, 10	C7	1, 2, 3, 7, 9	1, 5, 6, 7	1, 5, 8	1, 2, 5, 6	1, 2, 4, 5
18	Financial Management of the Medical Practice	1, 8	2, 4, 5, 6		1, 3, 4	5, 7	1, 5		3, 4
19	Seeking a Position As an Administrative Medical Assistant	1			1, 2, 3, 9	2, 4, 5, 6			3

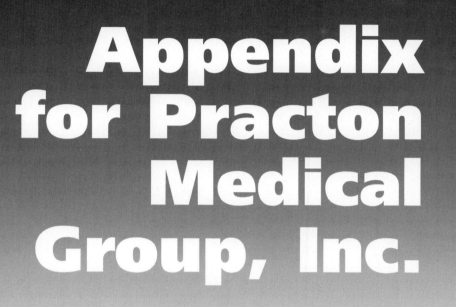

Appendix
for Practon
Medical
Group, Inc.

- **Introduction**
- **Medical Practice Reference Material**
- **Office Policies**
- **Payment Policies and Health Insurance Protocol**
- **Fee Schedule**
- ***CPT* Modifiers**
- ***HCPCS Level II* Codes**

INTRODUCTION

To gain practical experience and put theory to work, assume that you have been hired to work as an administrative medical assistant for a husband-and-wife team; Dr. Fran T. Practon is a family practitioner (FP) and Dr. Gerald M. Practon is a general practitioner (GP). Their practice is called Practon Medical Group, Inc., and they are on the staff of College Hospital. You will be presented with realistic scenarios and will perform tasks in the *Workbook* Job Skills as if you were employed in their office. Use this reference material for data required in the assignments.

MEDICAL PRACTICE REFERENCE MATERIAL

Practon Medical Group, Inc.
4567 Broad Avenue
Woodland Hills, XY 12345-4700
Telephone Number: (555) 486-9002
Fax Number: (555) 488-7815
Group National Provider Identification Number (NPI):
    36640210XX
Group Tax Identification Number (EIN): 20-8765432
Medicare Durable Medical Equipment (DME) Supplier
    Number: 33420985XX

Fran T. Practon, MD
State License Number: C 1503X
National Provider Identification (NPI) Number:
    65499947XX
Federal Tax Identification Number (EIN): 73-40313XX

Gerald M. Practon, MD
State License Number: C 1402X
National Provider Identification (NPI) Number:
    46278897XX
Federal Tax Identification Number: 78-51342XX

College Hospital
4500 Broad Avenue
Woodland Hills, XY 12345-4700
Telephone Number: (555) 487-6789
Fax Number: (555) 487-6790
Hospital National Provider Identification Number:
    54378601XX

OFFICE POLICIES

The office policies set by Drs. Fran and Gerald Practon appear on the next several pages. Refer to them for daily routine, office appointment scheduling, telephone procedures, and filing practices as you complete the *Workbook* Job Skills. Account information is also included to help determine fees and office policies regarding charges.

Daily Routine

Both physicians prefer that the medical assistant call the answering service for messages right after the office is opened and office machines turned on. Incoming mail should be opened and sorted when it arrives. Correspondence is to be mailed the same day it is dictated. Chart notes are to be placed in each patient's medical record as soon as possible after the dictation is received, typically within 72 hours.

Office Hours

Office hours are 9:00 a.m. to 5:00 p.m. Monday through Friday. The lunch hour is from 12:00 noon to 1:00 p.m. Both physicians leave the office at 3:00 p.m. on Wednesdays and reserve one morning each week for surgery and additional hospital responsibilities; Gerald reserves Tuesday mornings and Fran Thursday mornings. Each physician covers the office while the other is at the hospital. No elective appointments are scheduled between 11:30 a.m. and noon or between 4:30 p.m. and 5:00 p.m. to allow time for call-backs, work-ins, emergencies, and dictation. An asterisk (*) distinguishes Fran's patients from Gerald's when physician verification is necessary. Record office hours information on a 3″ by 5″ card for easy reference.

Appointments

Both physicians work by appointment. New patients receiving a complete physical examination or consultation are scheduled for one hour. Routine follow-up appointments for established patients are scheduled for half an hour. Brief office visits for services such as suture removals, cast checks, dressing changes, injections, and blood pressure checks are scheduled for 15-minute appointments. Appointments should be scheduled at the earliest time available and consecutively when possible. Check with the physician regarding time frames for office procedures and hospital surgeries. House calls are discouraged but, if necessary, are made after 5:00 p.m.

Patients should be specific in outlining the nature of their medical problem so appropriate time is allowed. If multiple problems exist and are made known by the patient, additional time will be allotted. There is no charge if appointments are cancelled 24 hours in advance; uncancelled appointments are billed at one-half the usual fee. Record appointment information on the back of the office hours 3″ by 5″ card for easy reference.

Telephone Calls

The medical assistant answers most inquiries so the physicians need not leave patients during examinations to answer the telephone. When a medical emergency arises or a telephone call is received from another physician, it may be necessary to knock on the door of the treatment room and advise the physician of the urgency of the telephone call or ask the physician if he or she wishes to take the call. When the assistant is unable to give a complete answer to a question asked via telephone, the physician is consulted and typically reviews the chart and either calls back the same day or has a member of the staff make the call-back. Routine calls that the physicians personally return are made after 11:30 a.m., during the lunch hour, or after 4:30 p.m. Generally, there is no charge for telephone calls.

Filing

The Patient Information (registration) form is stapled to the left inside area of the file folder. Correspondence in reference to a patient is filed under the patient's name. Folders are filed alphabetically according to rules established by the Association of Records Managers and Administrators (ARMA), and material is filed chronologically within each section of the file folder. Sections include (starting from the front of the chart):

> Progress notes
> Consultations
> Operative reports
> Laboratory test reports
> Radiology reports

In lieu of file folder dividers, sections may be indicated with a colored sheet of paper, titled according to the section. The history and physical report, as well as the discharge summary are filed along with the operative report for the patient's hospital encounter.

History and physical reports for new patients or yearly examinations and progress notes for established patients are filed under Progress Notes in the right portion of the file folder in chronological order. Ledger cards are kept alphabetically in a special file container; however in our mock situation, place them in front of the patient's file folder behind the Patient Information form.

PAYMENT POLICIES AND HEALTH INSURANCE PROTOCOL

After a patient is seen, the fee is determined by referring to the *CPT** code listing and the correct column in the fee schedule. The fee is posted to the patient's led-

ger card and entered on the daily journal (daysheet). All monies received by mail are posted in the same manner on the day they arrive. The first statement is given to the patient at the time of service or sent shortly thereafter. Successive statements are sent every 30 days according to a schedule set by the first date of service.

Noninsured patients are expected to pay at the time of service. Professional discounts are not typically allowed; however, uninsured or cash patients who pay the entire bill in cash at the time of service are allowed a 20% discount. If either physician treats an uninsured physician, a professional discount or no charge is considered. Financial hardship cases are reviewed case by case.

Patients who have health insurance coverage are expected to pay copayments prior to services being rendered. Insured patients are responsible for the total amount of the bill at the time services are rendered and will receive regular statements after the date of service; however, their insurance company is billed by Practon Medical Group, Inc., and patients can wait until the insurance company pays their portion before paying the coinsurance amount. If the insurance payment is delayed, the patient is responsible for paying the bill and contacting the insurance company to help resolve the problem.

When coding insurance claims, use codes from a Standard Code Set, which has been developed by the Centers for Medicare and Medicaid Services (CMS), formerly known as the Health Care Financing Administration (HCFA). Codes in this standard that apply to billing outpatient medical claims include:

- *International Classification of Diseases—9th Revision—Clinical Modification (ICD-9-CM)* [diagnostic codes]
- *Current Procedural Terminology (CPT)** [also referred to as *HCPCS* Level I codes for procedures and services]
- *Healthcare Common Procedure Coding System (HCPCS)* [*HCPCS Level II* codes]

When coding diagnoses using *ICD-9-CM*, refer to the following example, which illustrates how to locate a code by the main term found in the diagnostic statement.

Note: To identify the main term, ask, "What is wrong with the patient?" The additional term may state *where* the problem is (anatomic site), the *time frame* in which

Example of Main Terms			
Diagnostic Statement	Main Term	Code Selection*	Additional Term
muscle atrophy	atrophy	728.2	muscle—where
chronic bronchitis	bronchitis	491.9	chronic—time frame
allergic conjunctivitis	conjunctivitis	372.14	allergic—type
recurrent depression	depression	296.30	recurrent—time frame
nasal (bone) fracture	fracture	802.0	nasal—where

the patient is experiencing the problem (e.g., acute, subacute, chronic), or further define the *type* of problem (e.g., *alcoholic* liver disease).

For information regarding filing health insurance claim forms, refer to Chapter 16 and the CMS-1500 Field-by-Field Instructions in the textbook Appendix A. Both physicians bill using their group national provider identification number (see Field 33), not independently.

FEE SCHEDULE

Figure IV-1 is the fee schedule for Practon Medical Group, Inc. Fees are listed numerically according to *CPT** code number as found in the codebook. Sections of the codebook and subsections of the Surgery Section are included for easy reference. All fees listed are examples only. Fees can vary according to the region of the United States (West, Midwest, South, and East), the type of community (urban, suburban, or rural), the type of practice (solo, group, and so forth), and the specialty of the practitioner, as well as the practice overhead, expense, and a number of other factors.

The seven columns in the fee schedule are as follows:

- **Column 1 (*CPT* Code Number)** lists selected code numbers from 2007 *Current Procedural Terminology.**
- **Column 2 (*CPT* Code Description)** contains abbreviated descriptions of procedures and services.

- **Column 3 (Mock Fee)** shows the physician's standard fees. These are used to bill private patients as well as those on Medicaid, TRICARE, and workers' compensation.
- **Column 4 (Medicare—Participating)** lists the allowed amounts Medicare approves for a physician with a contract. Medicare pays 80%, the patient pays 20%, and the difference between the allowed amount and the charged amount is written off the books as a courtesy adjustment.
- **Column 5 (Medicare—Nonparticipating)** shows the allowed amounts Medicare approves for non-contracted physicians. Medicare pays 80%, and 20% is collected from the patient (see comments under Limiting Charge).
- **Column 6 (Limiting Charge)** lists the highest amounts that a nonparticipating physician is allowed to bill for the service rendered. In addition to the 20% collected from the nonparticipating physician's allowed amount, the noncontracted physician can also collect the difference between the nonparticipating fee (charged amount) and the limiting charge from the patient.
- **Column 7 (Follow-Up Days)** lists the number of follow-up days included in a surgical package.

Drs. Gerald and Fran Practon are both contracted with Medicare and use the participating fee unless otherwise stated.

Figure IV-1 Fee schedule for Practon Medical Group, Inc., for reference when doing the *Workbook* Job Skills.

FRAN T. PRACTON, M.D.	GERALD M. PRACTON, M.D.
Family Practice	General Practice

Practon Medical Group, Inc.
4567 Broad Avenue
Woodland Hills, XY 12345-4700

FEE SCHEDULE

		Medicare		
CPT Code No. and Description	Mock Fees	Participating	Nonparticipating	Limiting Charge
EVALUATION AND MANAGEMENT*				
OFFICE New Patient				
99201 Level I	33.25	30.43	28.91	33.25
99202 Level II	51.91	47.52	45.14	51.91
99203 Level III	70.92	64.92	61.67	70.92
99204 Level IV	106.11	97.13	92.27	106.11
99205 Level V	132.28	121.08	115.03	132.38
Established Patient				
99211 Level I	16.07	14.70	13.97	16.07
99212 Level II	28.55	26.14	24.83	28.55
99213 Level III	40.20	36.80	34.96	40.20
99214 Level IV	61.51	56.31	53.49	61.51
99215 Level V	96.97	88.76	84.32	96.97
HOSPITAL Observation Services (new or est pt)				
99217 Discharge	66.88	61.22	58.16	66.88
99218 D hx/exam SF/LC DM	74.22	67.91	64.54	74.22
99219 C hx/exam MC DM	117.75	107.78	102.39	117.75
99220 C hx/exam HC DM	147.48	134.99	128.24	147.48
Initial Hospital Care (new or est pt)				
99221 30 MIN	73.00	66.82	63.48	73.00
99222 50 MIN	120.80	110.57	105.04	120.80
99223 70 MIN	152.98	140.03	133.03	152.98
Subsequent Hospital Care				
99231 15 min	37.74	34.55	32.82	37.74
99232 25 min	55.56	50.85	48.31	55.56
99233 35 min	76.97	70.45	66.93	76.97
99238 Discharge	65.26	59.74	56.75	65.26
CONSULTATIONS office (new or est pt)				
99241 Level I	51.93	47.54	45.16	51.93
99242 Level II	80.24	73.44	69.77	80.24
99243 Level III	103.51	94.75	90.01	103.51
99244 Level IV	145.05	132.77	126.13	145.05
99245 Level V	195.48	178.93	169.98	195.48
Inpatient (new/est pt)				
99251 Level I	53.29	48.78	46.34	53.29
99252 Level II	80.56	73.74	70.05	80.56
99253 Level III	106.10	97.12	92.26	106.10
99254 Level IV	145.26	132.96	126.31	145.26
99255 Level V	196.55	179.91	170.91	196.55

*See Tables 16-5 and 16-6 in the textbook for more descriptions on E/M codes 99201 through 99255.

Figure IV-1 Fee schedule (*continued*)

CPT Code No. and Description		Mock Fees	Medicare		
			Participating	Nonparticipating	Limiting Charge
EMERGENCY DEPARTMENT (new/est pt)					
99281	PF hx/exam SF DM	24.32	22.26	21.15	24.32
99282	EPF hx/exam LC DM	37.02	33.88	32.19	37.02
99283	EPF hx/exam MC DM	66.23	60.62	57.59	66.23
99284	D hx/exam MC DM	100.71	92.18	87.57	100.71
99285	C hx/exam HC DM	158.86	145.41	138.14	158.86
CRITICAL CARE SERVICES					
99291	First hour	208.91	191.22	181.66	208.91
99292	Each addl. 30 min	102.02	92.46	87.84	102.02
NEONATAL INTENSIVE CARE					
99295	Initial	892.74	817.16	776.30	892.74
99296	Subsequent	418.73	383.27	364.11	418.73
NURSING FACILITY (initial new/est pt)					
99304	D/C hx/exam SF/LC DM	64.11	58.68	55.75	64.11
99305	C hx/exam MC DM	90.55	82.88	78.74	90.55
99306	C hx/exam HC DM	136.76	125.18	118.92	136.76
Subsequent (new/est pt)					
99307	PF hx/exam SF DM	37.95	34.74	33.00	37.95
99308	EPF hx/exam LC DM	55.11	50.44	47.92	55.11
99309	D hx/exam MC DM	69.61	63.72	60.53	69.61
99310	C hx/exam HC DM	83.12	77.11	74.88	83.12
DOMICILIARY, REST HOME, CUSTODIAL CARE New patient					
99324	PF hx/exam SF DM	46.10	42.20	40.09	46.10
99325	EPF hx/exam LC DM	65.02	59.52	56.54	65.02
99326	D hx/exam MC DM	86.18	78.88	74.94	86.18
99327	C hx/exam MC DM	105.77	113.54	109.40	105.77
99328	C hx/exam HC DM	123.98	131.06	127.62	123.98
Established patient					
99334	PF hx/exam SF DM	37.31	34.15	32.44	37.31
99335	EPF hx/exam LC DM	49.22	45.05	42.80	49.22
99336	D hx/exam MC DM	60.61	55.47	52.70	60.61
99337	C hx/exam MC/HC DM	72.03	77.65	74.12	72.03
HOME SERVICES New patient					
99341	PF hx/exam SF DM	70.32	64.37	61.15	70.32
99342	EPF hx/exam LC DM	91.85	84.07	79.87	91.85
99343	D hx/exam MC DM	120.24	110.06	104.56	120.24
Established patient					
99347	PF hx/exam SF DM	54.83	50.19	47.68	54.83
99348	EPF hx/exam LC DM	70.06	64.13	60.92	70.06
99349	D hx/exam MC DM	88.33	80.85	76.81	88.33
PROLONGED SERVICES WITH CONTACT Outpatient					
99354	First hour	96.67	88.76	84.32	96.97
99355	Each addl. 30 min	96.97	88.76	84.32	96.97
Inpatient					
99356	First hour	96.42	88.25	83.84	96.42
99357	Each addl. 30 min	96.42	88.25	83.84	96.42
PROLONGED SERVICES WITHOUT DIRECT CONTACT					
99358	First hour	90.00			
99359	Each addl. 30 min	90.00			

(*continues*)

Figure IV-1 Fee schedule (*continued*)

CPT Code No. and Description	Mock Fees	Medicare* Participating	Nonparticipating	Limiting Charge
PHYSICIAN STANDBY SERVICE				
99360 Each 30 min	95.00			
CASE MANAGEMENT SERVICES				
Team Conferences				
99361 30 min	85.00			
99362 60 min	105.00			
Telephone Calls				
99371 Simple or brief	30.00			
99372 Intermediate	40.00			
99373 Complex	60.00			
CARE PLAN OVERSIGHT SERVICES				
99374 15–29 min	93.40	85.49	81.22	93.40
99375 Greater than 30 min	118.00			
PREVENTIVE MEDICINE New Patient				
99381 Infant under age 1 year	50.00			
99382 1–4 years	50.00			
99383 5–11 years	45.00			
99384 12–17 years	45.00			
99385 18–39 years	50.00			
99386 40–64	50.00			
99387 65 yrs and over	55.00			
Established Patient				
99391 Infant under age 1 year	35.00			
99392 1–4 years	35.00			
99393 5–11 years	30.00			
99394 12–17 years	30.00			
99395 18–39 years	35.00			
99396 40–64 years	35.00			
99397 65 yrs & over	40.00			
COUNSELING (new/est pt)				
Individual—Preventive				
99401 15 min	35.00			
99402 30 min	50.00			
99403 45 min	65.00			
99404 60 min	80.00			
Group—Preventive				
99411 30 min	30.00			
99412 60 min	50.00			
Other Preventive Medicine Services				
99420 Health hazard appraisal	50.00			
99429 Unlisted preventive med serv	variable			
NEWBORN CARE				
99431 Hosp. & birthing room delivery	102.15	93.50	88.83	102.15
99432 Other than hosp. or birthing room	110.16	100.83	95.79	110.16
99433 Subsequent hospital care	54.02	49.44	46.97	54.02
99345 History & exam; discharge same day	240.55	220.18	209.17	240.55
99440 Newborn resuscitation	255.98	234.30	222.59	255.98

*Some services and procedures may not be considered a benefit under the Medicare program, and when listed on a claim form, no reimbursement may be received. However, it is important to include these codes when billing because Medicare policies may change without an individual knowing of a new benefit. For this reason, some of the services shown in this mock fee schedule do not have any amounts listed under the three Medicare columns.

Figure IV-1 Fee schedule (*continued*)

CPT Code No. and Description	Mock Fees	Medicare* Participating	Nonparticipating	Limiting Charge

ANESTHESIOLOGY

Anesthesiology fees are presented here for *CPT* codes. However, each case would require unit values indicating time, e.g., every 15 minutes would be worth $55. Some anesthetists may list a surgical code with modifier indicating anesthesiologist for carriers that do not acknowledge anesthesia codes.

QUALIFYING CIRCUMSTANCES

99100 Anes for pt under 1 yr/over 70	55.00	
99116 Anes complicated by use of total hypothermia	275.00	
99135 Anes complicated by use of hypotension	275.00	
99140 Anes complicated by emer cond	110.00	

PHYSICAL STATUS MODIFIER CODES

P-1 Normal healthy patient	variable	
P-2 Patient with mild systemic disease	variable	
P-3 Patient with severe systemic disease	55.00	
P-4 Patient with severe systemic disease (constant threat to life)	110.00	
P-5 Moribund pt not expected to survive for 24 hr without operation	165.00	
P-6 Declared brain-dead pt. organs being removed for donor	variable	

HEAD

00160 Anes for proc nose & accessory sinuses: NOS	275.00	
00172 Anes repair cleft palate	165.00	

THORAX

00400 Anes for proc integumentary system extremities, ant. trunk, and perineum	165.00	
00402 Anes breast reconstruction	275.00	
00546 Anes pulmonary resection with thoracoplasty	275.00	

SPINE & SPINAL CORD

00600 Anes cervical spine and cord	550.00	

LOWER ABDOMEN

00800 Anes for proc lower ant abdominal wall	165.00	
00840 Anes intraperitoneal proc lower abdomen: NOS	330.00	
00842 Amniocentesis	220.00	

PERINEUM

00914 Anes TURP	275.00	
00942 Anes colporrhaphy, colpotomy, vaginectomy	220.00	

UPPER LEG

01210 Anes open proc hip joint: NOS	330.00	
01214 Total hip replacement	440.00	

UPPER ARM AND ELBOW

01740 Anes open/arthroscopic proc elbow; NOS	220.00	
01758 Exc cyst/tumor humerus	275.00	

RADIOLOGIC PROCEDURES

01922 Anes noninvasive imaging/rad. therapy	385.00	

(continues)

*Some services and procedures may not be considered a benefit under the Medicare program, and when listed on a claim form, no reimbursement may be received. However, it is important to include these codes when billing because Medicare policies may change without an individual knowing of a new benefit. For this reason, some of the services shown in this mock fee schedule do not have any amounts listed under the three Medicare columns.

Figure IV-1 Fee schedule (*continued*)

CPT Code No. and Description	Mock Fees	Medicare Participating	Non-participating	Limiting Charge	Follow-Up Days[1]
INTEGUMENTARY SYSTEM					
10060 I & D furuncle, cyst, paronychia; single	75.92	69.49	66.02	75.92	10
11040 Debridement; skin, partial thickness	79.32	75.60	68.97	79.32	0
11044 Debridement; skin, subcu. muscle, bone	269.28	246.48	234.16	269.28	10
11100 Biopsy of skin, SC tissue &/or mucous membrane; 1 lesion	65.43	59.89	56.90	65.43	0
11200 Exc. skin tags; up to 15	55.68	50.97	48.42	55.68	10
11401 Exc. benign lesion, 0.6–1.0 cm trunk, arms, legs	95.62	87.53	83.15	96.62	10
11402 1.1–2.0 cm	121.52	111.23	105.67	121.52	10
11403 2.1–3.0 cm	151.82	138.97	132.02	151.82	10
11420 Exc. benign lesion. 0.5 cm or less scalp, neck, hands, feet, genitalia	75.44	69.05	65.60	75.44	10
11422 1.1–2.0 cm	131.35	120.23	114.22	131.35	10
11441 Exc. benign lesion face, ears, eyelids, nose, lips, or mucous membrane; 0.6–1.0 cm dia or less	119.08	109.00	103.55	119.08	10
11602 Exc. malignant lesion, trunk, arms, or legs; 1.1–2.0 cm dia	195.06	178.55	169.62	195.06	10
11720 Debridement of nails; 1–5	32.58	29.82	28.33	32.58	0
11721 6 or more	32.58	29.82	28.33	32.58	0
11730 Avulsion nail plate, partial or complete, simple repair; single	76.91	70.40	66.88	76.91	0
11750 Exc. nail or nail matrix, partial or complete; permanent	193.45	177.07	168.22	193.45	10
12001 Simple repair (scalp, neck, axillae, ext genitalia, trunk, or extremities incl hands & feet): 2.5 cm or less	91.17	83.45	79.82	91.17	10
12011 Simple repair (face, ears, eyelids, nose, lips or mucous membranes); 2.5 cm or less	101.44	92.85	88.21	101.44	10

Global Period

Various services are associated with an operative procedure when they are considered integral parts of that procedure. The global period refers to the time frame during which all services integral to the surgical procedure are covered by a single payment.

0	Services provided the day of the procedure are included in the fee schedule amount.
10	Services provided the day of and during the 10-day period following the surgical procedure are included in the fee schedule amount.
90	Services provided the day before, the day of, and during the 90-day period following the surgical procedure are included in the fee schedule amount.
INC	Services are included in the global period of another related service.
N/A	Not applicable

[1]Data for the surgical follow-up days from Ingenix St. Anthony Publishing, *Medicode Coding & Payment Manual for Procedures and Services*, 2003

Figure IV-1 Fee schedule (*continued*)

CPT Code No. and Description	Mock Fees	Medicare Partici-pating	Non-participating	Limiting Charge	Follow-Up Days[1]
INTEGUMENTARY SYSTEM (*continued*)					
12013 2.6–5.0 cm	123.98	113.48	107.81	123.98	10
12032 Repair, scalp axillae, trunk (intermediate) 2.6–7.5 cm	169.73	155.36	147.59	169.73	10
12034 7.6–12.5 cm	214.20	196.06	186.26	214.20	10
12051 Repair, intermediate, layer closure of wounds (face, ears, eyelids, nose, lips, or mucous membranes); 2.5 cm	167.60	153.41	145.74	167.60	10
17000 Destruction benign or premalignant lesion, first	37.38	34.58	32.85	37.38	10
17003 2–14 lesions, each	19.41	17.77	16.88	19.41	NA
17110 Destruction benign lesions, other than skin tags (laser, electro-, cryo-, chemosurgery, curettement); up to 14 lesions	77.05	70.53	67.00	77.05	10
17111 15 or more lesions	88.92	81.39	77.32	88.92	10
19020 Mastotomy, drainage/exploration; deep	237.36	217.26	206.40	237.36	90
19100 Biopsy, breast, needle core	96.17	88.03	83.63	96.17	0
19101 Biopsy, breast, incisional	281.51	257.67	244.79	281.51	10
MUSCULOSKELETAL SYSTEM					
20610 Arthrocentesis, aspiration, or injection joint (should, hip, knee) or bursa	52.33	47.89	45.50	52.33	0
21330 Nasal fracture, open treatment complicated	599.46	548.71	521.27	599.46	90
24066 Biopsy, deep, soft tissue, upper arm, elbow	383.34	350.88	333.34	383.34	90
27455 Osteotomy, proximal tibia	1248.03	1142.36	1085.24	1248.03	90
27500 Treatment closed femoral shaft fracture without manipulation	554.90	507.92	482.52	554.90	90
27530 Treatment closed tibial fracture, proximal, without manipulation	344.24	315.90	299.34	344.24	90
27750 Treatment closed tibial shaft fracture without manipulation	400.94	366.99	348.64	400.94	90
27752 with manipulation	531.63	486.62	462.29	531.63	90
29345 Appl long leg cast (thigh to toes)	123.23	112.80	107.16	123.23	0
29355 walker or ambulatory type	133.75	122.42	116.30	133.75	0
29425 Appl short leg walking cast	102.10	93.45	88.78	102.10	0
RESPIRATORY SYSTEM					
30110 Excision, simple nasal polyp	145.21	132.92	126.27	145.21	10
30520 Septoplasty	660.88	604.93	574.68	660.88	90
30903 Control nasal hemorrhage; anterior; complex	118.17	108.17	102.76	118.17	0
30905 Control nasal hemorrhage, posterior with posterior nasal packs; initial	190.57	174.43	165.71	190.57	0
30906 subsequent	173.01	158.36	150.44	173.01	0
31625 Bronchoscopy with biopsy	312.87	286.38	272.06	312.87	0
32310 Pleurectomy, parietal	1234.79	1130.24	1073.73	1234.79	90
32440 Pneumonectomy, total	1972.10	1805.13	1714.87	1972.10	90

(continues)

[1]Data for the surgical follow-up days from Ingenix St. Anthony Publishing, *Medicode Coding & Payment Manual for Procedures and Services*, 2003

Figure IV-1 Fee schedule (*continued*)

CPT Code No. and Description	Mock Fees	Medicare Partici-pating	Medicare Non-participating	Medicare Limiting Charge	Follow-Up Days[1]
CARDIOVASCULAR SYSTEM					
33020 Pericardiotomy	1289.25	1180.09	1121.09	1289.25	90
33206 Insertion of pacemaker; atrial	728.42	666.75	633.41	728.42	90
33208 AV	751.57	687.89	653.50	751.57	90
35301 Thromboendarterectomy with or without patch graft; carotid, vertebral, subclavian by neck incision	1585.02	1450.82	1378.28	1585.02	90
36005 Intravenous injection for contrast venography; extremity	59.18	54.17	51.46	59.18	0
36245 Catheter placement (selective) arterial system, ea first order	68.54	62.74	59.60	68.54	NA
36415 Routine venipuncture for collection of specimen(s)	10.00	—	—	—	XXX
38101 Splenectomy, partial	994.44	910.24	864.73	994.44	90
38510 Biopsy/excision deep cervical lymph node(s)	327.42	299.69	284.71	327.42	10
MEDIASTINUM/DIAPHRAGM/DIGESTIVE SYSTEM					
39520 Repair diaphragmic hernia	1436.50	1314.87	1249.13	1436.50	90
42820 T & A under age 12 years	341.63	312.71	297.07	341.63	90
42821 T & A over age 12 years	410.73	375.96	357.16	410.73	90
43234 Upper GI endoscopy, simple primary exam	201.86	184.77	175.53	201.86	0
43235 Upper GI endoscopy incl esophagus, stomach, duodenum, or jejunum; diagnostic	238.92	218.69	207.76	238.92	0
43456 Dilation esophagus	254.52	232.97	221.32	254.52	0
43820 Gastrojejunostomy	971.86	889.58	845.10	971.86	90
44150 Colectomy, total, abdominal	1757.81	1608.98	1528.53	1757.81	90
44320 Colostomy or skin cecostomy	966.25	884.44	840.22	966.25	90
44950 Appendectomy	568.36	520.24	494.23	568.36	90
45308 Proctosigmoidoscopy for removal of single tumor/polyp	135.34	123.88	117.69	135.34	0
45315 multiple tumors/polyps	185.12	169.44	160.97	185.12	0
45330 Sigmoidoscopy, diagnostic (for biopsy or collection of specimen by brushing or washing)	95.92	87.80	83.41	95.92	0
45380 Colonoscopy with biopsy	382.35	349.98	332.48	382.35	0
46255 Hemorrhoidectomy int & ext, simple	503.57	460.94	437.89	503.57	90
46258 with fistulectomy	636.02	582.17	553.06	636.02	90
46600 Anoscopy; diagnostic	32.86	30.07	28.57	32.86	0
46614 with control of hemorrhage	182.10	166.68	158.35	182.10	0
46700 Anoplastic, for stricture, adult	657.39	601.73	571.64	657.39	90
47600 Cholecystectomy	937.74	858.35	815.43	937.74	90
49505 Inguinal hernia repair, age 5 or over	551.07	504.41	479.19	551.07	90
49520 Repair, inguinal hernia, any age; recurrent	671.89	615.00	584.25	671.89	90

[1]Data for the surgical follow-up days from Ingenix St. Anthony Publishing, *Medicode Coding & Payment Manual for Procedures and Services*, 2003

Figure IV-1 Fee schedule (*continued*)

| CPT Code No. and Description | Mock Fees | Medicare | | | |
		Partici-pating	Non-participating	Limiting Charge	Follow-Up Days[1]
URINARY SYSTEM					
50080 Nephrostolithotomy, percutaneous	1323.93	1211.83	1151.24	1323.93	90
50780 Ureteronecystostomy	1561.23	1429.84	1357.59	1561.23	90
51900 Closure of vesicovaginal fistula abdominal approach	1196.32	1095.48	1040.71	1196.82	90
52000 Cystourethroscopy	167.05	152.90	145.26	167.05	0
52601 Transurethral electrosurgical resection of prostate	888.87	813.61	772.93	888.87	90
53040 Drainage of deep periurethral abscess	520.11	476.07	452.27	520.11	90
53230 Excision, female diverticutum (urethral)	859.69	786.91	747.56	859.69	90
53240 Marsupialization of urethral diverticulum, M or F	520.11	476.07	452.27	520.11	90
53620 Dilation, urethra, male	100.73	92.20	87.59	100.73	0
53660 Dilation, urethra, female	48.32	44.23	42.02	48.32	0
MALE/FEMALE GENITAL SYSTEM					
54150 Circumcision—clamp type	111.78	102.32	97.20	111.78	10
54520 Orchiectomy, simple	523.92	479.56	455.58	523.92	90
55700 Biopsy of prostate, needle or punch	156.22	142.99	135.84	156.22	0
55801 Prostatectomy, perineal subtotal	1466.56	1342.39	1275.27	1466.56	90
57265 Colporrhaphy AP with enterocele repair	902.24	825.85	784.56	902.24	90
57452 Colposcopy	84.18	77.05	73.20	84.18	0
57511 Cryocauterization of cervix	195.83	179.25	170.29	195.83	10
57520 Circumferential (cone) of cervix with or without D & C, cold knife or laser	387.08	354.30	336.59	387.08	90
58100 Endometrial biopsy	71.88	65.79	62.50	71.88	0
58120 D & C diagnostic and/or therapeutic (nonOB)	272.83	249.73	237.24	272.83	10
58150 TAH w/without salpingo-oophorectomy	1167.72	1068.85	1015.41	1167.72	90
58200 TAH, extended, corpus cancer, including partial vaginectomy	1707.24	1562.69	1484.56	1707.24	90
58210 with bilateral radical pelvic lymphadenectomy	2160.78	1977.83	1878.94	2160.78	90
58300 Insertion of intrauterine device	100.00	—	—	—	NA
58340 Hysterosalpingography with inj proc	73.06	66.87	63.53	73.06	0
58720 Salpingo-oophorectomy, complete or partial, unilateral or bilateral	732.40	670.39	636.87	732.40	90
MATERNITY CARE AND DELIVERY					
59120 Surgical treatment of ectopic pregnancy; salpinectomy and/or oophorectomy	789.26	722.43	686.31	789.26	90
59121 without salpingectomy and/or oophorectomy	638.84	584.75	555.51	638.84	90
59130 abdominal pregnancy	699.12	639.93	607.93	699.12	90
59135 total hysterectomy, interstitial, uterine pregnancy	1154.16	1056.44	1003.62	1154.16	90
59136 partial uterine resection, interstitial uterine pregnancy	772.69	707.26	671.90	772.69	90
59140 cervical, with evacuation	489.68	448.22	425.81	489.68	90

(continues)

[1]Data for the surgical follow-up days from Ingenix St. Anthony Publishing, *Medicode Coding & Payment Manual for Procedures and Services*, 2003

Figure IV-1 Fee schedule (*continued*)

CPT Code No. and Description	Mock Fees	Medicare Partici-pating	Medicare Non-participating	Medicare Limiting Charge	Follow-Up Days[1]
59160 Curettage; postpartum hemorrhage	293.46	268.61	255.18	293.46	10
59400 OB care—routine with vag dlvy, inc. antepartum/postpartum care	1864.30	1706.45	1621.13	1864.30	NA
59510 C-section, including antepartum and postpartum care	2102.33	1924.33	1828.11	2102.33	NA
59515 include postpartum care	1469.80	1345.36	1278.09	1469.80	NA
59812 Treatment of incompl abortion, any trimester; completed surgically	357.39	327.13	310.77	357.39	90
NERVOUS SYSTEM					
61314 Craniotomy infratentorial	2548.09	2332.35	2215.73	2548.09	90
62270 Spinal puncture, lumbar; diagnostic	77.52	70.96	67.41	77.52	0
EYE AND OCULAR ADNEXA					
65091 Excision of eye, without implant	708.22	648.25	615.84	708.22	90
65205 Removal of foreign body, ext eye	56.02	51.27	48.71	56.02	0
65222 corneal, with slit lamp	73.81	67.56	64.18	73.81	0
69420 Myringotomy	97.76	89.48	85.01	97.76	10
RADIOLOGY, NUCLEAR MEDICINE, AND DIAGNOSTIC ULTRASOUND					
70120 X-ray mastoids, 1/2 views p/side	38.96	35.66	33.88	38.96	
70130 X-ray mastoids, 3 views p/side	56.07	51.33	48.76	56.07	
71010 X-ray chest, 1 view	31.95	29.24	27.78	31.95	
71020 Chest x-ray, 2 views	40.97	37.50	35.63	40.97	
71030 Chest x-ray, compl, 4 views	54.02	49.44	46.97	54.02	
71060 Bronchogram, bilateral	143.75	131.58	125.00	143.75	
72100 X-ray spine, 2–3 views	43.23	39.57	37.59	43.23	
72114 complete, incl bending views	74.97	68.62	65.19	74.97	
73100 X-ray wrist, 2 views	31.61	28.94	27.49	31.61	
73500 X-ray hip, 1 view	31.56	28.88	27.44	31.56	
73540 X-ray pelvis & hips, infant or child, 2 views	37.94	34.73	32.99	37.94	
73590 X-ray tibia & fibula, 2 views	33.35	30.53	29.00	33.35	
73620 Radiologic exam, foot; 2 views	31.61	28.94	27.49	31.61	
73650 X-ray calcaneus, 2 views	30.71	28.11	26.70	30.71	
74241 Radiologic exam, upper gastrointestinal tract, with/without delayed films with KUB	108.93	99.71	94.72	108.93	
74245 with small bowel	161.70	148.01	140.61	161.70	
74270 Barium enema	118.47	108.44	103.02	118.47	
74290 Oral cholecystography	52.59	48.14	45.73	52.59	
74400 Urography (pyelography), intravenous, with or without KUB	104.78	95.90	91.11	104.78	
74410 Urography, infusion	116.76	106.87	101.53	116.76	
74420 Urography, retrograde	138.89	127.13	120.77	138.89	
75982 Percutaneous placement of drainage catheter	359.08	328.67	312.24	359.08	
76805 Ultrasound, pregnant uterus, B-scan or real time; after first trimester	154.18	141.13	134.07	154.18	
+76810* each additional gestation	306.54	280.59	266.56	306.54	

[1]Data for the surgical follow-up days from Ingenix St. Anthony Publishing, *Medicode Coding & Payment Manual for Procedures and Services*, 2003
*The symbol + designates an add-on code in *CPT*, 2007.

Figure IV-1 Fee schedule (*continued*)

| CPT Code No. and Description | Mock Fees | Medicare* | | |
		Participating	Nonparticipating	Limiting Charge
RADIOLOGY, NUCLEAR MEDICINE, AND DIAGNOSTIC ULTRASOUND (*continued*)				
76946 Ultrasonic guidance for amniocentesis	91.22	83.49	79.32	91.22
77055 Mammography, unilateral	62.57	57.27	54.51	62.57
77056 Mammography, bilateral	82.83	75.82	72.03	82.83
77300 Radiation dosimetry	97.58	89.32	84.85	97.58
77315 complex	213.59	195.51	185.73	213.59
78104 Bone marrow imaging, whole body	230.56	211.04	200.49	230.56
78215 Liver and spleen imaging	160.44	146.85	139.51	160.44
78800 Tumor localization, limited area	191.53	175.32	166.55	191.53
PATHOLOGY AND LABORATORY[1]				

Laboratory tests done as groups or combination "profiles" performed on multichannel equipment should be billed using the appropriate code number (80048 through 80076). Following is a list of the panels.

CPT Code No. and Description	Mock Fees	Participating	Nonparticipating	Limiting Charge
80048 Basic metabolic panel	75.00			
80050 General health panel	50.00			
80051 Electrolyte panel	50.00			
80053 Comprehensive metabolic panel	200.00			
80055 Obstetric panel	75.00			
80061 Lipid panel	50.00			
80069 Renal function panel	150.00			
80074 Acute hepatitis panel	50.00			
80076 Hepatic function panel	75.00			
81000 Urinalysis, non-automated, with microscopy	8.00	7.44	5.98	8.84
81001 Urinalysis, automated, with microscopy	8.00	7.44	5.98	8.84
81002 Urinalysis, non-automated, without microscopy	8.00	7.44	5.98	8.84
81015 Urinalysis, microscopy only	8.00	7.44	5.98	8.84
81025 Urine pregnancy test	10.00			
82565 Creatinine; blood	10.00	9.80	8.88	12.03
82951 Glucose tol test, 3 spec	40.00	41.00	36.80	45.16
82952 each add spec beyond 3	30.00	28.60	25.97	32.16
83020 Hemoglobin, electrophoresis	25.00	20.00	19.94	23.93
83700 Lipoprotein, blood; electrophoretic separation	25.00	20.00	19.94	23.93
84478 Triglycerides, blood	20.00	19.20	15.99	21.87
84480 Tribodothyronine (T-3)	20.00	19.20	15.99	21.87
84520 Urea nitrogen, blood (BUN); quantitative	25.00	20.99	19.94	23.93
84550 Uric acid, blood	20.00	19.20	15.99	21.87
84702 Gonadotropin, chorionic; quantitative	20.00	19.20	15.99	21.87
84703 qualitative	20.00	19.20	15.99	21.87
85018 Blood count, hemoglobin	20.00	19.20	15.99	21.87
85025 Complete blood count (CBC, Hgb, RBC, WBC, and platelet count), automated, differential WBC count	25.00	20.00	19.94	23.93
85032 manual count (each)	25.00	20.00	19.94	23.93
85097 Bone marrow, smear interpretation	73.52	67.29	63.93	73.52
85345 Coagulation time; Lee & White	20.00	19.20	15.99	21.87

(continues)

[1]Mock fees for laboratory tests presented in this schedule may not be representative of fees in your region due to the variety of capitation and managed care contracts as well as discount policies made by laboratories. At the time of this edition, Medicare guidelines may or may not pay for automatic multichannel tests where a large number of tests are performed per panel. Some cases require documentation and a related diagnostic code for each test performed. Providers must have the CLIA level of licensure to bill for tests, and test results must be documented.

Figure IV-1 Fee schedule (*continued*)

CPT Code No. and Description		Mock Fees	Medicare* Participating	Medicare* Nonparticipating	Medicare* Limiting Charge
86038	Antinuclear antibodies (ANA)	25.00	20.00	19.94	23.93
87081	Culture, screening for single organisms	25.00	20.00	19.94	23.93
87181	Sensitivity studies, antibiotic; per agent	20.00	19.20	15.99	21.87
87184	disk method, per plate (12 disks or less)	20.00	19.20	15.99	21.87
87210	Smear, primary source, wet mount with simple stain, for infectious agents	35.00	48.35	45.93	55.12
88150	Papanicolaou cytopath, manual screen (vag. or cerv.) under phys. sup.	35.00	48.35	45.93	55.12
88302	Surgical pathology (level II), gross & micro exam (skin, fingers, nerve, testis)	24.14	22.09	20.99	24.14
88305	Surgical pathology (level IV); bone marrow, interpret	77.69	71.12	67.56	77.69

MEDICINE SECTION

Immunization Injections

90471	Immunization admin. (inj.); one (single or combination)	2.50			
90473	Immunization admin. intranasal/oral; one (single or combination)	2.50			
90701	Diphtheria, tetanus, pertussis	34.00			
90703	Tetanus toxoid	28.00			
90712	Poliovirus vaccine, oral	28.00			

Therapeutic Injections

90772	Therapeutic, prophylactic, or diagnostic; IM or SC	4.77	4.37	4.15	4.77
90774	IV	21.33	19.53	18.55	21.33

Psychiatry

90804	Ind. Psychotherapy 20–30 min	73.70	67.46	64.09	73.30
90805	with E/M service	82.88	75.86	72.07	82.88
90806	Psychotherapy 45–50 min	110.23	100.89	95.98	110.23
90853	Group therapy	29.22	26.75	25.41	29.22

Hemodialysis

90935	Hemodialysis with physician eval.	117.23	107.31	101.94	117.23
90937	Hemodialysis with repeat eval.	206.24	188.78	179.34	206.24

Gastroenterology

91000	Esophageal intubation	69.82	63.91	60.71	69.82
91055	Gastric intubation	87.41	80.01	16.01	87.41

Opthalmologic Services

92004	Comprehensive eye exam	90.86	83.17	79.01	90.86
92100	Tonometry (serial)	47.31	43.31	41.14	47.31
92230	Fluorescein angloscopy	55.49	50.79	48.25	55.49
92275	Electroretinography	81.17	74.29	70.58	81.17
92531	Spontaneous nystagmus	26.00			

Audiologic Function Tests

92557	Basic comprehensive audiometry	54.33	49.73	47.24	54.33
92596	Ear protector measurements	26.81	24.54	23.31	26.81

Cardiovascular Therapeutic Services

93000	Electrocardiogram (ECG)	34.26	31.36	29.79	34.26
93015	Treadmill ECG	140.71	128.80	122.36	140.71
93040	Rhythm ECG; 1–3 leads	18.47	16.90	16.06	18.47

Figure IV-1 Fee schedule (*continued*)

CPT Code No. and Description		Mock Fees	Medicare*		
			Participating	Nonparticipating	Limiting Charge
Pulmonary					
94010	Spirometry	38.57	35.31	33.54	38.57
94060	Spirometry before and after bronchodilator	71.67	65.60	62.32	71.67
94150	Vital capacity, total	13.82	12.65	12.02	13.82
Allergy and Clinical Immunology					
95024	Intradermal tests	6.58	6.02	5.72	6.58
95044	Patch tests	8.83	8.08	7.68	8.83
95115	Treatment for allergy, single inj.	17.20	15.75	14.96	17.20
95117	two or more inj.	22.17	20.29	19.28	22.17
95165	Prof. service for super. of preparation and antigens for allergen immunotherapy, single or multiple antigens, multiple-dose vials	3.63	3.33	3.16	3.63
Neurology					
95812	Electroencephalogram, 41–60 min	129.32	118.37	112.45	129.32
95819	awake and asleep	126.81	116.07	110.27	126.81
95860	Electromyography, 1 extremity	88.83	81.31	77.24	88.83
95864	Electromyography, 4 extremities	239.99	219.67	208.69	239.99
96102	Psychological testing (per hour)	80.95	74.10	70.39	80.95
Physical Medicine					
97024	Diathermy	14.27	13.06	12.41	14.27
97036	Hubbard tank, each 15 min	24.77	22.67	21.54	24.77
97110	Physical therapy, one or more areas; 15 min	23.89	21.86	20.77	23.89
97140	Manual therapy, one or more areas; 15 min	16.93	15.49	14.72	16.93
Special Services and Reports					
99000	Handling of specimen (transfer from Dr.'s office to lab)	5.00			
99050	Services requested after office hours in addition to basic service	25.00			
99056	Services normally provided in office requested by pt inlocation other than office	20.00			
99058	Office services provided on an emergency basis	65.00			
99070	Supplies and materials over and above those usually required (itemize drugs and materials provided)	25.00			
99080	Special reports:				
	Insurance forms	10.00			
	Review of data to clarify pt's status	20.00			
	WC reports	50.00			
	WC extensive review report	250.00			

*Some services and procedures may not be considered a benefit under the Medicare program, and when listed on a claim form, no reimbursement may be received. However, it is important to include these codes when billing because Medicare policies may change without an individual knowing of a new benefit. For this reason, some of the services shown in this mock fee schedule do not have any amounts listed under the three Medicare columns.

CPT MODIFIERS

-21 Prolonged evaluation and management services (attach report to claim)
-22 Unusual procedural services (attach report to claim)
-23 Unusual anesthesia (pt requires general anesthetic instead of none or local anesthesia)
-24 Unrelated evaluation and management service by the same physician during a postoperative period
-25 Significant, separate identifiable evaluation and management service by the same physician on the day of a procedure
-26 Professional component (physician interpretation only, not technical component)
-32 Mandated services (e.g., consult requested by a third party payor)
-47 Anesthesia by surgeon
-50 Bilateral procedure
-51 Multiple procedures performed on the same day or at the same session
-52 Reduced services
-53 Discontinued procedure
-54 Surgical care only
-55 Postoperative care only
-56 Preoperative care only
-57 Decision for surgery (use with E/M service performed just prior to surg)
-58 Staged or related procedure or service by the same physician during the postoperative period
-59 Distinct procedural service
-62 Two surgeons (usually with different skills)
-63 Procedure performed on infants
-66 Surgical team
-76 Repeat procedure by the same physician
-77 Repeat procedure by another physician
-78 Return to the operating room for a related procedure during the postoperative period
-79 Unrelated procedure or service by the same physician during the postoperative period
-80 Assistant surgeon
-81 Minimum assistant surgeon
-82 Assistant surgeon (when qualified resident surgeon not available)
-90 Reference (outside) laboratory procedures performed by a lab other than the treating physician
-91 Repeat clinical diagnostic laboratory test
-99 Multiple modifiers (use of two or more modifiers for a service)

HCPCS LEVEL II CODES*

These codes have been selected from many HCPCS codes as examples. The fees stated are only examples.

		FEES
A0422	Ambulance service, oxygen supplies, life sustaining situation	$600
A4206	Syringe with needle; 1cc	$10
A5051	Ostomy pouch; one piece with barrier attached	$15
A6410	Eye pad, sterile	$15
A9150	Nonprescription drugs	$10
B4034	Enteral feeding supply kit syringe; per day	$25
E0100	Cane; any material, adjustable or fixed	$60
E0114	Crutches; underarm, other than wood	$100
G0008	Administration, influenza virus vaccine	$10
H0001	Alcohol and/or drug assessment	$75
J0120	Injection, tetracycline, up to 250 mg	$25
J0170	Injection, adrenalin, up to 1 ml ampule	$25
J0540	Injection, penicillin G, up to 1,200,000 units	$25
J1460	Injection, gamma globulin, intramuscular, 1cc	$20
J1470	Injection, gamma globulin, intramuscular, 2cc	$25
L0180	Cervical, multiple post collar	$50
L3209	Surgical boot, child	$50
M0075	Cellular therapy	$70
P3001	Papanicolaou smear screening (up to 3), interpretation by physician	$25

*2007 *HCPCS Level II* codes used.

V

Abbreviation Tables

TABLE V-1
Address Abbreviations

Alley	ALY	Center	CTR	Lakes	LKS	Rapids	RPDS	Terrace	TER
Annex	ANX	Circle	CIR	Lane	LN	Ridge	RDG	Track	TRAK
Apartment	APT	Cliffs	CLFS	Mall	MALL	River	RIV	Trail	TRL
Arcade	ARC	Club	CLB	Manager	MGR	Road	RD	Tunnel	TUNL
Association	ASSN	Court	CT	Manor	MNR	Room	RM	Turnpike	TPKE
Avenue	AVE	Drive	DR	Mount	MT	Route	RT	Union	UN
Bayou	BYU	East	E	Mountain	MTN	Row	ROW	Valley	VLY
Beach	BCH	Estates	ESTS	North	N	Run	RUN	Viaduct	VIA
Bend	BND	Expressway	EXPY	Northeast	NE	Rural	R	Vice President	VP
Bluff	BLF	Extension	EXT	Northwest	NW	Secretary	SECY	View	VW
Bottom	BTM	Freeway	FWY	Orchard	ORCH	Shoal	SHL	Village	VLG
Boulevard	BLVD	Grove	GRV	Palms	PLMS	Shore	SH	Ville	VL
Branch	BR	Harbor	HBR	Park	PK	South	S	Vista	VIS
Bridge	BRG	Heights	HTS	Parkway	PKWY	Southeast	SE	Walk	WALK
Brook	BRK	Hill	HL	Place	PL	Southwest	SW	Way	WAY
Burg	BG	Hospital	HOSP	Plaza	PLZ	Spring	SPG	Wells	WLS
Bypass	BYP	Institute	INST	Point	PT	Square	SQ	West	W
Camp	CP	Isle	ISLE	Port	PRT	Station	STA		
Canyon	CYN	Island	IS	Prairie	PR	Street	ST		
Cape	CPE	Junction	JCT	President	PRES	Suite	STE		
Causeway	CSWY	Lake	LK	Ranch	RNCH	Summit	SMT		

TABLE V-2
Appointment and Patient Care Abbreviations

A	allergy; abortion	comp	comprehensive
AB	antibiotic	compl	complete
abd, abdom	abdominal, abdomen	Con, CON, Cons, consult	consultation
abt	about	Cont.	continue
Acc, acc	accommodation	COPD	chronic obstructive pulmonary disease
accid	accident		
adm	admit; admission; admitted	CPE, CPX	complete physical examination
adv	advice	C section, C/S	cesarean section
aet.	at the age of	CT	computerized tomography
AgNO$_3$	silver nitrate	CV	cardiovascular
AIDS	acquired immune deficiency syndrome	CVA	costovertebral angle; cardiovascular accident; cerebrovascular accident
alb	albumin		
ALL	allergy		
a.m., AM	before noon	CXR	chest x-ray
AMA	American Medical Association	Cysto, cysto	cystoscopy
an ck	annual check	D & C	dilatation and curettage
an PX	annual physical examination	dc	discontinue
ant	anterior	DC	discharge, dressing change
ante	before	del	delivery
A & P	auscultation and percussion	Dg, dg, Dx, dx	diagnosis
AP	anterior posterior; anteroposterior; antepartum care	diag.	diagnosis, diagnostic
		diam.	diameter
AP & L	anteroposterior and lateral	diff.	differential
approx	approximate	dilat	dilate
apt	apartment	disch.	discharged
ASA	acetylsalicylic acid	DNA	does not apply
asap, ASAP	as soon as possible	DNKA	did not keep appointment
ASCVD	arteriosclerotic cardiovascular disease	DNS	did not show
ASHD	arteriosclerotic heart disease	DOB	date of birth
asst	assistant	dr, drsg	dressing
auto	automobile	DSHA	does she have appointment
Ba	barium	DTaP*	diphtheria, tetanus, and pertussis (vaccine)
BI	biopsy		
BM	bowel movement	Dx, Dg, dx	diagnosis
BMR	basal metabolic rate	E	emergency
BP, B/P	blood pressure	ECG	electrocardiogram; electrocardiograph
BP ck, BP ✓	blood pressure check		
breast ck	breast check	ED	emergency department
Brev	Brevital	EDC	estimated date of confinement; due date for baby
BUN	blood urea nitrogen		
Bx, BX	biopsy	EEG	electroencephalogram; electroencephalograph
C	cervical; centigrade; celsius		
C & S	culture and sensitivity	EENT	eye, ear, nose, and throat
Ca, CA	cancer, carcinoma	EKG	electrocardiogram; electrocardiograph
canc, cncl	cancel, canceled		
cast ck	cast check	EMG	electromyogram, electromyelogram
Cauc	Caucasian		
CBC	complete blood count	epith.	epithelial
CC	chief complaint	ER	emergency room
CDC	calculated date of confinement	ESR	erythrocyte sedimentation rate
chem	chemistry		
CHF	congestive heart failure	est.	established; estimated
chr	chronic	etiol.	etiology
ck, ✓	check	EU	etiology unknown
CI	color index	Ex, exam.	examination
cm	centimeter	exc.	excision
CNS	central nervous system	ext	external
CO, C/O	complains of	F	Fahrenheit; French (catheter)
CO$_2$, CO2	carbon dioxide		

*Abbreviation approved by the Joint Commission as the preferred abbreviation.

TABLE V-2
Appointment and Patient Care Abbreviations (*continued*)

FH	family history	JVD	jugulovenous distention
FHS	fetal heart sounds	K35	Kollmann (dilator)
flu syn	influenza syndrome	KUB	kidneys, ureters, bladder
fluor	fluoroscopy	L	left; laboratory; living children; liter
ft	foot; feet	lab, LAB	laboratory
FU, F/U	follow-up (visit)	lac	laceration
FUO	fever of unknown/undetermined origin	L&A, l/a	light and accommodation
FX, Fx	fracture	L&W	living and well
G	gravida (number of pregnancies)	lat, LAT	lateral
g, gm	gram	LBP	low back pain
GA	gastric analysis	lb(s)	pound(s)
GB	gallbladder	LLL	left lower lobe
GC	gonorrhea	LLQ	left lower quadrant
GGE	generalized glandular enlargement	LMP	last menstrual period
GI	gastrointestinal	lt., LT	left
GTT	glucose tolerance test	ltd.	limited
GU	genitourinary	LUQ	left upper quadrant
Gyn, GYN	gynecology	M	medication; married
H	hospital call	MA	mental age
HA	headache	med., MED	medicine
HBP	high blood pressure	mg	milligram(s)
HC	house call; hospital call; hospital consultation	MH	marital history
		ml	milliliter(s)
HCD	house call, day	mm	millimeter(s)
HCl	hydrochloric acid	MM	mucous membrane
HCN	house call, night	MMR	measles, mumps, rubella (vaccine)
hct	hematocrit	mo	month(s)
HCVD	hypertensive cardiovascular disease	MRI	magnetic resonance imaging
HEENT	head, eyes, ears, nose, and throat	N	negative
Hgb, Hb	hemoglobin	NA, N/A	not applicable
hist	history	NaCl	sodium chloride
H_2O, H2O	water	NAD	no appreciable disease
hosp	hospital	neg.	negative
H&P	history and physical	New OB	new obstetric patient
HPI	history of present illness	NFA	no future appointment
hr, hrs	hour, hours	NP, N/P, (N)	new patient
HS	hospital surgery	NPN	nonprotein nitrogen
Ht, ht	height	N/S, NS	no-show
HV	hospital visit	NTRA	no telephone requests for antibiotics
HX	history	N&V	nausea and vomiting
HX PX	history and physical examination	NYD	not yet diagnosed
I	injection	O_2, O2	oxygen
I&D	incision and drainage	OB	obstetrical patient, obstetrics; prenatal care
IC	initial consultation		
i.e.	that is	OC	office call
IM	intramuscular	occ	occasional
imp., IMP	impression	ofc	office
inc	include	OH	occupational history
inf, INF	infection, infected	OP, op.	operation, operative, outpatient
inflam., INFL	inflammation	OPD	outpatient department
init	initial	OR	operating room
inj., INJ	injection	orig.	original
int, INT	internal	OT	occupational therapy
intermed	intermediate	OTC	over the counter
interpret	interpretation	OV	office visit
IPPB	intermittent positive pressure breathing	P	pulse; preterm parity or deliveries before term
IQ	intelligence quotient		
IUD	intrauterine device	PA	posterior anterior, posteroanterior
IV, I.V.	intravenous	P&A	percussion and auscultation
IVP	intravenous pyelogram	PAP, Pap	Papanicolaou (test/smear)

(continues)

TABLE V-2
Appointment and Patient Care Abbreviations (*continued*)

Para I	woman having borne one child (Para II, two children, and so on)	SE	special examination
PBI	protein-bound iodine	sed rate	sedimentation rate
PC	present complaint; pregnancy confirmation	sep.	separated
PD	permanent disability	SH	social history
PE	physical examination	SIG, sigmoido	sigmoidoscopy
perf.	performed	SLR	straight leg raising
PERRLA, PERLA	pupils equal, round, react to light and to accommodation	slt	slight
		Smr, sm.	smear
pH	hydrogen ion concentration	S, M, W, D	single, married, widowed, divorced
PH	past history	SOB	shortness of breath
Ph ex	physical examination	sp gr	specific gravity
phys.	physical	SubQ*	subcutaneous
PI	present illness	SR	suture removal; sedimentation rate
PID	pelvic inflammatory disease	STAT, stat.	immediately
p.m., PM	after noon	STD	sexually transmitted disease
PMH	past medical history	strab	strabismus
PND	postnasal drip	surg.	surgery
PO	postoperative check, phone order	Sx.	symptoms
P Op, Post-op	postoperative check	T	temperature; term parity or deliveries at term
pos.	positive	T&A	tonsillectomy and adenoidectomy
post.	posterior	Tb, tbc, TB	tuberculosis
postop	postoperative	TD	temporary disability
PP	postpartum care	temp.	temperature
Pre-op, preop	preoperative (office visit)	TIA	transient ischemic attack
prep	prepare, prepared	TMs	tympanic membranes
PRN, p.r.n.	as necessary	TPR	temperature, pulse, respiration
procto	proctoscopic (rectal) examination	Tr.	treatment
prog	prognosis	TTD	total temporary disability
P&S	permanent and stationary	TURB	transurethral resection of bladder
PSP	phenolsulfonphthalein	TURP	transurethral resection of prostate
Pt, pt	patient	TX, Tx	treatment
PT	physical therapy	U	unit
PTR	patient to return	UA, U/A	urinalysis
PX	physical examination	UCHD	usual childhood diseases
R	right; residence call; report	UCR	usual, customary, and reasonable
RBC, rbc	red blood cell	UGI	upper gastrointestinal
rec	recommend	UPJ	ureteropelvic junction or joint
re ch	recheck	UR, ur	urine
re-exam, reex	reexamination	URI	upper respiratory infection
REF, ref	referral	UTI	urinary tract infection
reg.	regular	vac	vaccine
ret, retn	return	VD	venereal disease
rev	review	VDRL	Venereal Disease Research Laboratory (test for syphilis)
Rh-	Rhesus negative (blood)		
RHD	rheumatic heart disease	W	work; white
RLQ	right lower quadrant	WBC, wbc	white blood cell or count; well baby care
RO, R/O	rule out	WF	white female
ROS	review of systems	WI, W/I	walk-in, work-in
rt., R	right	wk	week; work
RT	respiratory therapy	wks	weeks
RTC	return to clinic	WM, W/M	white male
RTO	return to office	WNL	within normal limits
RUQ	right upper quadrant	WR	Wassermann reaction
RV	return visit	WT, Wt, wt	weight
Rx, RX, ℞	prescription; any medication or treatment ordered	x, X	x-ray(s); multiplied by
		XR	x-ray(s)
S	surgery	yr	year
SD	state disability		

*Abbreviation approved by the Joint Commission on Accreditation wof Healthcare Organizations (JCAHO) as the preferred abbreviation.

TABLE V-2
Appointment and Patient Care Abbreviations (*continued*)

Symbols	
*	birth
c̄, /c, w/	with
P̄	after
s̄, /s, w/o	without
c̄c, c̄/c	with correction (eyeglasses)
s̄c, s̄/c	without correction (eyeglasses)
+	positive
−, ō	negative
±	negative or positive; indefinite
Ⓛ	left
ⓜ	murmur
Ⓡ	right
♂	male
♀	female
μ	micron

TABLE V-3
Appointment Terms and Their Abbreviations

Medical Term	Abbreviation	Medical Term	Abbreviation
abdominal	abd, abdom	immediately	stat
accident	accid	infection	inf
annual check	an ck	influenza syndrome	flu syn
annual physical examination	an PX/PE	injection	inj, INJ
antepartum care	AP	intrauterine device	IUD
blood pressure check	BP	laboratory follow-up	Lab FU, Lab F/U
breast check	breast ck	laceration	lac
cancel, canceled	canc	low back pain	LBP
cast check	cast ck	measles, mumps, rubella vac.	MMR
check	ck	new patient	(N), N/P, NP
chest x-ray	CXR, PA chest, AP chest	new obstetric patient	New OB
complete blood count	CBC	no future appointment	NFA
complete physical examination	CPX, CPE	no-show	N/S, NS
consultation	consult, cons, con	obstetric patient	OB
cystoscopy	cysto	office visit	OV
diagnosis	Dx, dx, dg, diag.	Papanicolaou smear	Pap
did not keep appointment	DNKA	physical examination	PE, PX, Ph ex, phys
did not show	DNS	postoperative check	PO, Post-op
dressing	dr, drsg	postpartum care	PP
dressing change	DC	pregnancy confirmation	PC
electrocardiogram	EKG, ECG	prenatal care	OB
electromyogram,		preoperative office visit	Pre-op, preop
electromyelogram	EMG	proctoscopic examination	procto
emergency	E	referral	REF, ref
emergency room	ER	return to clinic	RTC
follow-up visit	FU	return to office	RTO
fracture	FX, Fx	return visit	RV, ret, retn
glucose tolerance test	GTT	sigmoidoscopy	SIG, sigmoido
gynecological check	Gyn ck, GYN	suture removal	SR
headache	HA	walk-in, work-in	WI, W/I
house call	HC	weight	WT

TABLE V-4
Bookkeeping Abbreviations and Definitions

AC or acct	account	EC, ER	error corrected	PVT CK	private check
A/C	account current	Ex MO	express money order	recd, recv'd	received
adj	adjustment	FLW/UP	follow-up	ref	refund
A/P	accounts payable	fwd	forward	req	request
A/R	accounts receivable	IB	itemized bill	ROA	received on account
B/B	bank balance	I/f	in full	snt	sent
Bal fwd, B/F	balance forward	ins, INS	insurance	T	telephoned
BD	bad debt	inv	invoice	TB	trial balance
BSY	busy	J/A	joint account	UCR	usual, customary, and reasonable
c/a, CS	cash on account	LTTR	letter		
cc	credit card	MO	money order	w/o	write off
ck	check	mo	month	$	money/cash
COINS	coinsurance	msg	message	—	charge already made
Cr	credit	NC, N/C	no charge		
CXL	cancel	NF	no funds	0	no balance due (zero balance)
DB	debit	NSF	not sufficient funds		
DED	deductible	PD	paid	✔	posted
def	charge deferred	pmt	payment	<$0.00>	credit
disc, discnt	discount	pt	patient		

TABLE V-5
Collection Abbreviations

B	bankrupt	N1, N2	note one, note two (sent)	S	she or wife
BLG	belligerent	NA	no answer	SEP	separated
EOM	end of month	NF/A	no forwarding address	SK	skip or skipped
EOW	end of week	NI	not in	SOS	same old story
FN	final notice	NLE	no longer employed	STO	she telephoned office
H	he or husband	NR	no record	T	telephoned
HHCO	have husband call office	NSF	not sufficient funds (check)	TB	telephoned business
HTO	he telephoned office	NSN	no such number	TR	telephoned residence
L1, L2	letter one, letter two (sent)	OOT	out of town	U/Emp	unemployed
LB	line busy	OOW	out of work	UTC	unable to contact
LD	long distance	Ph/Dsc	phone disconnected	Vfd/E	verified employment
LMCO	left message, call office	POW	payment on way	Vfd/I	verified insurance
LMVM	left message voice mail	PP	promise to pay		

TABLE V-6
Physician Specialist and Health Care Professional Abbreviations

Physician Specialist	Abbreviation	Health Care Professional	Abbreviation
Doctor of Chiropractic	DC	Certified First Assistant (surgical)	CFA
Doctor of Dental Surgery	DDS	Certified Laboratory Assistant; certified by Registry of American Society of Clinical Pathologists	CLA (ASCP)
Doctor of Dental Science	DD Sc		
Doctor of Emergency Medicine	DEM		
Doctor of Hygiene	D Hy	Certified Medical Assistant	CMA
Doctor of Medical Dentistry	DMD	Certified Medical Transcriptionist	CMT
Doctor of Medicine	MD	Certified Nurse Midwife	CNM
Doctor of Optometry	OD	Certified Professional Coder	CPC
Doctor of Ophthalmology	OphD	Certified Registered Nurse Anesthetist	CRNA
Doctor of Osteopathy	DO	Certified Surgical Technician (2nd surgical asst.)	CST
Doctor of Pharmacy	Pharm D	Emergency Medical Technician	EMT
Doctor of Podiatry	DPM	Health Information Management	HIM
Doctor of Public Health	DPH	Inhalation Therapist	IT
Doctor of Tropical Medicine	DTM	Laboratory Technician Assistant	LTA
Doctor of Veterinary Medicine	DVM	Licensed Practical Nurse	LPN
Doctor of Veterinary Surgery	DVS	Licensed Vocational Nurse	LVN
Fellow of the American Academy of Pediatrics	FAAP	Master of Public Health	MPH
Fellow of the American College of Obstetricians and Gynecologists	FACOG	Medical Technologist	MT (ASCP)
		Physician's Assistant—Certified	PA–C
Fellow of the American College of Surgery	FACS	Public Health Nurse	PHN
Senior Fellow	SF	Registered Dietitian	RD
		Registered Nurse	RN
		Registered Nurse First Assistant (surgical)	RNFA
		Registered Nurse Practitioner	RNP
		Registered Occupational Therapist	ROT
		Registered Physical Therapist	RPT
		Registered Respiratory Therapist	RRT
		Registered Technologist (Radiology)	RT (R)
		Registered Technologist (Therapy)	RT (T)
		Visiting Nurse	VN

TABLE V-7
Prescription Abbreviations* and Symbols

ā	before	o.m.	every morning
āā	of each	o.n.	every night
a.c.	before meals	OTC	over-the-counter (drugs)
ad lib.	as much as needed	oz	ounce
a.m. or AM	morning	p̄	after
ante	before	p.c.	after meals
aq.	aqueous/water	p.o.	by mouth (per os)
b.i.d.	two times a day	p.r.	per rectum
caps	capsule	p.r.n. or PRN	whenever necessary
c̄	with	q.	every
c̄c̄	with meals	q.a.m.	every morning
comp. or comp	compound	q.h.	every hour
d	day	q.h.s.	every night
DC or D/C	discontinue	q.i.d.	four times a day (not at night)
dos.	doses	q.n.	every night
DS	double strength	q.p.m.	every night
DSD	double starting dose	q.2 h.	every two hours
elix.	elixir	q.3 h.	every three hours
emul.	emulsion	q.4 h.	every four hours
et	and	rep, REP	let it be repeated; Latin repeto
ext.	extract	Rx	take (recipe), prescription
garg.	gargle	s̄	without
gm or g	gram	SC or subq	subcutaneous
gr	grain	sat.	saturated
gt.	drop	Sig.	write on label; give directions on prescription
gtt.	drops		
h.	hour	SL	sublingual
h.s.	before bedtime (hour of sleep)	sol.	solution
ID	intradermal	SR	sustained release
IM	intramuscular	ss	one-half
inj.	injection; to be injected	stat or STAT	immediately
IV or I.V.	intravenous	syr.	syrup
kg	kilogram	tab.	tablet
liq	liquid	t.i.d.	three times a day
M or m.	mix	top	topically
mcg	microgram	Tr. or tinct.	tincture
mg or mgm	milligram (used instead of "cc" for cubic centimeter)	tsp	teaspoon
		vag.	vagina
ml	milliliter	X or x	times (X10d/times ten days)
N.E. or ne	negative	i, ii, iii, iv; viii, etc.	1, 2, 3, 4; 8, etc.
noct.	night	5″, 10″, 15″	5, 10, 15 minutes, etc.
NPO or n.p.o.	nothing by mouth	5°, 10°, 15°, or 5′, 10′, 15′, etc.	5 hours, 10 hours, 15 hours, etc.
O₂	oxygen		
o.d.	once a day	ʒ or dr.	dram (drachm)
o.h.	every hour	℥ or oz.	ounce
oint	ointment		

*Many of these abbreviations are derived from Latin; they are usually typed in lowercase and with periods. Periods are especially important, if without periods an abbreviation would spell a word; for example, b.i.d. without periods is bid.

TABLE V-8
Two-Letter Abbreviations for the United States and Territories and Canadian Provinces

United States and Territories

Alabama	AL	Kentucky	KY	Ohio	OH
Alaska	AK	Louisiana	LA	Oklahoma	OK
Amer. Samoa	AS	Maine	ME	Oregon	OR
Arizona	AZ	Marshall Islands	MH	Palau	PW
Arkansas	AR	Maryland	MD	Pennsylvania	PA
California	CA	Massachusetts	MA	Puerto Rico	PR
Colorado	CO	Michigan	MI	Rhode Island	RI
Connecticut	CT	Minnesota	MN	South Carolina	SC
Delaware	DE	Mississippi	MS	South Dakota	SD
District of Columbia	DC	Missouri	MO	Tennessee	TN
Federated States of Micronesia	FM	Montana	MT	Texas	TX
Florida	FL	Nebraska	NE	Utah	UT
Georgia	GA	Nevada	NV	Vermont	VT
Guam	GU	New Hampshire	NH	Virginia	VA
Hawaii	HI	New Jersey	NJ	Virgin Islands, U.S.	VI
Idaho	ID	New Mexico	NM	Washington	WA
Illinois	IL	New York	NY	West Virginia	WV
Indiana	IN	North Carolina	NC	Wisconsin	WI
Iowa	IA	North Dakota	ND	Wyoming	WY
Kansas	KS	No. Mariana Islands	MP		

Canadian Provinces

Alberta	AB	Northwest Territories	NT	Quebec	QC
British Columbia	BC	Nova Scotia	NS	Saskatchewan	SK
Manitoba	MB	Nunavut	NU	Yukon Territory	YT
New Brunswick	NB	Ontario	ON		
Newfoundland and Labrador	NL	Prince Edward Island	PE		